....

Atherosclerosis, Large Arteries and Cardiovascular Risk

Advances in Cardiology

Vol. 44

Series Editor

Jeffrey S. Borer　*New York, N.Y.*

KARGER

Atherosclerosis, Large Arteries and Cardiovascular Risk

Volume Editors

Michel E. Safar   Paris
Edward D. Frohlich   *New Orleans, La.*

63 figures, 1 in color, and 29 tables, 2007

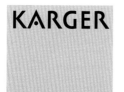

KARGER

Basel · Freiburg · Paris · London · New York ·
Bangalore · Bangkok · Singapore · Tokyo · Sydney

Advances in Cardiology

·······················

Prof. Dr. Michel E. Safar
Hôpital Hôtel-Dieu
Centre de Diagnostic
1 place du Parvis Notre-Dame
F–75181 Paris Cedex (France)

Prof. Dr. Edward D. Frohlich
Ochsner Clinic Foundation
1514 Jefferson Highway
New Orleans, LA 70121 (USA)

Library of Congress Cataloging-in-Publication Data

Atherosclerosis, large arteries, and cardiovascular risk / volume editors,
   Michel E. Safar, Edward D. Frohlich.
      p. ; cm. – (Advances in cardiology ; v. 44)
   Includes bibliographical references and index.
   ISBN-13: 978-3-8055-8176-9 (hard cover : alk. paper)
   1. Atherosclerosis–Pathophysiology.   2. Arteriosclerosis–Pathophysiology.
   3. Coronary heart disease–Etiology.   I. Safar, Michel.   II. Frohlich, Edward D., 1931-   .
   III. Series.
   [DNLM: 1. Atherosclerosis–physiopathology. 2. Arteries–physiopathology.
   3. Atherosclerosis–complications. 4. Cardiovascular Diseases–etiology. 5. Risk Factors.
   W1 AD53C v.44 2007 / WG 550 A8694 2007]
   RC692.A6748 2007

                                                            2006030607

Bibliographic Indices. This publication is listed in bibliographic services, including Current Contents® and Index Medicus.

© Copyright 2007 by S. Karger AG, P.O. Box, CH–4009 Basel (Switzerland)
www.karger.com
Printed in Switzerland on acid-free paper by Reinhardt Druck, Basel
ISSN 0065–2326
ISBN-10: 3–8055–8176–9
ISBN-13: 978–3–8055–8176–9

Contents

Preface

In recent years, our fundamental knowledge of atherosclerosis in the human being has dramatically increased, not only from a better understanding of the pathophysiological information, but also from the clinical use of new hypolipidemic agents which are so very different from the traditional therapeutic mechanisms directed toward atherosclerotic disease. This advance was exceedingly important for all clinical investigators since their clinical approach to atherosclerotic disease has changed, particularly regarding its links with hypertension and the aging process.

Moreover, as a consequence of new epidemiological findings, we have divided the well-established vascular 'diseases' into two pedagogic categories: those related to cardiovascular risk factors (hypertension, diabetes mellitus, dyslipidemia, obesity and smoking) and those related to specific clinical events affecting the target organ circulations (i.e., brain, kidney, heart, and lower limbs). Furthermore, because of increased longevity in recent years, a dissociation of atherosclerosis from the effects of aging per se has been a major effort in presenting the concept of this textbook. Another important point needed to be clarified: in understanding the different clinical and hemodynamic features of atherosclerosis, it was important to present a current means of evaluating cardiovascular risk as well as a practical rationale for developing a therapeutic strategy.

Finally, in arriving at a dissociation and understanding of the mechanisms of hypertensive disease and of the aging process, the structural and functional changes of the vessels of each must be recognized as clearly as possible with respect to how they involve the totality of the arterial and arteriolar system. Thus, it is necessary to comprehend both the aging phenomenon and the pathophysiology of hypertension and their respective global impacts on arterial stiffness, especially involving the aorta and its major large arterial branches. In this regard, the clinical aspects of arterial stiffness have been widely developed in hypertensive subjects over the last 10 years. In contrast, in patients with atherosclerosis, the distribution of arterial rigidity on large vessels is much more patchy and predominates in certain arteries – for example the coronary arteries and at the level of the arterial bifurcations. In these vessels, non-fibrous and non-calcified plaques do not necessarily contribute to increased vessel stiffness. Therefore, the problem of arterial rigidity in atherosclerosis is more difficult to resolve than in hypertension. For these reasons, the principal purpose of this book was to respond to the following questions: In which conditions does the atherosclerosis process contribute to the development of vascular stiffness and to vascular calcifications since both of these factors independently participate in determining cardiovascular risk and, possibly, in modifying therapeutic strategy?

This book is composed of four sections. First, the definition and measurement of arterial stiffness are described with respect to the pathophysiological aspects of atherosclerosis. Second, the mechanisms underlying arterial stiffness are described successively in the major territories involved with atherosclerosis, particularly the coronary arteries. Third, arterial stiffness is discussed with respect to its relation with other cardiovascular factors such as diabetes mellitus or hyperlipidemia. Finally, in the fourth section the therapeutic means of approaching arterial stiffness are analyzed in detail. We hope this approach to the effects of arterial stiffness involving hypertension, atherosclerosis, and aging is now better understood and that it will, in turn, result in a more clearly developed concept for therapy in the future.

Michel E. Safar, Paris
Edward D. Frohlich, New Orleans, La.

Safar ME, Frohlich ED (eds): Atherosclerosis, Large Arteries and Cardiovascular Risk.
Adv Cardiol. Basel, Karger, 2007, vol 44, pp 1–18

······················

Arterial Stiffness: A Simplified Overview in Vascular Medicine

Michel E. Safar

Diagnosis Center, Hôtel-Dieu Hospital, Paris, France

Abstract

Arterial elasticity is a common index of medical semiology, easier to understand than blood pressure measurement. This chapter summarizes the most classical aspects which are important to understand in vascular medicine.

In biophysics, the theory of elasticity deals with the relations between the forces applied to a body and its subsequent deformations [1–3]. The force per unit area is called the 'stress'. The deformation, described as the ratio of the deformation to its original form, is called the 'strain'. Because it is a ratio, strain is dimensionless. The slope of the strain-stress relationship is called 'elastic modulus'.

When forces act on a given solid body without displacing it, they will deform it, that is, cause a movement of the various parts of the body relative to one another. If the body regains its original form exactly when the force is removed it is said to be 'perfectly elastic'. If the body retains the deformation, then it is said to be 'plastic'. A large number of substances exhibit properties appropriate to both an elastic solid and a viscous liquid, and the deformation suffered by such a material will depend on both the magnitude of the stress and on the rate at which it is applied. Such substances are called 'visco-elastic'. It is to this large class that the arterial wall belongs.

In the case of biology of arterial vessels, the stress-strain relationship is simplified in terms of pressure relationship applied to a cylindrical vessel of constant length. The mechanical stress is represented by pressure and the strain by the change in 'diameter' (or volume). Because the relationship is non-linear, the slope of the curve at a given pressure represents the elasticity (or its inverse, the stiffness) of the system. Elasticity and stiffness are both qualitative terms. The corresponding establishing quantitative values are called 'compliance' or 'distensibility'. The purpose of this chapter is to define the visco-elastic properties of the large artery walls in relation to their principal applications in vascular medicine, mainly in subjects with atherosclerosis. Arterial stiffness is the qualitative and most widely used term to define the visco-elastic properties of the vascular wall.

Blood Pressure and the Mechanical Behavior of the Arterial Wall

The elastic thoracic aorta takes origin from the left ventricle and almost immediately curves, in a three-dimensional way, dividing into musculo-elastic and muscular branches to the heart, head, and upper and lower limbs (macro-circulation). Beyond the early branches, the total cross-sectional area of the arterial tree begins to expand markedly. Whereas total cross-section increases, the average diameter is reduced, reflecting the increased number of bifurcations toward arterioles and capillary network [1, 2] (fig. 1). The microcirculation begins when the arteriolar diameter is <150 μm (fig. 1). Along the arterial and arteriolar tree, the forces governing flow are exclusively interested in the pressure generated by the heart. This quantity, which is the difference between the actual pressure and its hydrostatic component, is commonly referred to as 'blood pressure' (BP) [1]. It is the gradient of excess pressure which drives the flow. The distribution of this excess pressure through the circulation, which is largely dissipated in forcing the blood through the microcirculation, is at the origin of the so-called 'vascular resistance'. The behavior of BP along the arterial tree and its consequences on the arterial wall is the first objective of this chapter, taking into account that the heart is an intermittent and not a steady pump.

Cardiac Contraction and Aortic Consequences of Intermittent Ventricular Ejection [1–3]

There are three main consequences on large vessels of the intermittent ventricular ejection of the heart: (1) as a result of the systolic contraction of the left ventricle, coronary blood flow is interrupted and the coronary arteries are perfused only during diastole [1–3]; (2) the thoracic aorta during systole acts

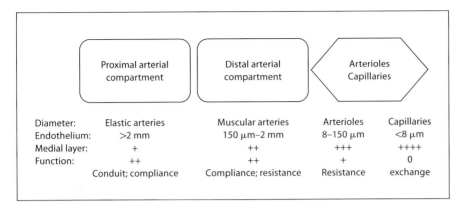

Fig. 1. Oversimplified description of the macro- and microcirculation. A semiquantitative evaluation of the extent of endothelium and medial layer function is indicated from + to +++ [1–4].

as an elastic reservoir (Windkessel function), and (3), following the systolic ejection of blood on the aortic wall, a shock wave acutely develops, resulting in the rapid propagation of this wave along the arterial tree. Only points 2 and 3 of this description are detailed in this paragraph.

At the end of ventricular ejection, the pressure in the aorta falls much more slowly than in the left ventricle because the large central arteries, and particularly the aorta, are elastic, and thus act as a reservoir during systole, storing part of the ejected blood, which is then forced out into the peripheral vessels, during diastole. More specifically, the pulsatile load is borne primarily by elastic-containing central arteries, which fulfill the bulk of the cushioning function by expanding during systole to store some, but not all, of each stroke volume, and then contracting during diastole to facilitate peripheral run-off of the stored blood. The cushioning function thus supports diastolic blood flow to peripheral tissues.

Then the pressure pulse generated by ventricular contraction travels along the aorta as a *wave* (fig. 2). It is possible to calculate the velocity of this wave (i.e., pulse wave velocity, PWV) from the delay between two BP curves located at two different sites of the arterial tree. Of course, the distance between measuring sites should be known. An example is given in figure 3. Because a fundamental principle is that pulse waves travel faster in stiffer arteries, the measurement of PWV is considered the best surrogate to evaluate arterial stiffness (fig. 3). Aortic PWV determines how quickly a disturbance of the arterial wall is moved away from the heart (up to 2 m/s with exercise). It approximates 3–5 m/s in young persons at rest, but increases considerably with age. Given that

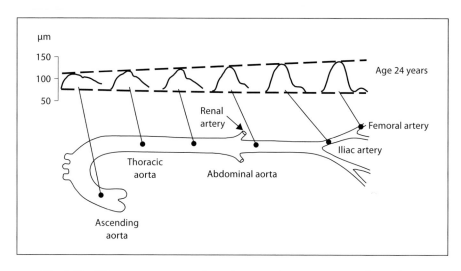

Fig. 2. The BP curve propagates along the arterial tree at a given velocity (PWV: see text). Note that, from central to peripheral arteries, SBP increases markedly while DBP is slightly reduced, and MAP (corresponding to the cross-sectional area under the BP curve) remains unmodified. With age, this amplification phenomenon, which is mainly due to wave reflections, tends to disappear [1–3].

peripheral arteries are markedly stiffer than central arteries, an important limitation of PWV measurements is the presence of a large heterogeneity of the arterial wall at its different sites.

BP Propagation and Amplification [2]

When several simultaneous BP measurements are done at different points all along the aorta, it appears that the pressure wave changes shape as it travels down the aorta. Whereas the systolic blood pressure (SBP) actually increases with distance from the heart, the *mean* level of the arterial pressure (MAP) slightly falls (about 4 mm Hg) during the same course along the length of the aorta (fig. 2). Thus the amplitude of the pressure oscillation between systole and diastole, which is pulse pressure (PP), nearly doubles (fig. 2). The SBP and PP amplification along the vascular tree is a physiological finding, which approximates 14 mm Hg between the origin of the thoracic aorta and the brachial artery, and continues in the branches of the aorta out to the level of about the third generation of branches. Thereafter, both PP and MAP decrease rapidly to the levels found in the microcirculation, a territory in which a nearly steady flow is achieved (fig. 4).

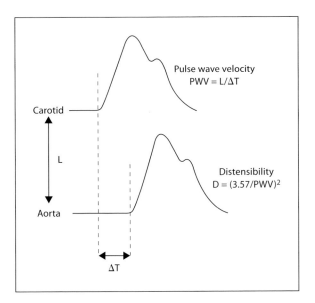

Fig. 3. Non-invasive determination of PWV between the carotid artery and the terminal aorta (i.e., the origin of femoral artery). The measured distance is L. If ΔT represents the time delay between the feet of the two waves, PWV equals L/ΔT. Distensibility may be then deduced from the Bramwell and Hill formula [1–3]. Automatic PWV measurements are widely used nowadays [1–3].

Transition from the Macro- to the Microcirculation [2]

Whereas the macrocirculation is characterized by pulsatile flow as well as by the propagation of pressure wave, PWV and PP amplification, the microcirculation is influenced by steady flow, and therefore by Poiseuille's law. At the arteriolar level, the pressure gradient becomes proportional to the rate of flow, the viscosity of blood, and the length of the arteriolar tree, and mostly is inversely proportional to the fourth power of vascular diameter.

In order to optimize the capillary exchanges, a low hydrostatic pressure profile is physiologically achieved in the microvascular network (fig. 4). The general consensus is that the resulting BP decrease occurs predominantly in precapillary vessels ranging from 10 to 300 μm [1–3]. Conversely, a very high vascular resistance (which represents, according to Poiseuille's law, the mechanical forces that are opposed to flow) builds up abruptly from larger to smaller arteries and capillaries, over a transitional short length of the path between arteries and veins, thus causing a steep decrease in MAP (fig. 4). At the same time, the PP amplitude decreases, resulting in almost completely steady flow through resistance vessels. However, a further contribution to opposition

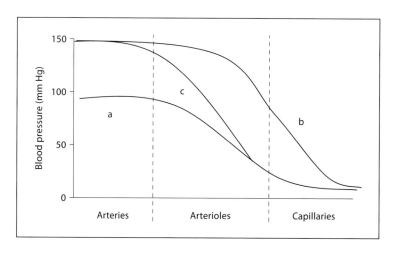

Fig. 4. Transition from the macrocirculation (large arteries) to the microcirculation (arterioles-capillaries). The decrease in BP along the vascular bed is represented under normal BP conditions (a), during arterial hypertensive without vasomotor adaptation (b), and after adaptation to the arterioles resulting in enhanced peripheral resistance but normal capillary pressure (c). During the same traject, the pulsatility disappears [1–3].

to flow is also derived from the reflection of arterial pulsations that cannot enter the high resistance vessels and are summated with pressure waves approaching the area of high resistance [1, 2]. This area of reflection, which is directly related to the number and geometrical properties of arteriolar bifurcations [1], contributes greatly to the hemodynamic profile of BP within large arteries (fig. 2).

Pulse Wave Morphology and Analysis (fig. 5)

If, in an individual, body length is 2 m at most and aortic PWV approximates 5 m/s, something must happen to the shape of the BP curve within the one beat if heart rate is 60/min. What happens is generation of wave reflections and their summation with the incident wave, as summarized in figure 5A and B. The incident wave passes away from the heart along the highly conductive arteries. There is a mismatch of impedance at the junction of a highly conductive artery and high resistance arterioles. So the wave cannot enter the arterioles and is repelled, traveling backward towards the heart. The morphology of any pulse wave results from the summation of incident (forward-traveling) and reflected (backward-traveling) pressure waves (fig. 5). Reflected waves may be initiated from any discontinuity of the arterial or arteriolar wall, but are mainly issued from high resistance vessels [2]. Pulse wave propagation and

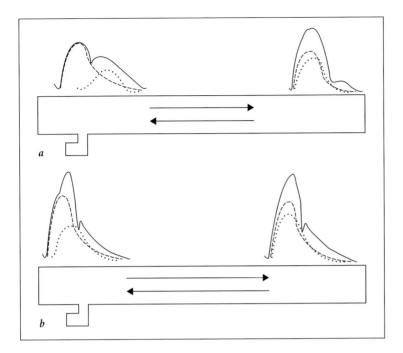

Fig. 5. Schematic representation of pressure-wave transmission and reflection in a tubular model of circulation. —— = Recorded pressure wave; – – – = incident/forward pressure wave; ····· = reflected pressure wave; → = PWV. On the right, pressure waves in the peripheral circulation are represented, while on the left, the pressure waves in the aorta and central arteries are represented. *a* Description of a distensible arterial system with a low PWV. In the peripheral circulation, the reflected wave occurs as an almost immediate response to the impact of incident pressure wave – the two waves are 'in phase' and their sum is the measured pressure wave. The reflected wave returns at a low PWV back to the central arteries and reaches the aorta after closure of the aortic valves or during the telesystole. The reflected wave is not 'in phase' with the incident wave and has no effect on SBP, but produces an additive 'boosting' effect on DBP. *b* Description of a stiff arterial system with increased PWV causing the reflected wave to return towards the central arteries and the aorta during ventricular ejection rather than during ventricular systole. In this situation the peripheral pressure amplification disappears. For *a* and *b*, the aortic BP curves are also represented in figure 6.

reflection varies considerably according to age. In young adults with full height and maximum elasticity of their central arteries (low PWV), the summation of the incident (forward-traveling) arterial pressure wave with the reflected (backward-traveling) wave results in progressive PP amplification so that SBP is higher at the brachial artery than at the ascending aorta (fig. 2 and 5a). This hemodynamic profile contrasts with MAP and DBP, which fall minimally

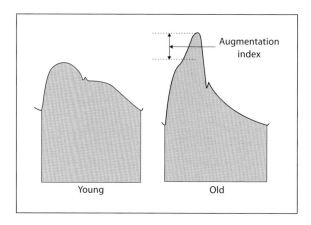

Fig. 6. BP curve in a younger and an older subject for the same cross-sectional area under the curve (i.e., the same heart rate and MAP) [1–3]. In younger subjects, the backward wave returns in diastole and participates to the diastolic perfusion, i.e., to the filling of coronary arteries. In older subjects, the backward wave returns earlier, i.e., in systole, causing an increase in 'augmentation index' and peak SBP, while diastolic perfusion is reduced, favoring myocardial ischemia [1–3]. 'Augmentation index' is the supplement of SBP due to the reflected wave and located between the two arrows indicated within the figure.

with distance from the heart in vessels at all ages (fig. 2). Note that, at the site of the thoracic aorta, as PWV is relatively low, the reflected wave comes back during diastole, thus maintaining DBP and boosting coronary perfusion (fig. 5a and 6). Thus an optimal arterial function is maintained, as well as an adequate coronary perfusion.

Wave Reflection, Arterial Stiffness and Ventricular Load [1–3]

The pattern of wave reflections and the pulse wave morphology are directly dependent on aging and arterial stiffness. The development of increasing arterial stiffness (high PWV) and altered wave reflections with aging and hypertension completely abolishes the differences between central and peripheral PP by age 50–60 years (fig. 5b and 6), with major consequences for ventricular load and coronary perfusion.

Arterial stiffness impacts the left ventricle into two ways: (1) the ejection of the stroke volume from the left ventricle into a stiff aorta generates a high early SBP, and (2) as mentioned earlier, the increased velocity of the aortic pulse wave allows the reflected waves to return to the aortic root earlier, during late systole (fig. 5 and 6). In that condition, the reflected waves summate with the forward-traveling wave to create an increase of 'augmentation' of central SBP (fig. 6) and ventricular load. In elderly persons with isolated systolic hypertension, aortic SBP can be increased by as much as 30–40 mm Hg as a result of the early return of wave reflection [1–3].

Furthermore, because the backward pressure returns in systole, and not in diastole, as a consequence of enhanced PWV (fig. 6), DBP and coronary blood flow tend to be reduced, a situation favoring coronary ischemia.

It is worth noting that the increased ventricular load is essentially 'wasted' cardiac work. Left ventricular workload is ultimately dependent on three major components: systemic vascular resistance; early systolic impedance, which increases the forward-traveling wave caused by proximal aortic stiffening; and finally, late systolic impedance, which influences the early return of the reflected (backward-traveling) pressure wave.

Vessel Wall and Mechanical Properties of Conduit Arteries

The vascular wall is composed of vascular smooth muscle (VSM) cells and extracellular matrix (ECM), which both contribute to the mechanical properties (i.e., arterial stiffness) of large vessels. The elastic behavior depends primarily on the composition and arrangement of the materials that make up the tunica media or middle layer of the vascular wall. In the media of the thoracic aorta and its immediate branches are large attachments of elastic lamellae to VSM cells, constituting the contractile-elastic units, which are arranged in an alternating oblique pattern that exerts maximum forces in a circumferential direction [4]. This arrangement is important for the balance of normal changes in intraluminal pressure and tension that occur during systole and diastole. In a normal young healthy person, the medial fibrous elements of the thoracic aorta contain a predominance of elastin over collagen, but as one proceeds distally along the arterial tree, there is a rapid reversal of the proportion with more collagen than elastin in the peripheral muscular arteries [2–4]. Thus, the thoracic aorta and its immediate branches show greater elasticity, whereas more distal vessels become progressively stiffer.

Close study of the infrastructure of the arterial media has shown that the structure is a composite of subunits, each comprising a group of fascicles of commonly oriented VSM cells surrounded by a similarly oriented array of interconnected elastic fibers [4]. The smooth cells of individual fascicles are bound together by a continuous intercellular and pericellular basal lamina (type IV collagen) and by a basketwork of fine collagen fibrils (type III), many of which are embedded in the basal lamina. Separately organized, coarser collagen fibers (type I) appear as bundles between adjacent musculo-elastic fascicles and only occasionally within them. The size, orientation and distribution of the musculo-elastic fascicles in relation to curves and branch regions suggest that they are aligned along lines of tensile force. The fiber bundles are crimped so that configurational rigidity may also contribute resistance to deformation or stretch. VSM cells are attached to the immediately surrounding elastin bars by a series of firm linear junctions. The collagen bundles are not attached to elastic fibers and are only occasionally attached to cells. This composite of stacked musculo-elastic fascicles results in a specific transmural distribution of aortic medial elements, not in layers of elastin-cells-elastin, but in layers of elastin-cells-elastin:collagen:elastin-cells-elastin:collagen, and so on [4].

The protein product of the elastin gene is synthesized by VSM cells and secreted as a monomer, tropoelastin [2–4]. After post-translational modification, tropoelastin is cross-linked and organized into elastin polymers that form concentric rings of elastic fenestrated lamellae around the arterial lumen. Elastin-deficient mice die from an occlusive fibrocellular pathology caused by subendothelial proliferation and accumulation of VSM cells in early neonatal life [5]. Thus, elastin is a crucial signaling molecule that directly controls VSM cell biology, and stabilizes arterial structure and resting vessel diameter. On the other hand, vascular collagen is determined at a very early developmental stage and thereafter remains quite stable, due to a very low turnover. Nevertheless, the proportion of collagen types I and III has a differential mechanical impact on stiffness of the vessel wall [6]. Furthermore, neurohumoral factors, particularly those related to angiotensin II and aldosterone, modulate collagen accumulation [1–3, 6, 7]. Finally, under the influence of several enzymes such as metalloproteinases, collagen is also subjected to important chemical modifications, such as breakdown, cross-linking or glycation, resulting in marked changes in stiffness along the vessel wall [3]. Several other molecules, such as connexins or desmins, may contribute to the three-dimensional distribution of mechanical forces within the arterial wall, acting on cell-cell and cell-matrix attachments and favoring resulting changes in arterial stiffness [8, 9]. Finally, ECM is mostly responsible for the passive mechanical properties of the arteries, in particular of the aorta and its main branches [1, 2]. These passive properties, which must to be studied in the absence of VSM tone (after poisoning VSM cells by potassium cyanide), are usually mathematically defined from a cylindrical model of the artery. When the transmural pressure rises, a curvilinear (and not a linear) pressure-diameter curve ensues, as a consequence of recruitment of elastin at low pressure and of collagen fibers at high pressure (fig. 7) [1, 2]. From this framework, various indices have been described to define arterial stiffness and are summarized in table 1.

Independently of ECM, VSM cells do not represent a homogenous population. For the same genomic background, they have different mixtures of phenotypes, involving not only contractile and secretory but also proliferative and

Table 1. Arterial stiffness indices [1–3, 12–14] (see also pp. 22–24)

Pulse wave velocity[1]	Speed of travel of the pulse along an arterial segment (fig. 3) Distance/Δt (cm/s)
Arterial distensibility[1]	Relative diameter (or area) change for a pressure increment; the inverse of elastic modulus (fig. 7) $\Delta D/(\Delta P \cdot D)$ (mm Hg^{-1})
Arterial compliance[1]	Absolute diameter (or area) change for a given pressure step at fixed vessel length $\Delta D/\Delta P$ (cm/mm Hg) (or cm^2/mm Hg) (fig. 7)
Elastic modulus	Intrinsic elastic properties of wall material $\Delta P \cdot V/\Delta V \cdot h$ (mm Hg/cm) (fig. 7)

Nowadays, most of these indices are measured non-invasively in vivo using echo-Doppler techniques with high resolution and high degree of reproducibility, particularly for D, ΔD and h. The most important difficulty is BP measurement, which may require local tonometry. The latter then requires calibration, which remains a difficult problem to resolve.

P = Pressure; D = diameter; V = volume; h = wall thickness; t = time.

[1] These indices are site-specific and vary with distending pressure (fig. 7). They may be measured in vivo (active properties in the presence of VSM tone) or in vitro (or even in vivo, in situ) (passive properties after poisoning VSM cells).

apoptotic properties [3, 10]. The distribution of these phenotypes is mainly influenced by age, by the location within the vascular tree, and the presence of underlying pathological factors. VSM contractile properties, which are mainly expressed in muscular arteries and arterioles, are responsible for the active mechanical properties of these vessels [1–3]. Changes in VSM tone may occur either directly or through signals arising from endothelial cells. Endothelium is a source of substances, particularly nitric oxide (NO), and of signal transduction mechanisms [11], that necessarily influence the biophysical properties of arteries and are defined according to the same mathematical formulas as passive mechanical properties (table 1, fig. 7) [1–3]. Many of these signals are influenced by blood flow through the mechanism of endothelium-dependent flow dilatation, which is observed for vessels of all sizes (muscular or musculo-elastic). In contrast, the role of mediators arising from endothelium predominates in muscular distal arteries and arterioles [3, 11, 12]. The wall-to-lumen ratio of such vessels is influenced by the local differential effects of NO and other vasodilating (bradykinin–prostaglandins) or vasoconstricting (norepinephrine, angiotensin, endothelin) compounds.

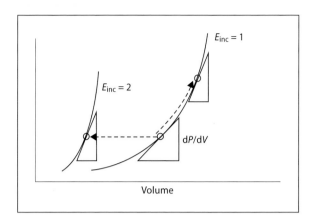

Fig. 7. Schematic representation of the pressure-volume relationship in CV structures with different incremental elastic modulus (E_{inc}: intrinsic stiffness of biomaterials)
(see table 1). Increasing E_{inc} shifts the pressure-volume (or diameter) curve to the left, increasing the pressure effect of volume changes [1–3]. Note that each pressure-volume
curve is curvilinear, due to the role of elastin at low pressure and collagen at high pressure. Thus, the slope dP/dV of the pressure-volume relationship is reduced when pressure
increases, and characterizes, at each given pressure, the elasticity of the system (called
also compliance or distensibility: see table 1). When the material of the arterial wall is
changed (i.e., when E_{inc} changes from position 1 to position 2; see table 1), the pressure-
volume curve is reset [1–3].

In muscular arteries, dilators such as nitroglycerine cause a large degree
of dilation but little change or even an increase in arterial stiffness, whereas
constrictors seem to have an opposite effect. Such hemodynamic profiles can
be explained on the basis of models connecting VSM cells to the stiff collagen
and less stiff elastin fibers [2]. It has been suggested that VSM cells are in series
with collagen but in parallel with elastin [2]. Hence, muscular contraction
makes an artery stiffer as well as more narrow, whereas muscular relaxation
makes the artery less stiff as well as wider. Nevertheless, the latter change may
not be apparent if collagenous fibers are modified by the passive increase in
diameter.

Finally, through their dilating properties, arteriolar vessels may contribute to change the pattern of wave reflections. Reflection sites are located at
any discontinuity of ECM and/or VSM cells. The reflectance properties of the
arterial and arteriolar system are nowadays the subject of emerging research.

Mechanical Stress and Arterial Remodeling

An arterial wall is a complex tissue composed of different cell populations capable of structural and functional changes, in response to direct injury and atherogenic factors, or to modifications of long-term hemodynamic conditions. The principal geometric modifications induced by hemodynamic alterations are changes of arterial lumen and/or arterial wall thickness due to activation, proliferation and migration of VSM cells, and rearrangements of cellular elements and ECM [12–18].

The mechanical signals for arterial remodeling associated with hemodynamic overload are cyclic tensile stress and shear stress [13–17]. BP is the principal determinant of arterial wall stretch and tensile stress, creating radial and tangential forces that counteract the effect of intraluminal pressure. Blood-flow alterations result in changes of shear stress, the dragging frictional force created by blood flow. While acute changes in tensile or shear stress induce transient adjustments in vasomotor tone and arterial diameter, chronic alterations of mechanical forces lead to modifications of the geometry and composition of the vessel walls [15].

According to Laplace's law, tensile stress (σ) is directly proportional to arterial transmural pressure (P) and radius (r), and inversely proportional to arterial wall thickness (h) according to the formula $\sigma = Pr/h$ [1–3, 14]. In response to increased BP or arterial radius, tensile stress is maintained within the physiological range by thickening of the heart and vessel walls, a process which is constantly observed in the cardiovascular (CV) system of atherosclerotic or hypertensive subjects [14–16, 18]. Due to a very low stress level, this process cannot be clearly observed or is even absent at the site of smaller arterioles or capillaries.

Shear stress is a function of the blood-flow pattern. In 'linear' segments of the vasculature, blood is displaced in layers moving at different velocities [1, 2]. The middle of the stream moves more rapidly than the side layers, generating a parabolic velocity profile. The slope of the velocity profile, i.e., the change of blood velocity per unit distance across the vessel radius, defines the shear rate. Shear stress is the product of the shear rate × blood viscosity. Thus, shear stress (τ) is directly proportional to blood flow (Q) and blood viscosity (η) and inversely proportional to the radius (r) of the vessel, according to the formula $\tau = Q\eta/\pi r^3$ [2, 14, 16]. Shear stress is often presented as the major mechanical factor acting in atherosclerosis while tensile stress is rather acting in hypertension. In fact, changes in shear and tensile stress are interconnected, because any modification of the arterial radius caused by alterations in blood flow and shear stress induces changes in tensile stress (unless the BP varies in the opposite direction).

The characteristics of arterial remodeling depend largely on the nature of hemodynamic stimuli applied to the vessel. To maintain tensile stress within physiological limits, arteries respond by thickening their walls (Laplace's law), but the increased tensile stress results from both the direct effect of high BP and the pressure-dependent passive distension of the arterial lumen. Studies in animals and humans have shown that this pressure-related distension of the arterial diameter is limited to central (elastic-type) arteries, being absent from peripheral (muscular-type) arteries, and causes an increase of the wall-to-lumen ratio which is proportional to the pressure [2, 3, 14]. The limitation or absence of a pressure-dependent diameter increase efficiently maintains tensile stress within normal limits. The nature of the mechanism(s) preventing the passive 'dilatory' effect of pressure is unknown but requires the presence of an intact endothelium [14]. Pertinently, but beyond the scope of this chapter, endothelial function is consistently altered in subjects with hypertension and/ or atherosclerosis [14, 15, 19].

Experimental and clinical data indicate that acute and chronic augmentations of arterial blood flow induce proportional increases in the vessel lumen, whereas decreasing flow reduces the arterial inner diameter [14, 15]. An example of flow-mediated remodeling associates arterial dilation and sustained high blood flow after the creation of an arteriovenous fistula [20]. Increased arterial inner diameter is usually accompanied by wall hypertrophy and increased intima-media cross-sectional area (following increases in the radius and wall tension). The presence of the endothelium is a prerequisite for normal vascular adaptation to chronic changes of blood flow, and experimental data indicate that flow-mediated arterial remodeling can be limited through inhibition of NO synthase [19]. Finally, although the alterations of tensile and shear stresses are interrelated, changes of tensile stress primarily induce alterations and hypertrophy of the arterial media, whereas changes of shear stress principally modify the dimensions and structure of the intima.

Pathophysiological Changes of Arterial Stiffness and Wave Reflections

Physiologically, MAP is quite similar throughout the arterial tree, while PP and vessel stiffness increases progressively from the proximal to the distal part of the vascular traject. These changes in elasticity result from the combination of the continuous decrease of the vessel cross-sectional area along the arterial tree, the progressive increased rigidity of vascular wall material, and the physiological rise in PP from central to peripheral arteries, which largely results from changes in wave reflections [2]. Because vascular elasticity is higher in proximal than in distal arteries, a progressive increase in the stiffness gradient of wall tissue is observed from proximal to distal arteries. In humans, the increase in stiffness between the carotid and the radial artery approximates 25% in normal subjects [3, 21]. With age, the difference in stiffness between proximal and distal arteries is significantly reduced, due to a more rapid increase in stiffness with age in the central than in the peripheral arteries [3, 21]. This rapid increase in stiffness of central (but not peripheral) arteries is largely independent of MAP and involves enlargement of mean diameter, reduction of pulsatile diameter, age-mediated reduction in endothelial function, development of connective tissue, early wave reflections and reduction of PP amplification [3]. The latter relates to the more rapid increase of aortic than peripheral PP with age, due both to increased stiffness and altered reflectance properties of the vessel wall.

Aging is the dominant process altering vascular stiffness, wave reflections, and PP. There is however an extreme variability of the age-mediated changes [21]. This variability is influenced by the histopathological particularities of arterial tissue (muscular or musculo-elastic), and mostly by the presence of other CV risk factors inside the microenvironment. In subjects with middle-age hypertension, when other CV risk factors (tobacco consumption, diabetes mellitus, dyslipidemia, obesity...) are not or minimally present, high MAP contributes dominantly to the increase of arterial stiffness, whereas MAP-independent structural and functional changes in stiffness play a more important role in older subjects, as described earlier [3, 21]. MAP-independent increase of arterial stiffness largely predominates in subjects with endothelial dysfunction as observed prematurely in the evolution of patients with diabetes mellitus, metabolic syndrome, obesity, end-stage renal disease or finally with multiple atherosclerotic alterations [3, 21].

Environmental (sodium) and genetic factors are now considered to play a major contribution in the mechanisms of changes in arterial wall mechanics [3, 7]. The mostly described gene polymorphisms are often related either to hypertension (as gene polymorphisms of the renin-angiotensin-aldosterone system), or to atherosclerosis, or to CV aging [3]. The combination of two or three specific polymorphisms can affect vessel wall properties more consistently than a single one. In particular, in elderly subjects with systolic hypertension, the DD genotype of the angiotensin-converting-enzyme gene polymorphism, mostly associated with specific genotypes of the aldosynthase and α-adducin genes, involves in men a consistent increase of arterial stiffness together with an increase of SBP and PP [22, 23].

Arterial Stiffness, Aging, Arteriosclerosis and Atherosclerosis

As described earlier, age is the major determinant of increased arterial stiffness. The CV risk factors mentioned earlier contribute greatly to arterial wall stiffening, even independently of MAP level. However, the most important connection of increased arterial stiffness is atherosclerosis.

Aging, Loss of Elastin and Fatigue [2]

Central artery elasticity is critically dependent on normal content and function of the matrix protein elastin, which with a half-life of 40 years, is one of the most stable proteins in the body. Despite this stability, fatigue of elastin fibers and lamellae can occur by the sixth decade of life from the accumulated cyclic stress of more than 2 billion aorta expansions during ventricular contraction. Long-standing cyclic stress in the media of elastic-containing arteries produces fatigue and eventual fracturing of elastin along with structural changes of the ECM that include proliferation of collagen and deposition of calcium [2]. Humoral factors, cytokines, and oxidative metabolites may also play a role. This degenerative process, classically termed *arteriosclerosis*, is the pathologic process that results in increased central arterial stiffness. In untreated, and even long-term treated hypertensive subjects, an acceleration of the rate of development of conduit artery stiffness is observed. This process in turn may perpetuate a vicious cycle of accelerated hypertension and further increase in aortic rigidity, particularly through the associated development of vascular calcifications.

Atherosclerosis versus Arteriosclerosis

Disease processes such as diabetes, chronic renal failure and generalized atherosclerosis can accelerate aging of the aorta and central arteries with earlier development of arterial stiffness. Arteriosclerosis is often confused with atherosclerosis, but these two disease states are independent, but frequently in overlapping, conditions (table 2) [1–4]. Atherosclerosis is primarily focal, starts in the intima, and tends to be occlusive. Arteriosclerosis tends to be diffuse, starts in the media, and frequently results in a dilated and tortuous aorta. Moreover, the pathophysiology of atherosclerosis is that of inflammatory disease with lipid-containing plaques and predominantly downstream ischemic disease, which results in increased thoracic aortic stiffness and elevated left ventricle workload.

Finally, the purpose of this book is not only to give some insight into the relationship between arterial stiffness and atherosclerosis, but also to establish the possible interactions with age and high BP, and therefore to define new therapeutic perspectives for CV prevention.

Table 2. Differential features of atherosclerosis and arteriosclerosis [2]

Feature	Atherosclerosis	Arteriosclerosis
Distribution	Focal	Diffuse
Location	Intima	Media, adventitia
Geometry	Occlusive	Dilatory
Pathology	Plaque	$\downarrow$Elastin, $\uparrow$collagen, Ca^{2+}
Physiology	Inflammation	Large artery stiffness
Hemodynamics	Ischemia	$\uparrow$Left ventricular workload

$\downarrow$ = Decrease; $\uparrow$ = increase.

Acknowledgments

This study was performed with the help of INSERM and GPH-CV (groupe de Pharmacologie et d'Hémodynamique Cardiovasculaire), Paris. We thank Dr. Anne Safar for helpful and stimulating discussions.

References

1 Caro CG, Pedley TJ, Schroter RC, Seed WA: The Mechanics of the Circulation. New York, Oxford University Press, 1978, pp 243–349.
2 Nichols WW, O'Rourke M: McDonald's Blood Flow in Arteries. Theoretical, Experimental and Clinical Principles, ed 4. London, Arnold, 1998, pp 54–401.
3 Safar ME, Levy BI, Struijker-Boudier H: Current perspectives on arterial stiffness and pulse pressure in hypertension and cardiovascular diseases. Circulation 2003;107:2864–2869.
4 Glagov S: Hemodynamic risk factors: mechanical stress, mural architecture, medial nutrition and vulnerability of arteries to atherosclerosis; in Wissler RW, Geer JC (eds): The Pathogenesis of Atherosclerosis. Baltimore, Williams & Wilkins, 1972, pp 164–199.
5 Li DY, Brooke B, Davis EC, Mecham RP, Sorensen LK, Boak BB, Eichwald E, Keating MT: Elastin is an essential determinant of arterial morphogenesis. Nature 1998;393:276–280.
6 Fleischmayer R, Perlish JS, Burgeson RE, Shaikh-Bahai F: Type I and type III collagen interactions during fibrillogenesis. Ann NY Acad Sci 1990;580:161–175.
7 Safar ME, Thuilliez C, Richard V, Benetos A: Pressure-independent contribution of sodium to large artery structure and function in hypertension. Cardiovasc Res 2000;46:269–276.
8 Ko YS, Coppen SR, Dupont E, Rothery S, Severs NJ: Regional differentiation of desmin, connexin43, and connexin45 expression patterns in rat aortic smooth muscle. Arterioscler Thromb Vasc Biol 2001;21:355–364.
9 Lacolley P, Challande P, Boumaza S, Cohuet G, Laurent S, Boutouyrie P, Grimaud JA, Paulin D, Lamaziere JM, Li Z: Mechanical properties and structure of carotid arteries in mice lacking desmin. Cardiovasc Res 2001;51:178–187.
10 Hamet P: Proliferation and apoptosis of vascular smooth muscle in hypertension. Curr Opin Nephrol Hypertens 1995;4:1–7.
11 Davies PF: Flow-mediated endothelial mechanotransduction. Physiol Rev 1995;75:519–560.
12 Levy BI, Ambrosio G, Pries AR, Struijker-Boudier HAJ: Microcirculation in hypertension. A new target for treatment? Circulation 2001;104:735–740.

13   Cohn JN, Finkelstein S, McVeigh G: Non-invasive pulse wave analysis for the early detection of vascular disease. Hypertension 1995;26:503–508.
14   Langille BL: Remodeling of developing and mature arteries: endothelium, smooth muscles, and matrix. J Cardiovasc Pharmacol 1993;21(suppl I):S11–S17.
15   Kamiya A, Togawa T: Adaptative regulation of wall shear stress to flow change in the carotid artery. Am J Physiol 1980;239:H14–H21.
16   Gibbons GH, Dzau VJ: The emerging concept of vascular remodeling. N Eng J Med 1994;330: 1431–1438.
17   Williams B: Mechanical influences on vascular smooth muscle cell function. J Hypertens 1998; 16:1921–1929.
18   Folkow B: Physiological aspects of primary hypertension. Physiol Rev 1982;62:347–504.
19   Pohl U, Holtz J, Busse R, Bassenge E: Crucial role of endothelium in the vasodilator response to the increased flow in vivo. Hypertension 1986;8:37–44.
20   Girerd X, London G, Boutouyrie P, Mourad JJ, Safar M, Laurent S: Remodeling of radial artery in response to a chronic increase in shear stress. Hypertension 1996;27:799–803.
21   Safar ME, Blacher J, Mourad JJ, London GM: Stiffness of carotid artery wall material and blood pressure in humans. Stroke 2000;31:782–790.
22   Balkenstein EJ, Staessen JA, Wang JG, van der Heijden-Spek JJ, van Bortel LM, Barlassina C, Bianchi G, Brand E, Herrmann SM, Struijker Boudier HA: Carotid and femoral artery stiffness in relation to three candidate genes in a white population. Hypertension 2001;38:1190–1197.
23   Safar ME, Lajemi M, Rudnichi A, Asmar R, Benetos A: Angiotensin-converting enzyme D/I gene polymorphism and age-related changes in pulse pressure in subjects with hypertension. Arterioscler Thromb Vasc Biol 2004;24:782–786.

Prof. Michel Safar
Centre de Diagnostic Hôtel-Dieu, 1, place du Parvis Notre-Dame
FR–75181 Paris Cedex 04 (France)
Tel. +33 1 4234 8025, Fax +33 1 4234 8632, E-Mail michel.safar@htd.ap-hop-paris.fr

Safar ME, Frohlich ED (eds): Atherosclerosis, Large Arteries and Cardiovascular Risk.
Adv Cardiol. Basel, Karger, 2007, vol 44, pp 19–34

....

Aging and Arterial Structure-Function Relations

Joseph L. Izzo, Jr.[a]   *Gary F. Mitchell*[b]

[a]State University of New York at Buffalo, Buffalo, N.Y., and
[b]Cardiovascular Engineering, Inc., Waltham, Mass., USA

Abstract

Aging and hypertension interact and are associated with long-term changes in arterial structure and function. Systolic BP is not constant along the arterial tree due to different proportional contributions of forward and reflected pressure waves. Brachial cuff BP values are inadequate to detect these changes. Increased PP is the result of an imbalance between arterial flow and arterial impedance, which can be due to increased effective arterial wall stiffness or to a smaller proportional arterial diameter. After middle age, there is both dilation and stiffening of large arteries, along with increased effective stiffness caused by the corresponding changes in content of collagen, elastin, and VSM in the vascular wall. Intermediate conduit arteries also dilate with age but their functional characteristics remain relatively preserved. In the microcirculation, vasoconstriction, VSM hypertrophy and rarefaction accompany and may contribute to changes in organ function.

Copyright © 2007 S. Karger AG, Basel

The last few years have witnessed a radical change in thinking about the syndrome of hypertension. Systolic blood pressure (BP) is widely accepted as the primary endpoint of clinical concern [1, 2] and it is now recognized that aging and hypertension interact to alter the relations between systolic and diastolic BP [3–6]. Although interrelated, it can even be argued that systolic and diastolic hypertension are two fundamentally different hemodynamic abnormalities [5, 7]. At the very least, the pathogenesis of essential hypertension is

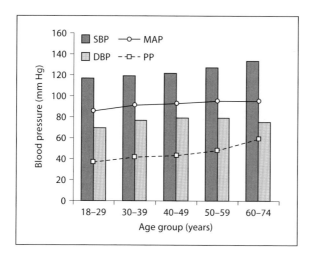

Fig. 1. Age and blood pressure. In the 3rd National Health and Nutrition Examination Survey (NHANES III) of the US population, there was a trend for systolic blood pressure (SBP) to increase with age, while diastolic (DBP) increased until about age 50 and then declined. Mean arterial pressure (MAP) reached a plateau at about age 50, while pulse pressure (PP) continued to increase in later years. Data shown are for white males; trends are similar for all races and both genders. Adapted from Burt et al. [18].

not described adequately by the historical model of increased distal vasoconstriction. This chapter reviews available epidemiologic and pathophysiologic studies that cast new light on the ventricular-vascular interactions that underlie wide pulse pressure (PP) and systolic hypertension [3–10].

Aging and Blood Pressure

Systolic hypertension is an acquired, age-related characteristic that has moderate and variable genetic contribution [11–15] but aging is not inexorably associated with systolic hypertension. In primitive or cloistered societies, there are no relations between age and BP and the incidence of hypertension at any age is very low [16, 17]. In industrialized societies, complex relations between age and BP are found (fig. 1) [6, 18], where systolic BP increases linearly with age, while diastolic BP increases until about age 50 then declines. Mean arterial pressure (MAP) increases until about age 50 then plateaus, while PP is constant until age 50 then increases. In adults, systolic hypertension is thus the predominant form of the condition and the percent with diastolic hypertension rapidly dwindles with aging. Furthermore, systolic hypertension is not a

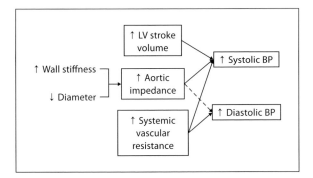

Fig. 2. Pathogenesis of systolic and diastolic BP elevations. Increased systemic vascular resistance (SVR) causes parallel elevations in diastolic, mean arterial, and systolic BP. Rarely, increased left ventricular (LV) stroke volume can cause elevated systolic BP. The determinant of wide pulse pressure is increased aortic impedance, either due to a smaller aortic diameter or increased effective wall stiffness. At older ages, high aortic impedance is usually associated with wide pulse pressure due to increased aortic stiffness, which acts to reduce diastolic BP even when SVR is moderately elevated (see text).

consequence of longstanding diastolic hypertension, as once thought. Systolic hypertension arises de novo at any age, and often preceding diastolic hypertension [6]. What is usually different from a pathophysiologic viewpoint is that the underlying hemodynamic mechanisms of systolic BP elevation and wide PP vary considerably as systolic hypertension presents itself in various clinical populations.

BP Components and Risk

The information conveyed by PP is fundamentally different from that conveyed by MAP, the product of cardiac output and systemic vascular resistance (SVR). While MAP is closely related to SVR, PP is determined principally by flow-impedance relations in large arteries, often called 'ventricular-vascular interactions'. When the aorta cannot optimally accommodate the degree of pulsatile flow, either due to an inappropriately small aortic diameter [19] or increased aortic wall stiffness [7, 8, 20], PP and systolic BP inevitably increase (fig. 2). Increased SVR can further exacerbate increased systolic BP (fig. 2) because PP and MAP have additive effects on systolic BP. In contrast, these two physiologically and anatomically distinct components of BP have opposing effects on diastolic BP. An increase in MAP is associated with higher DBP, while an increase in PP is generally associated with a lower DBP.

To make matters more confusing, higher MAP and higher PP are each independently associated with increased cardiovascular disease risk. The contrasting effects of MAP and PP on diastolic DBP contribute to the frequently described and often misunderstood non-linear (U- or J-shaped) relation between diastolic BP and cardiovascular events. For example, low diastolic BP and wide PP are associated with increased risk of mortality [21] yet high diastolic BP independently increases risk [22]. The problem is in the confounding caused by the use of diastolic BP as a risk surrogate. The situation becomes much clearer if risk is attributed to *either* elevated MAP *or* elevated PP. Hypertension as a clinical condition is thus intrinsically heterogeneous, and is perhaps best considered as an admixture of disordered large artery function (generating systolic hypertension) and disordered microcirculatory function (generating diastolic hypertension). Understanding which form of hypertension to treat and how to improve therapy begins with a discussion of normal and abnormal vascular function.

Arterial Wall Structure-Function Relations

Changes in the structure and function of the aorta and to a lesser extent the central arteries are the principal features underlying changes in PP. Large 'elastic arteries' are composed of three layers: the intima, the tunica media, and the adventitia [23]. In the proximal (thoracic) aorta, elastic lamellae are normally attached to smooth muscle cells to form 'contractile-elastic units' [24] that damp pulsation. Collagen is found in the adventitia and media, while elastin is located in the tunica media, not only in the internal and external elastic laminae, but also throughout the interstitial spaces surrounding the vascular smooth muscle (VSM) cells. Collagen fibers are oriented longitudinally, elastin forms a trabeculated sheath, and VSM are oriented in a spiral pattern. This geometric pattern contributes to the sequence of loading of the arterial wall that generally begins at low pressure with VSM, then shifts at higher pressures to elastin, and finally at the highest pressures to collagen. Overall, this sequence creates a non-linear loading response of arterial diameter and wall tension that limits pressure-dependent arterial dilation. Farther down the arterial tree, the proportion of wall constituents changes substantially. Elastin decreases markedly and the proportion of VSM cells increases. Distal arteries function less as dampers and more as 'conduits'. In resistance arterioles, there is little elastin and a markedly reduced proportion of collagen; the function of these microvessels is highly dependent on the tonic state of contraction of VSM and its relation with the endothelium.

The combined effects of wall thickness (h), wall stiffness (Young's modulus, E) and lumen radius (R) determine the impedance and compliance properties of large arteries. Changes in smooth muscle tone and remodeling in response to alterations in ambient flow can modulate each of the foregoing properties of the artery. The slope of the non-linear relation between arterial wall stress and strain (load) is the elastic modulus (E) of the vessel. The effective elastic modulus at any given distending pressure depends on the composition of the arterial wall (i.e., relative content of the three major structural elements – elastin, collagen and VSM), the state of smooth muscle activation, the extent of cross-linking within and between collagen and elastin fibers and the content and properties of other matrix components including various proteoglycans. Vascular loading characteristics also vary within the cardiac cycle, with contractile-elastic units being preferentially loaded during diastole, while elastin and collagen are loaded more fully in systole.

Stiffness of a given artery is pressure-dependent and non-linear, and varies according to the stiffness measure evaluated. Measures of arterial stiffness have differing dependencies on the three independent and interdependent determinants (E, h and R) that combine differently in various settings. Clinical estimation of aortic stiffness usually involves measurement of pulse wave velocity (PWV), which determines the speed of wave propagation in an artery, or characteristic impedance (Zc), which determines the early systolic pressure rise associated with a given pulsatile flow prior to the return of any reflected waves. These related measures of arterial function differ considerably in their relation to arterial lumen radius:

$$PWV = k(Eh/R)^{1/2} \qquad Zc = k(Eh/R^5)^{1/2}$$

where E = elastic modulus, h = arterial thickness, and R = arterial radius.

An increase in smooth muscle tone generally has little effect on PWV because the reduction in R (which reduces wall tension) is counteracted by the increases in medial thickness (h) and the intrinsic increase in E caused by VSM contraction. In contrast, Zc invariably increases substantially with local VSM activation because of the amplified (fivefold greater) dependency of Zc on R. Any process that primarily increases effective arterial wall stiffness (Eh) will limit the increase in R at a given distending pressure and will therefore have a greater effect on Zc than PWV.

Each artery has a range of maximum compliance (or minimum Zc) that usually corresponds to the physiologic operating range of pressures occurring in that vessel [25]. Relative to this nominal value, physiologic systems (e.g. sympathetic nervous and renin-angiotensin or local nitric oxide generative) that control vascular tone have relatively complex effects on local and systemic vascular elastic properties as described above. The in vivo regional response to increased VSM tone is further complicated by the associated changes in MAP. A localized increase in smooth muscle tone will tend to increase Zc as noted above. However, when MAP increases because of associated changes in resistance vessel tone, large artery diameter and Zc may remain unchanged (or may increase) while PWV is likely to be increased because of the attenuated dependency of PWV on R. Thus, PWV is also more dependent on diastolic BP than is Zc.

Arterial Changes in Aging and Hypertension

Arteriosclerosis is the process of age-related large artery stiffening usually found in individuals with wide PP or systolic hypertension. This adventitial and medial process must be differentiated from atherosclerosis, the occlusive low-grade endovascular inflammatory process that results from endothelial dysfunction and lipid oxidation. Arteriosclerosis often coexists with atherosclerosis but is worth differentiating from the former because prevention and treatment of the two conditions probably differ significantly. Histopathologically, arteriosclerosis is a diffuse non-inflammatory fibrotic process affecting primarily the adventitia and media, with breakdown of elastin, increased collagen and matrix deposition, and VSM hypertrophy [23]. Changes in other arterial wall components such as the vasa vasora may contribute to arteriosclerosis because occlusion of these adventitial vessels tends to increase the collagen:elastin ratio and arterial stiffness [26].

The difference between 'usual' and 'optimal' aging and the related question of the etiology of arteriosclerosis remain unclear. Nevertheless, over a lifetime, excessive burdens of pressure (causing cellular deformation and hypertrophy) and pulsatile flow (cyclic shear stress) are likely contributors to reduced elasticity and increased wall stiffness. Age-related dilation usually occurs in large arteriosclerotic arteries [27, 28], increasing PWV, while it minimally affects Zc [9, 10, 19]. Metabolic phenomena, including oxidative burden and different forms of cross-linking of proteins in the arterial wall, may be important as well. Overstimulation of physiologic systems can also influence arterial structure and function. In rats, chemical sympathectomy acutely increases aortic diameter and compliance but chronically reduces elastin content, vessel diameter and distensibility [29]. Exercise conditioning in rats reduces sympathetic nervous activity and lowers BP but does not affect the proportion of elastin or arterial wall constituents [30]. There are several lines of evidence that suggest a role for the renin-angiotensin-aldosterone system as an important modulator of arterial properties. Angiotensin II increases aortic wall thickness and stiffness in rats [31, 32]. Aldosterone administration reversibly increases rat aortic stiffness and fibronectin content in dose-dependent fashion independent of wall stress, with no changes in collagen or elastin [33]. Arterial stiffness in humans has been related to genetic variation in components of the renin-angiotensin-aldosterone system. Variability in PWV has been related to polymorphisms in the angiotensin II receptor (AGTR1) [34, 35], while variation in PP has been related to genetic variation in the angiotensin-converting enzyme gene [36].

Chronic structural changes are at least partially reversible, suggesting a tonic dependence on mechanical and neurohumoral inputs. Compared to angiotensin-converting enzyme inhibition alone, there are greater improvements in human Zc caused by neutral endopeptidase inhibition (which increases atriopeptins and further augments bradykinin) [37]. Matrix metalloproteinases are sensitive to nitric oxide, so neutral endopeptidase inhibition inhibitors may directly affect remodeling of vessels. The idea that aortic stiffness is largely independent of distal vascular resistance has practical applications for the future in the form of drugs that may reduce aortic stiffness by affecting large arterial wall components, especially those that block or disrupt collagen cross-links without affecting arteriolar function [38].

Wide Pulse Pressure: Stiffness vs. Diameter

As introduced in the foregoing discussion, the relation between large arteries and BP involves age-dependent and BP-dependent changes in arterial diameter, wall thickness, and wall composition that are themselves interdependent. The problem in understanding these complex associations begins with the many observations that MAP and PP are remarkably constant across the animal kingdom and throughout growth and development, despite wide variations in body size and heart rate. This relative constancy of MAP in normal animals is due to the proportional scaling of flow and impedance. There is a similar 'built-in' proportional scaling between arterial radius and effective stiffness (Eh), where both the numerator and the denominator of the impedance equation move in the same direction with aging. In humans, population variation and a long life span lead to differences between biologic and chronologic aging and in turn to greater variation in BP between individuals.

It has long been assumed that systolic hypertension simply represents 'burned out' diastolic hypertension and that the age-related widening of PP in older age is simply the result of 'normal' aging. There is no doubt that there is increased aortic stiffness, wall thickness, and elastic modulus with age and that wide PP can arise from the loss of aortic storage capacity (or compliance) and the concomitant loss of elastic recoil function. In a sense, the proximal aorta is the third pumping chamber of the heart. Although its function is largely passive, an elastic aorta dampens and sustains pulsatile flow throughout the cardiac cycle. If the aorta is not sufficiently elastic to expand during systole, Zc is increased, a reduced fraction of each cardiac stroke volume is retained in the central arteries during systole, and there is increased peak systolic flow velocity with systolic BP elevation. In diastole, lessened aortic retention of the 'residual' fraction of the stroke volume and diminished aortic elastic recoil leads to reduced diastolic flow and pressure. Thus with a stiff aorta, early systolic BP and flow are proportionally higher, while diastolic BP and flow are proportionally lower, leading to increased PP, even if cardiac stroke volume remains normal.

Yet increased aortic wall stiffness does not explain the observation that elevated systolic BP is also the most common presentation of hypertension in middle age, when arterial elasticity is not necessarily abnormal [6, 9, 12, 19]. In these cases, increased aortic impedance is related primarily to smaller aortic diameter, not a stiffer aortic wall [19]. Inspection for the formula for Zc reveals that aortic diameter is profoundly important in the determination of systolic BP and PP because Zc varies inversely with $R^{2.5}$. Aortic diameter steadily increases with age in humans – a change that has been attributed in the past to 'breakdown' of elastic elements in the aortic wall. However, increasing aortic diameter with advancing age may also be viewed as a maladaptive attempt by the aorta to limit the age-related increase in aortic impedance that would otherwise accompany age-related stiffening of the aortic wall. Age-related arterial dilation tends to reduce (not increase) arterial impedance, thereby reducing systolic BP and PP [39]. The idea that systolic hypertension can be caused by a disproportionately small aortic diameter runs counter to older thinking and has been attacked on the basis of studies showing increased PWV, elastic modulus, and aortic wall thickness in convenience samples of older people [40–42]. However, two large, community-based studies have shown an inverse relation between aortic diameter and PP [43, 44], adding support for the hypothesis that a mismatch between (inappropriately low) aortic diameter and resting flow contributes to elevated Zc and PP in humans.

The roles of the two competing phenomena in arterial impedance (decreased radius vs. increased effective stiffness) can be fully reconciled if one accepts that systolic hypertension is a heterogeneous condition dictated primarily by the aorta (and to a lesser degree other large central arteries), with modification by increased distal vasoconstriction (fig. 2). It is most likely that the well-documented age-related increase in aortic diameter [27, 28] represents the mechanical impact of the lifetime BP burden, as modified by genetic predispositions at multiple loci on several chromosomes [12]. In this context, aortic dilation may be a maladaptive response that tries to lower central PP at the expense of increased aortic wall tension, which presumably induces structural

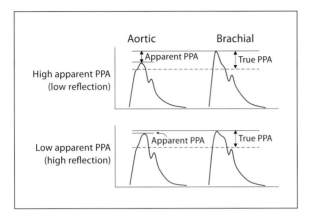

Fig. 3. Pulse pressure amplification (PPA). In healthy individuals, peripheral systolic BP is usually higher than central systolic BP because increased impedance in vessels of decreasing caliber causes true PPA (and high apparent PPA) of the forward pressure wave. True PPA, the difference between the forward pressure wave peak centrally (first central systolic peak, horizontal dotted lines) and peripherally, is almost always due to intrinsic vascular properties affecting forward wave alone. Current custom is to report 'apparent PPA,' which is confounded by the fact that peak central SBP includes components related to both forward and reflected waves (the second systolic peak, horizontal solid lines). When there is a substantial component of wave reflection, apparent PPA declines and measured central and peripheral systolic BP values are more equal.

changes in the arterial wall that increase effective stiffness. Individuals with smaller initial aortic diameters simply begin at a different starting point in the relation between radius and Eh. It is entirely possible that individuals with initially smaller aortic diameters 'age' faster than their counterparts in that they make a more rapid transition to a stiffer aortic wall. A study of the natural history of the functional changes that occur with age and hypertension is underway in the third-generation cohort of the Framingham Heart Study.

Pulse Transmission in Conduit Arteries

There has been a long tradition of assuming that changes in brachial cuff BP are similar to those at the heart or in peripheral target organs. As discussed, this is simply not the case due to intra- and interindividual differences in forward wave transmission and wave reflection [45, 46]. Differences in systolic BP from one site to another can be traced to alterations in the timing and amplitude of the forward and reflected pressure waves (fig. 3). Unlike diastolic or mean BP, systolic BP is thus not constant throughout the arterial tree. Within an individual, smaller distal arteries have higher input impedances than large central arteries because of the combined impact of decreasing lumen diameter and increasing effective wall stiffness. This increasing arterial stiffness gradient leads to the phenomenon of true pulse pressure amplification (PPA), where the amplitude of the forward wave increases within large and medium-sized arteries, so that systolic BP is normally higher in the peripheral arteries than in the aorta. PPA is variable between individuals but follows certain rules [47]. With normal aging, there is a reversal of the normal tendency for distal arterial stiffness (PWV) to exceed central arterial stiffness, a phenomenon that would be expected to lower the degree of PPA observed [9]. Muscular conduit arteries (e.g. brachial or femoral arteries) in hypertension do not usually differ from normal arteries in their stiffness, probably due in large measure to the fact that they also dilate with age, presumably by the same pressure-dependent mechanisms that affect the aorta [39]. Age-adjusted compliance of conduit arteries is also higher in hypertension compared to normals, another result of the generalized increase in arterial diameter.

Amplification and Reflection: Central vs. Peripheral BP

The morphology of a pulse contour at any point along the vascular tree represents the sum of the forward and reflected pressure waves at that point. Pulse wave morphology is unique in each artery because of differences in time of arrival of the forward and reflected pressure waves. Unlike diastolic or mean BP, systolic BP is thus not constant throughout the arterial tree.

In the arm, the amplitude of the forward wave is generally much greater than the amplitude of the reflected wave, so brachial cuff systolic BP conveys information primarily about the forward wave, including PPA, but is largely blind to changes in wave reflection (fig. 3). In contrast, peak central systolic BP is the result of a different admixture of the forward and reflected pressure waves, where the pulse pressure generated by the forward pressure wave may be augmented by as much as 100% by the reflected wave. In such cases, there may be very little difference between central and peripheral peak systolic pressure [40] and thus very little *apparent* PPA. This does not mean that *true* PPA of the forward wave is absent, just that the sum of the forward and reflected waves in the aorta is equal to the degree of true PPA of the forward wave in the arm. PPA tends to be greater in young individuals with isolated systolic hypertension despite lower SVR [47].

Relations between age and wave reflection are complex in normal and hypertensive individuals. Augmentation index (AI, the fractional increment of central PP caused by the principal reflected wave) is higher in hypertension but in the general population, AI increases until middle age, then plateaus or declines [9, 48]. There has also been significant confusion in the literature about the relation between AI and arterial stiffness. AI is only minimally related to the properties of central arteries [49–52] and is more governed by the degree of arteriolar narrowing of the distal circulation [52–54]. In contrast, widening of PP with age is almost always due to increased amplitude of the forward wave due to increased Zc in the central aorta.

Because the reflected wave is not apparent in the peak systolic BP measured by arm cuff, phenomena related to altered wave reflection go unnoticed in everyday clinical medicine. Newer techniques of pulse wave analysis offer new insight into this problem, however. The most popular method utilizes a generalized transfer function to derive central systolic BP from peripheral tonometric recordings of radial pressure. There is recurring debate regarding the reliability of the generalized transfer function in estimating central systolic BP [55], in part due to the need for different formulas for different disease states [56]. Nevertheless, the insensitivity of brachial cuff BP readings to detect clinically important changes in central systolic BP has been demonstrated in recent studies. For example, β-blockers have been found to be less effective than vasodilators in reducing augmentation pressures or central systolic BP [57–59]. Such studies suggest that non-invasive assessment of central systolic BP may be useful in assessing cardiac loading characteristics and the relative benefits of different antihypertensive drug classes [60].

Small Arteries and Arterioles

Aging and disease modify vascular structure and function. Hypertension is associated with vasoconstriction, VSM hypertrophy and rarefaction in the microcirculation. Pulse volume, pressure, and velocity are important physiological variables that may function as biologic signals to the endothelium and VSM of the microcirculation. The capillary pulse volume modifies and in turn is modified by microcirculatory structure and function. For example, both MAP and PP affect glomerular filtration rate independently, presumably through direct effects on glomerular filtration pressure [61]. Increased systolic BP or PP is associated with a variety of disorders related to aging, including atherosclerotic cardiovascular disease [62, 63], heart failure [64], stroke [65, 66], cognitive disorders [67–69], white matter lesions [70, 71], macular degeneration [72], renal dysfunction [73], osteoporosis [74], and glucose intolerance [75–77]. Abnormal microcirculatory pulsation may participate in the pathogenesis of organ dysfunction in these various disease states [7, 78–84]. Endothelial function in medium-sized and smaller arteries may also be impaired by increased pressure pulsatility [85, 86]. Capillary rarefaction has been demonstrated in young prehypertensive individuals with wide PP, suggesting a relation between PP and microcirculatory surface area [87, 88]. Wide PP is also associated with increased albuminuria, a marker of microcirculatory damage [89]. Since structure and function in small arteries may be adversely affected by exposure to high PP, the possibility exists that increased aortic stiffness and elevated PP may contribute directly to the pathogenesis of the various small vessel disorders and diseases described above, including hypertension.

References

1   Izzo JL Jr, Levy D, Black HR: Clinical Advisory Statement. Importance of systolic blood pressure in older Americans. Hypertension 2000;35:1021–1024.
2   Chobanian AV, Bakris GL, Black HR, Cushman WC, Green LA, Izzo JL Jr, Jones DW, Materson BJ, Oparil S, Wright JT Jr, Roccella EJ: Seventh Report of the Joint National Committee on Prevention, Detection, Evaluation, and Treatment of High Blood Pressure. Hypertension 2003;42: 1206–1252.
3   Galarza CR, Alfie J, Waisman GD, Mayorga LM, Camera LA, del Rio M, Vasvari F, Limansky R, Farias J, Tessler J, Camera MI: Diastolic pressure underestimates age-related hemodynamic impairment. Hypertension 1997;30:809–816.
4   Laurent S, Lacolley P, Girerd X, Boutouyrie P, Bezie Y, Safar M: Arterial stiffening: opposing effects of age- and hypertension-associated structural changes. Can J Physiol Pharmacol 1996;74: 842–849.
5   McEniery CM, Yasmin, Wallace S, Maki-Petaja K, McDonnell B, Sharman JE, Retallick C, Franklin SS, Brown MJ, Lloyd RC, Cockcroft JR, Wilkinson IB: Increased stroke volume and aortic stiffness contribute to isolated systolic hypertension in young adults. Hypertension 2005; 46:221–226.
6   Franklin SS, Pio JR, Wong ND, Larson MG, Leip EP, Vasan RS, Levy D: Predictors of new-onset diastolic and systolic hypertension: the Framingham Heart Study. Circulation 2005;111:1121–1127.
7   Izzo JL Jr: Arterial stiffness and the systolic hypertension syndrome. Curr Opin Cardiol 2004; 19:341–352.
8   Mitchell GF, Pfeffer MA: Pulsatile hemodynamics in hypertension. Curr Opin Cardiol 1999;14: 361–369.
9   Mitchell GF, Parise H, Benjamin EJ, Larson MG, Keyes MJ, Vita JA, Vasan RS, Levy D: Changes in arterial stiffness and wave reflection with advancing age in healthy men and women: the Framingham Heart Study. Hypertension 2004;43:1239–1245.
10 Mitchell GF, Lacourciere Y, Arnold JM, Dunlap ME, Conlin PR, Izzo JL Jr: Changes in aortic stiffness and augmentation index after acute converting enzyme or vasopeptidase inhibition. Hypertension 2005;46:1111–1117.
11 Hollenberg NK: Implications of species difference for clinical investigation: studies on the renin-angiotensin system. Hypertension 1999;35:150–154.
12 Mitchell GF, DeStefano AL, Larson MG, Benjamin EJ, Chen MH, Vasan RS, Vita JA, Levy D: Heritability and a genome-wide linkage scan for arterial stiffness, wave reflection, and mean arterial pressure: the Framingham Heart Study. Circulation 2005;112:194–199.
13 Camp NJ, Hopkins PN, Hasstedt SJ, Coon H, Malhotra A, Cawthon RM, Hunt SC: Genome-wide multipoint parametric linkage analysis of pulse pressure in large, extended Utah pedigrees. Hypertension 2003;42:322–328.

14 Caulfield M, Munroe P, Pembroke J, Samani N, Dominiczak A, Brown M, Benjamin N, Webster J, Ratcliffe P, O'Shea S, Papp J, Taylor E, Dobson R, Knight J, Newhouse S, Hooper J, Lee W, Brain N, Clayton D, Lathrop GM, Farrall M, Connell J: Genome-wide mapping of human loci for essential hypertension. Lancet 2003;361:2118–2123.

15 DeStefano AL, Larson MG, Mitchell GF, Benjamin EJ, Vasan RS, Li J, Corey D, Levy D: Genome-wide scan for pulse pressure in the National Heart, Lung and Blood Institute's Framingham Heart Study. Hypertension 2004;44:152–155.

16 Hollenberg NK, Martinez G, McCullough M, Meinking T, Passan D, Preston M, Rivera A, Taplin D, Vicaria-Clement M: Aging, acculturation, salt intake, and hypertension in the Kuna of Panama. Hypertension 1997;29:171–176.

17 Timio M, Saronio P, Venanzi S, Gentili S, Verdura C, Timio F: Blood pressure in nuns in a secluded order: a 30-year follow-up. Miner Electrolyte Metab 1999;25:73–79.

18 Burt VL, Whelton P, Roccella EJ, Brown C, Cutler JA, Higgins M, Horan MJ, Labarthe D: Prevalence of hypertension in the US adult population: results from the Third National Health and Nutrition Examination Survey, 1988–1991. Hypertension 1995;25:305–313.

19 Mitchell GF, Lacourciere Y, Ouellet JP, Izzo JL Jr, Neutel J, Kerwin LJ, Block AJ, Pfeffer MA: Determinants of elevated pulse pressure in middle-aged and older subjects with uncomplicated systolic hypertension: the role of proximal aortic diameter and the aortic pressure-flow relationship. Circulation 2003;108:1592–1598.

20 Kelly R, Hayward C, Avolio A, O'Rourke M: Noninvasive determination of age-related changes in the human arterial pulse. Circulation 1989;80:1652–1659.

21 Neaton JD, Wentworth D, Group MR: Serum cholesterol, blood pressure, cigarette smoking, and death from coronary heart disease: overall findings and differences by age for 316,099 white men. Arch Intern Med 1992;152:56–64.

22 Lewington S, Clarke R, Qizilbash N, Peto R, Collins R: Age-specific relevance of usual blood pressure to vascular mortality: a meta-analysis of individual data for one million adults in 61 prospective studies. Lancet 2002;360:1903–1913.

23 Avolio A, Jones D, Tafazzoli-Shadpour M: Quantification of alterations in structure and function of elastin in the arterial media. Hypertension 1998;32:170–175.

24 Bezie Y, Lacolley P, Laurent S, Gabella G: Connection of smooth muscle cells to elastic lamellae in aorta of spontaneously hypertensive rats. Hypertension 1998;32:166–169.

25 Shykoff BE, Hawari FI, Izzo JL Jr: Diameter, pressure and compliance relationships in dorsal hand veins. Vasc Med 2001;6:97–102.

26 Stefanadis C, Vlachopoulos C, Karayannacos P, Boudoulas H, Stratos C, Filippides T, Agapitos M, Toutouzas P: Effect of vasa vasorum flow on structure and function of the aorta in experimental animals. Circulation 1995;91:2669–2678.

27 Vasan RS, Larson MG, Levy D: Determinants of echocardiographic aortic root size. The Framingham Heart Study. Circulation 1995;91:734–740.

28 Agmon Y, Khandheria BK, Meissner I, Schwartz GL, Sicks JD, Fought AJ, O'Fallon WM, Wiebers DO, Tajik AJ: Is aortic dilatation an atherosclerosis-related process? Clinical, laboratory, and transesophageal echocardiographic correlates of thoracic aortic dimensions in the population with implications for thoracic aortic aneurysm formation. J Am Coll Cardiol 2003;42:1076–1083.

29 Lacolley P, Glaser E, Challande P, Boutouyrie P, Mignot JP, Duriez M, Levy B, Safar M, Laurent S: Structural changes and in situ aortic pressure-diameter relationship in long-term chemical-sympathectomized rats. Am J Physiol 1995;269:H407–H416.

30 Nosaka T, Tanaka H, Watanabe I, Sato M, Matsuda M: Influence of regular exercise on age-related changes in arterial elasticity: mechanistic insights from wall compositions in rat aorta. Can J Appl Physiol 2003;28:204–212.

31 Brouwers-Ceiler DL, Nelissen-Vrancken HJ, Smits JF, De Mey JG: The influence of angiotensin II-induced increase in aortic wall mass on compliance in rats in vivo. Cardiovasc Res 1997;33:478–484.

32 Ceiler DL, Nelissen-Vrancken HJ, Smits JF, De Mey JG: Pressure but not angiotensin II-induced increases in wall mass or tone influences static and dynamic aortic mechanics. J Hypertens 1999;17:1109–1116.

33   Lacolley P, Labat C, Pujol A, Delcayre C, Benetos A, Safar M: Increased carotid wall elastic modulus and fibronectin in aldosterone-salt-treated rats: effects of eplerenone. Circulation 2002;106: 2848–2853.

34   Benetos A, Topouchian J, Ricard S, Gautier S, Bonnardeaux A, Asmar R, Poirier O, Soubrier F, Safar M, Cambien F: Influence of angiotensin II type 1 receptor polymorphism on aortic stiffness in never-treated hypertensive patients. Hypertension 1995;26:44–47.

35   Benetos A, Gautier S, Ricard S, Topouchian J, Asmar R, Poirier O, Larosa E, Guize L, Safar M, Soubrier F, Cambien F: Influence of angiotensin-converting enzyme and angiotensin II type 1 receptor gene polymorphisms on aortic stiffness in normotensive and hypertensive patients. Circulation 1996;94:698–703.

36   Safar ME, Lajemi M, Rudnichi A, Asmar R, Benetos A: Angiotensin-converting enzyme D/I gene polymorphism and age-related changes in pulse pressure in subjects with hypertension. Arterioscler Thromb Vasc Biol 2004;24:782–786.

37   Mitchell GF, Izzo JL Jr, Lacourciere Y, Ouellet JP, Neutel J, Qian C, Kerwin LJ, Block AJ, Pfeffer MA: Omapatrilat reduces pulse pressure and proximal aortic stiffness in patients with systolic hypertension: results of the conduit hemodynamics of omapatrilat international research study. Circulation 2002;105:2955–2961.

38   Kass DA, Shapiro EP, Kawaguchi M, Capriotti AR, Scuteri A, deGroof RC, Lakatta EG: Improved arterial compliance by a novel advanced glycation end-product crosslink breaker. Circulation 2001;104:1464–1470.

39   Van Bortel LM, Spek JJ: Influence of aging on arterial compliance. J Hum Hypertens 1998;12: 583–586.

40   Kelly R, Hayward C, Avolio A, O'Rourke M: Noninvasive determination of age-related changes in the human arterial pulse. Circulation 1989;80:1652–1659.

41   O'Rourke MF, Nichols WW: Changes in wave reflection with advancing age in normal subjects. Hypertension 2004;44:e10.

42   O'Rourke MF, Nichols WW: Aortic diameter, aortic stiffness, and wave reflection increase with age and isolated systolic hypertension. Hypertension 2005;45:652–658.

43   Vasan RS, Larson MG, Benjamin EJ, Levy D: Echocardiographic reference values for aortic root size: the Framingham Heart Study. J Am Soc Echocardiogr 1995;8:793–800.

44   Bella JN, Wachtell K, Boman K, Palmieri V, Papademetriou V, Gerdts E, Aalto T, Olsen MH, Olofsson M, Dahlof B, Roman MJ, Devereux RB: Relation of left ventricular geometry and function to aortic root dilatation in patients with systemic hypertension and left ventricular hypertrophy (the LIFE study). Am J Cardiol 2002;89:337–341.

45   Karamanoglu M, O'Rourke MF, Avolio AP, Kelly RP: An analysis of the relationship between central aortic and peripheral upper limb pressure waves in man. Eur Heart J 1993;14:160–167.

46   O'Rourke MF, Vlachopoulos C, Graham RM: Spurious systolic hypertension in youth. Vasc Med 2000;5:141–145.

47   Wilkinson IB, Franklin SS, Hall IR, Tyrrell S, Cockcroft JR: Pressure amplification explains why pulse pressure is unrelated to risk in young subjects. Hypertension 2001;38:1461–1466.

48   McEniery CM, Yasmin, Hall IR, Qasem A, Wilkinson IB, Cockcroft JR: Normal vascular aging: differential effects on wave reflection and aortic pulse wave velocity: the Anglo-Cardiff Collaborative Trial (ACCT). J Am Coll Cardiol 2005;46:1753–1760.

49   Filipovsky J, Ticha M, Cifkova R, Lanska V, Stastna V, Roucka P: Large artery stiffness and pulse wave reflection: results of a population-based study. Blood Pressure 2005;14:45–52.

50   Woodman RJ, Kingwell BA, Beilin LJ, Hamilton SE, Dart AM, Watts GF: Assessment of central and peripheral arterial stiffness: studies indicating the need to use a combination of techniques. Am J Hypertens 2005;18:249–260.

51   Lacy PS, O'Brien DG, Stanley AG, Dewar MM, Swales PP, Williams B: Increased pulse wave velocity is not associated with elevated augmentation index in patients with diabetes. J Hypertens 1937;22:1937–1944.

52   Lemogoum D, Flores G, Van den Abeele W, Ciarka A, Leeman M, Degaute JP, van de Borne P, Van Bortel L: Validity of pulse pressure and augmentation index as surrogate measures of arterial stiffness during β-adrenergic stimulation. J Hypertens 2004;22:511–517.

53   Wilkinson IB, MacCallum H, Hupperetz PC, van Thoor CJ, Cockcroft JR, Webb DJ: Changes in the derived central pressure waveform and pulse pressure in response to angiotensin II and noradrenaline in man. J Physiol 2001;530:541–550.

54   Wilkinson IB, MacCallum H, Cockcroft JR, Webb DJ: Inhibition of basal nitric oxide synthesis increases aortic augmentation index and pulse wave velocity in vivo. Br J Clin Pharmacol 2002; 53:189–192.

55   Hope SA, Meredith IT, Cameron JD: Effect of non-invasive calibration of radial waveforms on error in transfer-function-derived central aortic waveform characteristics. Clin Sci 2004;107: 205–211.

56   Hope SA, Tay DB, Meredith IT, Cameron JD: Use of arterial transfer functions for the derivation of central aortic waveform characteristics in subjects with type 2 diabetes and cardiovascular disease. Diabetes Care 2004;27:746–751.

57   Morgan T, Lauri J, Bertram D, Anderson A: Effect of different antihypertensive drug classes on central aortic pressure. Am J Hypertens 2004;17:118–123.

58   Dhakam Z, McEniery CM, Yasmin, Cockcroft JR, Brown MJ, Wilkinson IB: Atenolol and eprosartan: differential effects on central blood pressure and aortic pulse wave velocity. Am J Hypertens 2006;19:214–219.

59   Williams B, Lacy PS, Thom SM, Cruickshank K, Stanton A, Collier D, Hughes AD, Thurston H, O'Rourke M: Differential impact of blood pressure-lowering drugs on central aortic pressure and clinical outcomes: principal results of the Conduit Artery Function Evaluation (CAFE) study. Circulation 2006;113:1213–1225.

60   Oparil S, Izzo JL Jr: Pulsology rediscovered: commentary on the Conduit Artery Function Evaluation (CAFE) study. Circulation 2006;113:1162–1163.

61   Loutzenhiser R, Bidani A, Chilton L: Renal myogenic response: kinetic attributes and physiological role. Circ Res 2002;90:1316–1324.

62   Mitchell GF, Moye LA, Braunwald E, Rouleau JL, Bernstein V, Geltman EM, Flaker GC, Pfeffer MA: Sphygmomanometrically determined pulse pressure is a powerful independent predictor of recurrent events after myocardial infarction in patients with impaired left ventricular function. SAVE investigators. Survival and Ventricular Enlargement. Circulation 1997;96:4254–4260.

63   Franklin SS, Khan SA, Wong ND, Larson MG, Levy D: Is pulse pressure useful in predicting risk for coronary heart disease? The Framingham Heart Study. Circulation 1999;100:354–360.

64   Chae CU, Pfeffer MA, Glynn RJ, Mitchell GF, Taylor JO, Hennekens CH: Increased pulse pressure and risk of heart failure in the elderly. JAMA 1999;281:634–639.

65   Domanski MJ, Davis BR, Pfeffer MA, Kastantin M, Mitchell GF: Isolated systolic hypertension: prognostic information provided by pulse pressure. Hypertension 1999;34:375–380.

66   Laurent S, Katsahian S, Fassot C, Tropeano AI, Gautier I, Laloux B, Boutouyrie P: Aortic stiffness is an independent predictor of fatal stroke in essential hypertension. Stroke 2003;34:1203–1206.

67   Kivipelto M, Helkala EL, Laakso MP, Hanninen T, Hallikainen M, Alhainen K, Iivonen S, Mannermaa A, Tuomilehto J, Nissinen A, Soininen H: Apolipoprotein E ε4 allele, elevated midlife total cholesterol level, and high midlife systolic blood pressure are independent risk factors for late-life Alzheimer disease. Ann Intern Med 2002;137:149–155.

68   Launer LJ, Masaki K, Petrovitch H, Foley D, Havlik RJ: The association between midlife blood pressure levels and late-life cognitive function. The Honolulu-Asia Aging Study. JAMA 1995; 274:1846–1851.

69   Freitag MH, Peila R, Masaki K, Petrovitch H, Ross GW, White LR, Launer LJ: Midlife pulse pressure and incidence of dementia: the Honolulu-Asia Aging Study. Stroke 2006;37:33–37.

70   Liao D, Cooper L, Cai J, Toole J, Bryan N, Burke G, Shahar E, Nieto J, Mosley T, Heiss G: The prevalence and severity of white matter lesions, their relationship with age, ethnicity, gender, and cardiovascular disease risk factors: the ARIC Study. Neuroepidemiology 1997;16:149–162.

71   Duprez DA, De Buyzere ML, Van den Noortgate N, Simoens J, Achten E, Clement DL, Afschrift M, Cohn JN: Relationship between periventricular or deep white matter lesions and arterial elasticity indices in very old people. Age Ageing 2001;30:325–330.

72   Klein R, Klein BE, Tomany SC, Cruickshanks KJ: The association of cardiovascular disease with the long-term incidence of age-related maculopathy: the Beaver Dam Eye Study. Ophthalmology 2003;110:1273–1280.

Aging and Arterial Structure-Function Relations

73   Safar ME, Blacher J, Pannier B, Guerin AP, Marchais SJ, Guyonvarc'h PM, London GM: Central pulse pressure and mortality in end-stage renal disease. Hypertension 2002;39:735–738.

74   Hirose K, Tomiyama H, Okazaki R, Arai T, Koji Y, Zaydun G, Hori S, Yamashina A: Increased pulse wave velocity associated with reduced calcaneal quantitative osteo-sono index: possible relationship between atherosclerosis and osteopenia. J Clin Endocrinol Metab 2003;88:2573–2578.

75   Salomaa V, Riley W, Kark JD, Nardo C, Folsom AR: Non-insulin-dependent diabetes mellitus and fasting glucose and insulin concentrations are associated with arterial stiffness indexes. The ARIC Study. Atherosclerosis Risk in Communities Study. Circulation 1995;91:1432–1443.

76   Henry RM, Kostense PJ, Spijkerman AM, Dekker JM, Nijpels G, Heine RJ, Kamp O, Westerhof N, Bouter LM, Stehouwer CD, Study H: Arterial stiffness increases with deteriorating glucose tolerance status: the Hoorn Study. Circulation 2003;107:2089–2095.

77   Mackey RH, Sutton-Tyrrell K, Vaitkevicius PV, Sakkinen PA, Lyles MF, Spurgeon HA, Lakatta EG, Kuller LH: Correlates of aortic stiffness in elderly individuals: a subgroup of the Cardiovascular Health Study. Am J Hypertens 2002;15:16–23.

78   Safar ME: Peripheral pulse pressure, large arteries, and microvessels. Hypertension 2004;44: 121–122.

79   O'Rourke MF, Safar ME: Relationship between aortic stiffening and microvascular disease in brain and kidney: cause and logic of therapy. Hypertension 2005;46:200–204.

80   Mitchell GF, Vita JA, Larson MG, Parise H, Keyes MJ, Warner E, Vasan RS, Levy D, Benjamin EJ: Cross-sectional relations of peripheral microvascular function, cardiovascular disease risk factors, and aortic stiffness: the Framingham Heart Study. Circulation 2005;112:3722–3728.

81   Baumbach GL, Siems JE, Heistad DD: Effects of local reduction in pressure on distensibility and composition of cerebral arterioles. Circ Res 1991;68:338–351.

82   Baumbach GL: Effects of increased pulse pressure on cerebral arterioles. Hypertension 1996;27: 159–167.

83   James MA, Watt PA, Potter JF, Thurston H, Swales JD: Pulse pressure and resistance artery structure in the elderly. Hypertension 1995;26:301–306.

84   Christensen KL: Reducing pulse pressure in hypertension may normalize small artery structure. Hypertension 1991;18:722–727.

85   Ryan SM, Waack BJ, Weno BL, Heistad DD: Increases in pulse pressure impair acetylcholine-induced vascular relaxation. Am J Physiol 1995;268:H359–H363.

86   Nigam A, Mitchell GF, Lambert J, Tardif JC: Relation between conduit vessel stiffness (assessed by tonometry) and endothelial function (assessed by flow-mediated dilatation) in patients with and without coronary heart disease. Am J Cardiol 2003;92:395–399.

87   Sullivan JM, Prewitt RL, Josephs JA: Attenuation of the microcirculation in young patients with high-output borderline hypertension. Hypertension 1983;5:844–851.

88   Ciuffetti G, Schillaci G, Innocente S, Lombardini R, Pasqualini L, Notaristefano S, Mannarino E: Capillary rarefaction and abnormal cardiovascular reactivity in hypertension. J Hypertens 2003;21:2297–2303.

89   Cirillo M, Stellato D, Laurenzi M, Panarelli W, Zanchetti A, De Santo NG: Pulse pressure and isolated systolic hypertension: association with microalbuminuria. The GUBBIO Study Collaborative Research. Kidney Int 2000;58:1211–1218.

Joseph L. Izzo, Jr.
Department of Medicine, State University of New York at Buffalo
3 Gates Circle, Buffalo, NY 14209 (USA)
Tel. +1 716 898 5653, Fax +1 716 887 5551, E-Mail jizzo@ams.ecmc.edu

Safar ME, Frohlich ED (eds): Atherosclerosis, Large Arteries and Cardiovascular Risk.
Adv Cardiol. Basel, Karger, 2007, vol 44, pp 35–61

....

Local Elasticity Imaging of Vulnerable Atherosclerotic Coronary Plaques

Radj A. Baldewsing[a]   *Johannes A. Schaar*[a]   *Frits Mastik*[a]
Antonius F.W. van der Steen[a, b]

[a]Biomedical Engineering, Thorax Center, Erasmus Medical Center, Rotterdam,
and [b]Interuniversity Cardiology Institute of the Netherlands,
Utrecht, The Netherlands

Abstract

The material composition and morphology of vulnerable atherosclerotic plaque components are considered to be more important determinants of acute coronary syndromes than the degree of stenosis. Rupture of a plaque causes thrombogenic material to contact the blood, resulting in a thrombus. Rupture-prone plaques contain an inflamed thin fibrous cap covering a large soft lipid pool. Mechanically, rupture occurs when plaques cannot withstand the internal stresses induced by the pulsating blood. These stresses concentrate within/around the cap/edge, since the lipid pool cannot bear much stress. During plaque development these stresses further increase when caps become thinner, lipid pools become larger, or the difference in stiffness (modulus) between the cap and the lipid pool increases. Intravascular ultrasound (IVUS) strain elastography/palpography and IVUS modulus elastography are imaging techniques that assess local plaque elasticity (strain and modulus) based on the principle that tissue deformation (strain) by a mechanical stress is a function of its elastic properties (modulus). Combined use of these techniques provides clinicians an all-in-one modality for detecting plaques, assessing their rupture proneness and imaging their elastic material composition. This chapter describes the terminology and pathophysiology of vulnerable plaques and discusses the techniques behind, the methods for and the validations of the elasticity imaging techniques.

Copyright © 2007 S. Karger AG, Basel

1. Vulnerable Plaque: Description and Pathophysiology

Introduction

Investigators, working in the field of identification and treatment of high-risk/vulnerable atherosclerotic plaques and patients, have recognized that an increased understanding of the pathophysiology of coronary thrombosis and onset of acute coronary syndromes has created the need for agreement on nomenclature [1]. This chapter gives a summary of that agreement.

Conceptual Terms

Overview
The terms in figure 1 are proposed for use on a conceptual basis. The progression from asymptomatic atherosclerosis, to a high-risk/vulnerable plaque, to a thrombosed plaque, and to clinical events is presented. It is of note that the later stages of the progression may be repeated in a relatively short time interval as documented by the high short-term risk of a recurrent event in patients with acute coronary syndromes. This may be caused by rethrombosis of the lesion causing the index event, and/or the simultaneous occurrence of multiple high-risk/vulnerable plaques and/or thrombosed plaques that have not previously caused symptoms. An acute coronary syndrome may be a clinical marker of widespread (multifocal) disease activity in the coronary arteries, possibly related to inflammation [2–9].

The Vulnerable Patient
The primary clinical and preventive goal is to identify patients who are vulnerable to acute coronary thrombosis. Such patients are likely to have a high atherosclerotic burden, high-risk/vulnerable plaques, and/or thrombogenic blood [2]. There is an important need to improve diagnostic methods to identify vulnerable patients, and the plaques, which contribute to their increased risk.

Vulnerable/High-Risk/Thrombosis-Prone Plaques
Studies indicate that there are plaques at increased risk of thrombosis and rapid stenosis progression, which often lead to symptomatic disease. Synonyms to be used for such plaques are 'vulnerable', 'high-risk', or 'thrombosis-prone' plaques.

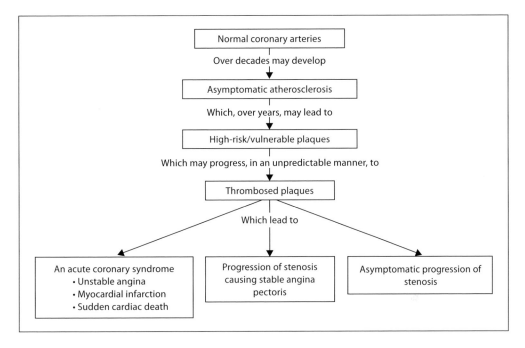

Fig. 1. Development of atherosclerosis and progression to thrombosis and clinical events.

At the present time, there is no widely accepted diagnostic method to prospectively identify these plaques. Until such information is provided, the suggested synonyms should only be used to describe the concept and function of these plaques, and not their histologic basis.

Histologic Features of Plaques Causing Coronary Artery Thrombosis

At present, the most detailed evidence concerning the plaques causing coronary thrombosis and rapid lesion progression, or symptomatic disease, is derived from autopsy studies [10–14].

In the acute coronary syndromes, the lesion causing most clinical events is often a plaque complicated by thrombosis extending into the lumen [12–15]. Such plaques are termed 'thrombosed plaques'. In some cases, multiple thrombosed plaques may exist, only one of which is acting as the culprit lesion. A plaque may also develop thrombosis, which remains asymptomatic due to the presence of collaterals, or failure of the thrombus to significantly impede blood

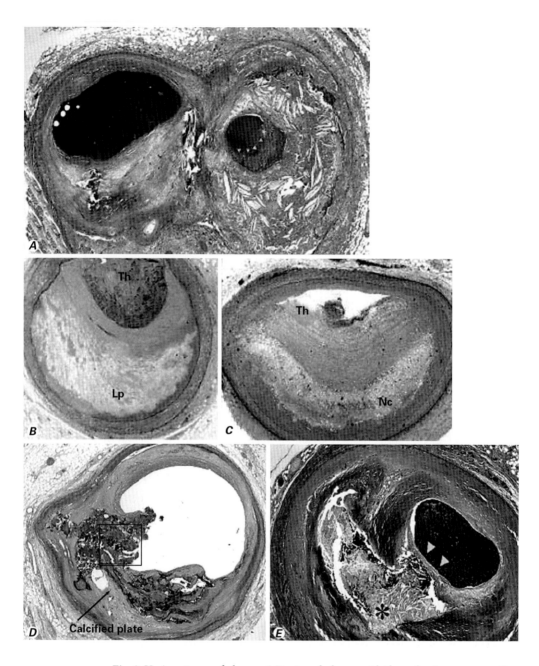

Fig. 2. Various types of plaque. *A* Ruptured plaque with thrombosis: a cross section of a coronary artery is cut just distal to a bifurcation. The atherosclerotic plaque to the left (circumflex branch) is fibrotic and partly calcified whereas the plaque to the right (marginal branch) is lipid-rich with a non-occluding thrombus superimposed. *B, C* Eroded

flow. However, such subclinical thrombosis may contribute to the rapid progression of stenosis [16, 17]. In cases of stable angina, the culprit lesion is often a non-thrombosed plaque.

The following terms are proposed to describe the thrombosed plaques causing the coronary syndromes: 'A *ruptured plaque*' – a plaque with deep injury with a real defect or gap in the fibrous cap that had separated its lipid-rich atheromatous core from the flowing blood, thereby exposing the thrombogenic core of the plaque (fig. 2A). This is the most common cause of coronary thrombosis [11–13]. '*An eroded plaque*' – a plaque with loss and/or dysfunction of the lumenal endothelial cells leading to thrombosis (fig. 2B, C). There is no structural defect (beyond endothelial injury) or gap in the plaque, which is often rich in smooth muscle cells and proteoglycans [14]. '*A plaque with a calcified nodule*' – a heavily calcified plaque with the loss and/or dysfunction of endothelial cells over a calcified nodule (fig. 2D). This is the least common of the three causes of thrombosis described here [14].

Prospective Identification of a Vulnerable Plaque

There is considerable interest in the identification of plaques prior to the occurrence of thrombosis. On the basis of knowledge of the types of plaques identified as causes of thrombosis (ruptured, eroded and calcific nodule plaques), the following types of plaques are suspected to be vulnerable plaques.

A Plaque Prone to Rupture
Retrospective pathologic studies of plaque rupture with thrombosis suggest that prior to the event, the plaque was an inflamed, thin-cap fibroatheroma (TCFA) (fig. 2E) [11–14, 18–20]. The major components of such TCFA are:

plaques with thrombosis: plaque erosion lesions from two different patients showing in *B* a lesion with lipid pool (Lp) and in *C* a necrotic core (Nc) with luminal thrombi (Th). Note a thick fibrous cap above the necrotic core in *C* and a lack of communication between it and the lumen. *D* Calcified nodule: a section of the mid right coronary artery shows an eccentric lesion with extensive calcification (calcified plate) and surface calcified nodules with loss of fibrous cap and luminal fibrin deposition. *E* Inflamed thin-cap fibroatheroma: a section of a coronary artery contains a large lipid-rich core that is covered by a thin fibrous cap (arrowheads). The lumen contains contrast medium injected postmortem. The fibrous cap is severely inflamed, containing many macrophage foam cells (asterisk), and extravasated erythrocytes within the necrotic and avascular core just beneath the cap, indicating that the cap is ruptured nearby.

(a) a lipid-rich, atheromatous core; (b) a thin fibrous cap, with (i) macrophage and lymphocyte infiltration and/or (ii) decreased smooth muscle cell content, and (c) expansive remodeling.

A Plaque Prone to Erosion

Retrospective pathologic studies of plaque erosion with thrombosis suggest that, prior to the event, the plaque was often rich in proteoglycans, but, in most cases, lacked a distinguishing structure such as a lipid pool or necrotic core. If a lipid-rich core is present, the fibrous cap is usually thick and rich in smooth muscle cells [14]. These plaques are often associated with constrictive remodeling.

A Plaque with a Calcified Nodule

Retrospective pathologic studies of plaques with thrombosis covering a calcified nodule suggest that, prior to the event, the plaque appeared to be heavily calcified with a calcified nodule protruding into the lumen [14].

While such plaques (an inflamed TCFA, a proteoglycan-rich plaque, and a plaque with a calcified nodule) are suspected to be vulnerable plaques, they cannot be designated as such until prospective studies provide the necessary supporting data. Hence, an inflamed TCFA is best described as a 'suspected' vulnerable plaque, since, while confirmatory data are lacking, its structure definitely resembles that of ruptured plaques.

Novel Imaging Techniques Will Provide Additional Information on Vulnerable Plaques

New technologies to improve characterization of plaque in patients are under development [19–29]. These techniques seek to identify the histologic features, discussed above, of plaques suspected to represent vulnerability, and provide additional information about plaques that has not heretofore been available (data on structure, composition, deformability, pathophysiology, metabolism, temperature, etc.). The novel information will expand the list of features suspected to represent vulnerability. These features need validation in longitudinal, prospective, clinical trials that will document the natural history of plaques. Once such trials are positive, it may then be possible to identify a vulnerable plaque prospectively in an individual patient.

Finally, it is the hope that widespread adoption of the terminology established in Schaar et al. [1], and briefly summarized in this chapter, will accelerate progress in the prevention of acute coronary events.

2. Vulnerable Plaque: Elasticity Imaging

Introduction

Intravascular ultrasound (IVUS) is the only commercially available clinical technique providing real-time cross-sectional images of the coronary artery in patients [30]. IVUS provides information on the severity of the stenosis and the remaining free luminal area. Furthermore, calcified and non-calcified plaque components can be identified. Although many investigators studied the value of IVUS to identify the plaque composition, identification of fibrous and fatty plaque components remains limited [31, 32]. IVUS radiofrequency (RF)-based tissue identification strategies appear to have better performance [32, 33]. However, none of them is yet capable of providing sufficient spatial and parametric resolution to identify a lipid pool covered by a thin fibrous cap.

Identification of different plaque components is of crucial importance to detect the vulnerable plaque since these are characterized by an eccentric plaque with a large lipid pool shielded from the lumen by a thin fibrous cap [13, 34]. Inflammation of the cap by macrophages further increases the vulnerability of these plaques [35]. The mechanical properties of fibrous and fatty plaque components are different [36–38]. Furthermore, fibrous caps with inflammation by macrophages are weaker than caps without inflammation [39].

The stress that is applied on an artery by the pulsating blood pressure must balance the circumferentially directed load integrated over the whole arterial wall. To maintain the connection between mechanically different tissue structures (like soft lipid pools and stiff fibrous caps) during arterial deformation, relatively soft regions will therefore carry only a fraction of the total circumferential load and the surrounding stiffer material a greater portion [40, 41]. This mechanism causes circumferential stress concentrations in and around the stiff cap, which will rupture if the cap is unable to withstand this stress. This increased circumferential stress will result in an increased radial deformation (strain) of the tissue due to the incompressibility of the material. Therefore, methods that are capable of measuring the radial strain provide information about plaques that may influence clinical decision-making.

In 1991, Ophir et al. [42] proposed a method to measure the elasticity (strain and modulus) of biological tissues using ultrasound. The tissue was deformed by externally applying a stress on it. Different strain values were found in tissues with different material properties. Implementing this method for intravascular purposes has potential to identify the vulnerable plaque by (i) identification of elastically different plaque components and (ii) detection of high radial strain/circumferential stress regions.

This chapter discusses the technique behind the method for and the validation of IVUS strain elastography, which is differentiated into IVUS strain elastography/palpography when the strain is imaged and IVUS modulus elastography when the modulus is imaged.

Elasticity Imaging

The Movement Begins
In 1991, Ophir and colleagues [42, 43] developed an elasticity imaging technique called elastography, which is based on (quasi-)static deformation of a linear elastic, isotropic material. The tissue under inspection is deformed by applying stress (i.e., force normalized by area) on a part of its boundary. The resulting distribution of strain (i.e., length of a small block of tissue after deformation, divided by its length before deformation) depends upon (i) the distribution of the tissue's material properties (Young's modulus and Poisson's ratio) and (ii) the displacement or stress conditions on the remaining tissue boundaries. The Young's modulus E [kPa] is a material property, which can be interpreted as the ratio between the normal stress S [kPa] (tensile or compressive) enforced upon a small block of tissue and its resulting strain (elongation or compression). The Poisson's ratio is also a material property and it quantifies a material's local volumetric compressibility. The resulting strain is determined, directly or indirectly using displacement, with ultrasound using two pairs of ultrasound signals, one signal obtained before and the other after deformation [44]. The method was initially developed for detection and characterization of tumors in breast. Nowadays, this principle is also applied to many other biological objects [45], including prostate, kidney, liver, myocardium, skin, coronary artery and superficial arteries.

Although Ophir et al. [42, 43] never explored the quasi-static approach for intravascular purposes, this approach seems to be the most fruitful concept. In this application, beside knowledge of the material properties of the different plaque components, the strain in itself may be an excellent diagnostic parameter. Furthermore, in intravascular applications, the arterial deformation is naturally present and is caused by the systemic blood pressure. Also user-controlled deformation is possible by inflating an intravascular balloon [46].

IVUS Strain Elastography/Palpography
The principle of IVUS strain elastography is illustrated in figure 3. An echogram of a vessel phantom with a stiff wall and a soft eccentric plaque is acquired at a certain intraluminal pressure using an IVUS catheter. Notice that there is no difference in echogenicity between the wall and the plaque, which

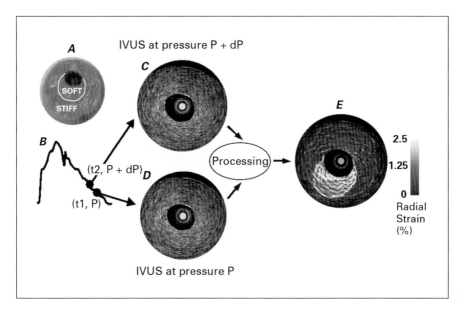

Fig. 3. Principle of intravascular ultrasound (IVUS) strain elastography measurement procedure. An IVUS catheter is inserted into an object, in this case a vessel-mimicking phantom with a soft plaque (***A***). Next, at two different intraluminal pressures (***B***), an IVUS echogram is acquired (***C, D***); in this case dP = 1 mm Hg. In each echogram, the gray circle indicates the catheter tip of 1.1 mm diameter. Finally, the local deformation (i.e., strain) of the tissue is determined using cross-correlation processing on the acquired IVUS RF data. This information is plotted as an additional image to the IVUS echogram and called a (strain) elastogram (***E***). In this example, the eccentric soft plaque of a vessel-mimicking phantom is clearly visible between 4 and 8 o'clock in the elastogram, as a region of high strain, whereas this plaque cannot be identified from the IVUS echograms.

results in a homogeneous echogram. A second acquisition at a higher pressure is obtained. The radial strain information is plotted as a complimentary image to the echogram and is called a (strain) elastogram. The elastogram reveals the presence of an eccentric region with increased strain values, thus identifying the soft eccentric plaque. The differences in strategies to perform IVUS strain elastography/palpography (i.e. assess the local deformation of the tissue) are due to (i) the way of detecting the strain and (ii) the type of source that deforms the vascular tissue.

The principle of IVUS strain palpography is similar to the principle of IVUS strain elastography. There are two minor differences that make palpography faster and more robust and, therefore, more suited for real-time in vivo applications. Firstly, palpography restricts its region of interest to the innermost layer of the arterial wall (first 450 μm), making it faster. Secondly, it uses a slightly larger amount of ultrasound signal making it more robust but at the expense of spatial resolution [47, 48]. A strain image obtained with IVUS strain palpography is called a (strain) palpogram.

Implementation of the Technique
Typically for in vivo IVUS strain elastography/palpography, intraluminal pressure differences in the order of 1–5 mm Hg are used. The strain induced by this pressure differential in vascular tissue is in the order of 2%. This means that a small block of tissue with an initial length of 100 μm will be deformed to 98 μm. To differentiate between strain levels, sub-micron estimation of the tissue displacement is required.

Envelope Based. Talhami et al. [49] and Ryan and Foster [50] introduced IVUS strain elastography using the envelope of the ultrasound RF signal. Although robust, their techniques do not provide sufficient resolution and signal-to-noise ratio for intravascular applications. Based on work of Varghese and Ophir [51], a smaller variance of the strain estimate and a higher spatial resolution is expected using the RF signal instead of its envelope.

Radiofrequency Based. Shapo et al. [52] developed a technique based on cross-correlation of A-lines. They aimed at maximizing the signal-to-noise ratio of the displacement and strain estimation. To achieve this, the artery had to be deformed much more that occurs in vivo. This high deformation was obtained by inflating a non-compliant balloon within the artery. So far, their technique has not yet been developed towards clinical applications.

De Korte et al. [53] incorporated 'correlation-based' elastography [42] for intravascular purposes and is called IVUS strain elastography/palpography. The intraluminal pressure strains the vascular tissue; this strain is calculated from local tissue displacements, as follows. First, the local tissue displacements are determined using cross-correlation analysis of the gated RF signals (fig. 4). A cross-correlation function between two signals will have its maximum if the signals are not shifted with respect to each other. If a shift between the signals is present, the peak of the cross-correlation function is found at the position representing the tissue displacement. For each angle, the tissue displacement at the lumen vessel-wall boundary is determined. Next, the displacement of the tissue at D micrometer from the vessel-wall boundary is determined. The strain of the tissue is then calculated by dividing the differential tissue displacement (displacement of tissue at boundary – displacement of tissue in wall) by the distance between these two locations (= D micrometer). Strain is thus dimensionless and it is common practice to multiply it by 100% to obtain strain values around 1%. The strain for each angle is color-coded and plotted as a ring on the IVUS echogram at the lumen vessel-wall boundary [47, 48, 54]

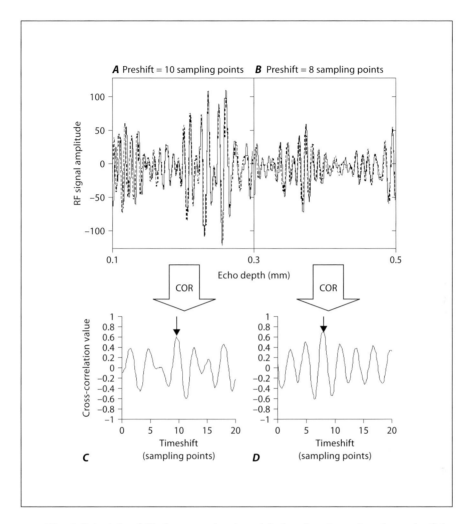

Fig. 4. Principle of displacement (or time delay) estimation using the peak of the cross-correlation coefficient function. In the upper part, two segments (*A*, *B*) of the pre-deformation (solid line) and post-deformation (dotted, and preshifted for better visual comparison) RF signals are shown. Both segments start at a different position in the tissue. For each segment, the cross-correlation coefficient function between the two signals is computed (*C*, *D*). The functions show a decreasing position of the peak with increasing echo depth. The difference in peak position represents the differential tissue displacement; normalizing this difference by the distance between the segments, i.e. 0.2 mm, gives the strain of the tissue between 0.2 and 0.4 mm.

and this ring is called a (strain) palpogram. If the strain is determined for multiple regions per angle, the strain for the whole vessel-wall cross section can be constructed; this additional image to the IVUS echogram is called a (strain) elastogram. For palpography, the value for D is approximately 450 μm and for elastography approximately 225 μm.

The used cross-correlation technique is suited for strain values smaller than 2.5%; these values are present during in vivo acquisitions when only a part of the heart cycle is used to strain the tissue [55].

Frequently used IVUS catheters are the 20-MHz phased-array catheter (Volcano Corp., Inc., Rancho Cordova, Calif., USA) and the 30-MHz mechanically rotating single-element catheter (ClearView, CVIS, Boston Scientific Corp., Watertown, Mass., USA).

IVUS Strain Elastography/Palpography: Results

In vitro Validation on Human Arteries
De Korte et al. [56] performed a validation study on excised human coronary (n = 4) and femoral (n = 9) arteries (fig. 5) to investigate the capability of IVUS strain elastography to characterize different plaque components. First, the elastographically imaged cross sections were segmented in regions (n = 125) based on the strain value in the elastogram. The dominant plaque types in these regions (fibrous, fibro-fatty or fatty) were obtained from histology (i.e., collagen, smooth muscle cells and macrophages) and correlated with the average strain and echo intensity.

Mean strain values of 0.27, 0.45 and 0.60% were found for fibrous, fibro/fatty and fatty plaque components (at a pressure differential of 20 mm Hg). The strain for the three plaque types as determined by histology differed significantly (p = 0.0002). This difference was independent on the type of artery (coronary or femoral) and was mainly evident between fibrous and fatty tissue (p = 0.0004). The plaque types did not reveal echo-intensity differences in the IVUS echogram (p = 0.992).

Since fibrous and fatty tissue resulted in different strain values and high strain values often co-localized with increased concentrations of macrophages, these results revealed the potential for identification of the vulnerable plaque.

Later, Schaar et al. [21] performed a study on excised human coronary arteries (n = 24) with IVUS strain elastography in order to: (i) quantify its predictive value for detecting vulnerable plaques, and (ii) use it for characterizing vulnerable plaque features.

In histology, a vulnerable plaque was defined as a plaque consisting of a thin cap (<250 μm) with moderate to heavy macrophage infiltration and at

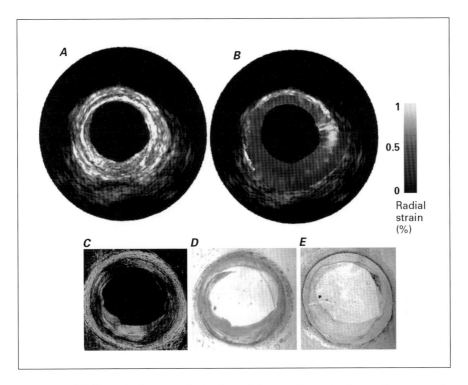

Fig. 5. IVUS strain elastography in vitro of a human femoral artery and corresponding histology. ***A*** IVUS echogram. ***B*** IVUS strain elastogram superimposed on the IVUS
echogram. ***C–E*** Histology: (***C***) collagen, (***D***) smooth muscle cells, and (***E***) macrophages.
The elastogram reveals that the plaque contains a region of high strain between 1 and 4
o'clock. Histology shows that this region is heavily infiltrated by macrophages and lacks
smooth muscle cells and collagen. Furthermore, the remaining plaque region between 4
and 1 o'clock shows low strain and at this region histology reveals that the plaque contains
much smooth muscle cells and collagen but no macrophages.

least 40% of atheroma. In a radial strain elastogram, a vulnerable plaque was
defined as a plaque with a high strain region at the surface with adjacent low
strain regions (fig. 6). 54 cross sections were studied. In histology, 26 vulnerable plaques and 28 non-vulnerable plaques were found. The sensitivity was
88% and the specificity 89% to detect vulnerable plaques. Linear regression
showed high correlation between the strain in caps and the amount of macrophages ($p < 0.006$) and an inverse relation between the amount of smooth
muscle cells and strain ($p < 0.0001$). Plaques, which were declared vulnerable
in IVUS strain elastography, had a thinner cap than non-vulnerable plaques
($p < 0.0001$).

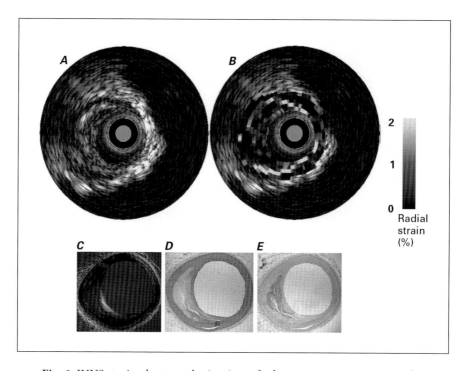

Fig. 6. IVUS strain elastography in vitro of a human coronary artery and corresponding histology. *A* IVUS echogram. *B* IVUS strain elastogram superimposed on the IVUS echogram. *C–E* Histology: (*C*) collagen, (*D*) smooth muscle cells, and (*E*) macrophages. Histology shows that the plaque consists of a homogeneous soft lipid pool covered by a stiff fibrous cap with much collagen and smooth muscle cells. Increased strain is found at both shoulders of the lipid pool. In the IVUS echogram, the gray circle defines the catheter tip of 1.1 mm diameter and the black circle removes part of the catheter ringdown diameter 2 mm.

This study showed that IVUS strain elastography has a high sensitivity and specificity to detect human vulnerable plaques in vitro and that strain in caps had a high correlation with vulnerable plaque features.

In vivo Animal Studies

IVUS strain elastography was also validated in vivo using iliac and femoral arteries of atherosclerotic Yucatan mini-pigs (n = 6) to investigate its potential for identifying different plaque components in vivo [57].

In total, 20 cross sections were investigated. Tissue was strained by the pulsatile blood pressure. Histology (collagen, fat (oil red O), and macrophages) was used to classify plaques as absent, as early fatty lesion, early fibrous lesion or as advanced fibrous plaque. The mean strain in these plaques and normal cross sections was determined.

Strains were similar in the plaque-free arterial wall and the early and advanced fibrous plaques. Cross sections with early fatty lesions had significantly higher strain values than those with fibrous plaques ($p = 0.02$). The presence of a high strain spot had a high predictive value to identify the presence of macrophages (sensitivity and specificity $= 92\%$). In case there was no high strain spot present, no fatty plaque was found.

In vivo Patient Studies

IVUS strain elastography was applied to patients ($n = 12$) during percutaneous transluminal coronary angioplasty procedures [58]. Tissue was strained by the pulsatile blood pressure. This strain was determined using cross-correlation analysis of sequential RF frames. A likelihood function was determined to obtain the frames with minimal motion of the catheter in the lumen, since motion of the catheter prevents reliable strain estimation. Minimal motion was observed near end-diastole. Reproducible strain estimates were obtained within one pressure cycle and over several pressure cycles. Validation of the results was limited to the information provided by the echogram. Strain in calcified material, as identified from the echogram was significantly lower than in non-calcified tissue. The elastogram of stented plaques revealed very low strain values, except for two regions: these are between the stent struts and at the shoulders of the plaque.

Recently, Schaar et al. [59] used 3D IVUS strain palpography in patients undergoing percutaneous intervention to assess the incidence of a specific high-strain pattern, which has shown in vitro to have a high sensitivity and specificity for detecting the TCFA. Furthermore, they explored the relation of such patterns to clinical presentation and to C-reactive protein levels.

3D strain palpograms were derived from continuous IVUS pullbacks through arteries (fig. 7). Patients ($n = 55$) were classified by clinical presentation as stable angina, unstable angina, or acute myocardial infarction (MI). In every patient, one coronary artery was scanned (culprit vessel in stable and unstable angina, non-culprit vessel in acute MI) and the number of plaques with a vulnerable plaque-specific strain pattern were assessed.

Stable angina patients had significantly less deformable plaques per vessel (0.6 ± 0.6) than unstable angina ($p = 0.0019$) patients (1.6 ± 0.7) or acute MI ($p < 0.0001$) patients (2.0 ± 0.7). Levels of C-reactive protein were positively correlated with the number of mechanically deformable plaques ($R^2 = 0.65$, $p < 0.0001$).

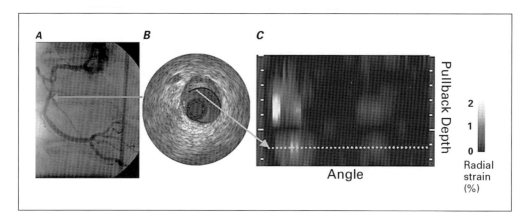

Fig. 7. 3D IVUS strain palpography of a patient in vivo. **A** Angiogram of the right coronary artery. **B** 2D IVUS strain palpogram superimposed on the IVUS echogram, which was taken at the location indicated by arrow in **A**. The echogram shows an eccentric plaque and the high strain regions with adjacent low strains at the shoulders of this plaque suggest that it is vulnerable. **C** A map of multiple 2D IVUS strain palpograms stacked after each other. The dotted line corresponds to the palpogram shown in **B**. This map provides an overview of the deformability of the inner layer of the arterial wall.

The main conclusion was that 3D IVUS palpography detects vulnerable plaque-specific strain patterns in human coronary arteries that correlated both with clinical presentation and levels of C-reactive protein.

Ultrasound Modulus Elastography

Motivation

IVUS strain elastography has proven to be a clinically available tool that is able to detect the presence of vulnerable plaques in vitro with high sensitivity and specificity [21]. In vivo animal experiments and in vitro human experiments demonstrated that discrimination between fibrous and fatty plaques is possible [56, 57].

However, a strain elastogram (and also a palpogram) cannot be interpreted directly as a morphology and material composition image of a plaque, since there is no one-to-one relation between the local radial strain value in a strain elastogram and the local plaque component type (calcified, fibrous, fatty or tissue weakened by macrophage inflammation). The underlying reason for this is that the stresses that induce local strain depend upon the structural build-up of the artery, the stiffness (i.e., Young's modulus) and geometry of its plaque components; furthermore, the radial component of the strain depends upon the catheter position used during imaging [60, 61]. Figure 6 exemplifies this. Histology shows a TCFA that consist of a soft homogeneous lipid pool covered by a stiff fibrous cap. Because the lipid pool is soft and homogenous, one would expect high radial strain throughout the same region in the IVUS strain elastogram. However, due to the stiffness of the cap and its circumferentially distributed geometry, stress concentrations occur at the shoulders of the lipid pool [41] resulting in local high strain. Furthermore, the presence of the cap hinders deformation behind it, which results in the low-strain region at the center of the lipid pool.

To overcome this limitation, one could image the Young's modulus distribution of a plaque. In general, modulus elastography (also called modulography) is the name for methods that compute a Young's modulus image (also called a modulogram) from a strain (or displacement) image. The Young's modulus E [kPa] is a material parameter, which can be loosely interpreted as the ratio between the normal stress S [kPa] (tensile or compressive) enforced upon a small block of tissue and its resulting strain (elongation or compression) [62]. The Young's modulus of soft tissue (e.g., lipid pool) is low and of stiff tissue (e.g., media or fibrous cap) high. There are two main reasons for performing modulography: (i) a modulogram can be interpreted as a material composition image because there is large difference between the Young's moduli of various tissue components, including plaque components [63], and (ii) a modulogram shows the modulus of tissue, which is a material property and, therefore, the appearance of the modulogram is independent of the geometry of tissue components, in contrast to strain.

In this section, the technique behind the methods and the results with IVUS modulus elastography are discussed.

Implementation of the Technique

The general approach to perform ultrasound modulus elastography is to firstly use ultrasound displacement/strain elastography to measure one or more components of the displacement vector and/or strain components of the deformed tissue. Next, a deformation model for computing the deformation, strain and/or stress of tissue is defined. This model consists of (i) a set of mathematical (partial differential) equations that describe the equilibrium of tissue, (ii) the relation between displacement and strain of tissue and, finally (iii) the constitutive equation, which defines the relation between stress and strain of tissue [62]. Many researchers approximate the behavior of biological tissue by a linear, isotropic, nearly incompressible (Poisson's ratio >0.49) elastic material. In those cases, the constitutive relation contains only one material parameter, namely the Young's modulus. Finally, the deformation model and the measured displacement/strain components are used to compute the modulogram by a 'direct reconstruction approach' or by an 'iterative reconstruction approach'.

Direct. In the direct approach the measured displacement/strain data are plugged in the deformation equations, which are mathematically manipulated so that the moduli can be considered and expressed as the unknowns. Next, the moduli are computed using a discretization [64] or numerical integration of the manipulated deformation equations [65, 66].

Iterative. In the iterative approach, the deformation model is treated as a finite element (computer) model (FEM). The FEM fills the space of the tissue with a mesh that consists of small discrete (finite) elements (e.g. triangles, bricks) and each element is given a constitutive relation, i.e. Young's modulus. Next, an initial modulus value for each element is defined. Finally, the modulus value of each individual mesh element or groups of mesh elements in the FEM are iteratively changed such that the computed FEM deformation output eventually closely matches the measured deformation (displacement/strain data). This matching is fully automatically performed by a minimization algorithm [67].

Much research has focused on applying these two approaches on non-vascular tissue geometries such as a cross section of a homogeneous rectangular medium with a circular or rectangular inclusion, or a breast, brain, heart. To date, only a few groups have investigated modulography for vascular geometries. Most of them used an adjusted iterative reconstruction method [68–71] and [72] some others an adjusted direct reconstruction method [73, 74]. All groups encountered difficulties in computing a modulus elastogram (related to uniqueness and continuity), which may be caused by noisy measurements, a limited number of measured displacement/strain components, type of boundary data [75], using an inadequate deformation model for the tissue, non-uniqueness of the inverse problem [76], converging to non-optimal local minima by the minimization algorithm.

IVUS Modulus Elastography
Baldewsing et al. [28] focused on performing modulography of atherosclerotic vascular geometries by using a newly developed iterative reconstruction approach with geometric constraints. To this end, they used the arterial radial strain, as measured with IVUS strain elastography, and an a priori parametric plaque geometry model. Their motivation for using a priori information is threefold. Firstly, they want to compute a modulogram of an atherosclerotic plaque that is diagnostically useful and easy to interpret in clinical settings. Secondly, the computation should suffer at least as possible from

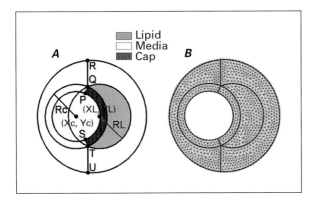

Fig. 8. Parametric finite element model for a vulnerable plaque. **A** Each circle is parameterized by its center (X, Y) and a radius R. The dynamic control points P, Q, R, S, T, and U are used to define the three plaque component regions. **B** Finite element mesh regions corresponding to geometry in **A**. Each finite element in a region has the same material property values as other elements in that region. L = Lipid, c = cap.

converging problems. Finally, they want to be able to investigate and quantify reconstruction difficulties (uniqueness and continuity) and limitations for computing a modulogram of plaques in a structured manner.

Their approach is specially suited for TCFAs [1, 77]. To this end, the deformation output calculated with a parametric finite element model (PFEM) representation of a TCFA (fig. 8) is matched to the plaque's radial strain, as measured with IVUS strain elastography. The PFEM uses only six morphology and three material composition parameters, but is still able to model a variety of these TCFAs. The computed modulogram of the TCFA shows both the morphology and Young's modulus values of three main plaque components, namely lipid, cap and media, and should therefore be easy to interpret.

In the next three subsections, the main parts of their iterative solution approach are discussed, namely the PFEM for a TCFA, the used deformation model, and used minimization algorithm.

PFEM Geometry for a Plaque. An idealized TCFA [77] is used as a model for a plaque and is an extension of the PFEM model used by Loree et al. [40]. The PFEM geometry consists of a media area containing a lipid pool, which is covered by a fibrous cap. The borders of the lipid, cap and media areas are defined using circles (fig. 8). Lipid is defined by region QTQ, cap by region PQTSP, and media by the remaining area. Each circle is parameterized by its center with cartesian coordinates (X, Y) and radius R, resulting in a total of six morphology parameters.

Material Deformation Model. Baldewsing et al. [78] used coronary arteries (n = 5) to demonstrate that radial strain elastograms measured in vitro using IVUS strain elastography could be simulated with a (finite-element) computer model. Their material deformation model treated the arterial tissue as a linear elastic, isotropic, plane strain, nearly incompressible material with a Poisson's ratio of 0.4999 [79].The computer-model geometry and material properties were determined from histology (collagen, smooth muscle cells and macro-phages). The agreement between a simulated and measured elastogram was performed upon features of high-strain regions. Statistical tests showed that there was no significant difference between simulated and corresponding measured elastograms in location, surface area and mean strain value of a high strain region (n = 8).

The same material deformation model is used for the PFEM. Lipid, cap and media region are assumed to have a constant Young's modulus value E_L, E_C, and E_M, respectively. This results in a total of only three material composition parameters.

The PFEM radial strain deformation is computed using the finite element package SEPRAN (Sepra Analysis, Technical University Delft, The Nether-lands), with the catheter center as origin. This radial strain field is called a PFEM elastogram. The whole process from defining the PFEM morphology and material composition parameters up to the calculation of the PFEM strain elastogram is fully automatic.

Minimization Algorithm. The modulus elastogram of a plaque is deter-mined by a minimization algorithm. This algorithm tries to find values for the six morphology and three modulus parameters of the PFEM such that the cor-responding PFEM elastogram 'looks similar' to the measured IVUS strain elastogram. The similarity between elastograms is quantified as the root-mean-squared (RMS) error, between PFEM strain elastogram and measured IVUS strain elastogram. The sequential-quadratic-programming minimiza-tion algorithm fully automatically searches a local minimum of the RMS by iteratively updating the nine PFEM parameters. Each update gives a lower RMS error. The algorithm stops when the either the RMS itself or each of a few consecutive RMS values is below a threshold value. When the resulting final PFEM elastogram has qualitatively enough strain pattern features in common with the measured elastogram, the corresponding modulus elastogram is con-sidered as a good approximation of the real plaque.

IVUS Modulus Elastography of Vulnerable Plaques: Results

Baldewsing et al. [28, 80] have shown the feasibility and robustness of their approach by successfully applying their modulography approach to ra-dial strain elastograms of vulnerable plaques that were (a) simulated, (b) mea-

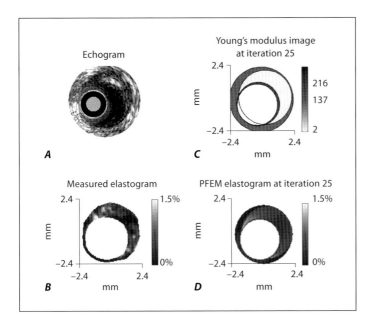

Fig. 9. Modulography of a patient in vivo: a Young's modulus image is computed from an IVUS strain elastogram that was measured in vivo from a patient with a vulnerable plaque. *A* IVUS echogram. *B* In vivo measured compounded strain elastogram. *C* Computed Young's modulus image in kPa. *D* PFEM strain elastogram computed from *C*.

sured in vitro and (c) measured in vivo in a patient. Two computer-simulated plaques, a plaque-mimicking phantom and two human coronary plaques (in vitro and in vivo) were used. FEMs were used to simulate strain elastograms for two plaque geometries, both having a lipid pool covered by a cap; one geometry was defined by circles, the other by tracing arterial histology. For their in vitro phantom and coronary artery, strain elastograms were processed from RF data obtained with a 20-MHz 64-element phased-array IVUS catheter. For the patient's case, multiple in vivo strain elastograms, obtained during the diastolic phase of a cardiac cycle where catheter motion was minimal, were averaged into one in vivo compounded strain elastogram to increase the signal-to-noise ratio. All the computed modulus elastograms approximated the geometry and material properties of the real plaque composition. Figure 9 shows computation of an IVUS in vivo modulus elastogram from the in vivo measured compounded IVUS strain elastogram of the patient. The echogram (fig. 9A) reveals the presence of a large eccentric plaque between 10 and 5 o'clock, but cannot discriminate between the possible cap and lipid component of the plaque. The in vivo measured compounded IVUS strain elastogram (fig. 9B) suggests the presence of a soft lipid pool covered by a stiff cap by means of a typical high radial strain region at the shoulders of the plaque and mechanical shadowing, which causes the low strain at the center of the plaque. The computed Young's modulus elastogram (fig. 9C) with ($E_L = 2$, $E_C = 216$, and $E_M = 137$ kPa) is a likely candidate for the real underlying plaque composition, since the measured compounded IVUS strain elastogram (fig. 9B) and the PFEM strain elastogram (fig. 9D) show two co-localizing high-strain regions and mechanical shadowing.

IVUS Modulus Elastography of Arbitrary Atherosclerotic Plaques

Atherosclerotic plaques can have a complex, heterogeneous material composition consisting of a mixture of plaque components, like lipids, fibrotic tissue, calcified nodules or tissues weakened by extracellular matrix breakdown caused by macrophages. Imaging of such complexes may require a different, more local approach, e.g., like that used by Soulami et al. [71], which does not enforce a restriction on the plaque structure. Although their approach does not require a priori information, the large number of moduli to be computed might prevent a successful convergence of the minimization algorithm.

Recently, Baldewsing et al. [80] extended their modulography approach [28] so that it also works for arbitrary atherosclerotic plaques. To this end, they first developed a deformable plaque geometry model, which (i) has deformable curves as distal borders of the PFEM lipid pool and cap region, instead of circle borders, and (ii) uses the true lumen and media contours, as extracted from the IVUS echogram. This deformable model led to a more accurate and reliable modulogram, for a much larger collection of complicated TFCA plaque component morphologies, than the TCFA plaque geometry model did. They then combined this deformable model with a compounding procedure to obtain a heterogeneous modulogram from various individual modulograms [29]. The preliminary results showed that the modulogram of a TCFA or heterogeneous plaque can be well approximated using their compounding procedure.

Discussion and Conclusion

Identification of plaque components and the proneness of a lesion to rupture is a major issue in interventional cardiology. IVUS echography is a real-time, clinically available technique capable of providing cross-sectional images and identifying calcified plaque components.

IVUS strain elastography/palpography are clinically available IVUS-derived techniques capable of mechanically identifying the rupture-prone plaque.

This is of paramount importance to investigate the underlying principle of plaque rupture, the effectiveness of pharmaceutical treatments and, in the long term, preventing sudden cardiac deaths. Since palpography is a faster and more robust technique, its introduction in the catheterization laboratory is easier. Although palpography reveals no information on the composition of material deeper in the plaque, it identifies the weak, soft spots in an artery. If a plaque ruptures, this rupture will start at the lumen vessel wall boundary, the region imaged by palpography. Clinical studies have been (and are being) performed to assess the potential role of palpography to identify patients at risk of future clinical events and to quantify the effect of pharmaceutical drugs and circulating biomarkers on reduction of these events [81].

Modulography is a new method for plaque-tissue characterization. It can be used in combination with other imaging modalities that are capable of measuring deformation, e.g. (intra)vascular OCT elastography or MRI elastography. Since modulography only needs a deformation elastogram as input, it may also be applied to other organs from which deformation can be measured, such as the breast, prostate, femoral or carotid. Finally, modulography, in combination with IVUS strain elastography, provides in vivo plaque morphology, strain and Young's modulus, therefore, one can perform an in vivo finite element-based stress analysis. This may be a more reliable analysis than when a priori Young's modulus values, plaque model or plaque structure obtained from tracing histology are used. Furthermore, it may aid the development and validation of plaque vulnerability indices, which are defined from local strain, stress and Young's modulus information.

In conclusion, the combined use of IVUS, IVUS strain elastography/palpography and modulography provides clinicians/researchers an all-in-one modality for detecting plaques, assessing information related to their rupture proneness and imaging their elastic material composition.

Acknowledgements

The research discussed in this chapter has been funded by grants from the Dutch Technology Foundation (STW), the Netherlands Organization for Scientific Research (NWO), Deutsche Herzstiftung (DHS), Dutch Heart Foundation (NHS). Feedback by Volcano Corp., Inc., Rancho Cordova, Calif., USA, was greatly appreciated.

References

1   Schaar JA, Muller JE, Falk E, Virmani R, Fuster V, Serruys PW, Colombo A, Stefanadis C, Ward Casscells S, Moreno PR, Maseri A, van der Steen AF: Terminology for high-risk and vulnerable coronary artery plaques. Report of a meeting on the vulnerable plaque, June 17 and 18, 2003, Santorini, Greece. Eur Heart J 2004;25:1077–1082.
2   Maseri A, Fuster V: Is there a vulnerable plaque? Circulation 2003;107:2068–2071.
3   Asakura M, Ueda Y, Yamaguchi O, Adachi T, Hirayama A, Hori M, Kodama K: Extensive development of vulnerable plaques as a pan-coronary process in patients with myocardial infarction: an angioscopic study. J Am Coll Cardiol 2001;37:1284–1288.
4   Goldstein JA: Multifocal coronary plaque instability. Prog Cardiovasc Dis 2002;44:449–454.
5   Rioufol G, Finet G, Ginon I, Andre-Fouet X, Rossi R, Vialle E, Desjoyaux E, Convert G, Huret JF, Tabib A: Multiple atherosclerotic plaque rupture in acute coronary syndrome: a three-vessel intravascular ultrasound study. Circulation 2002;106:804–808.
6   Buffon A, Biasucci LM, Liuzzo G, D'Onofrio G, Crea F, Maseri A: Widespread coronary inflammation in unstable angina. N Engl J Med 2002;347:5–12.
7   Casscells W, Naghavi M, Willerson JT: Vulnerable atherosclerotic plaque: a multifocal disease. Circulation 2003;107:2072–2075.
8   Krams R, Segers D, Gourabi BM, Maat W, Cheng C, van Pelt C, van Damme LC, de Feyter P, van der Steen T, de Korte CL, Serruys PW: Inflammation and atherosclerosis: mechanisms underlying vulnerable plaque. J Interv Cardiol 2003;16:107–113.
9   Libby P: Inflammation in atherosclerosis. Nature 2002;420:868–874.
10 Van der Wal AC, Becker AE, van der Loos CM, Das PK: Site of intimal rupture or erosion of thrombosed coronary atherosclerotic plaques is characterized by an inflammatory process irrespective of the dominant plaque morphology. Circulation 1994;89:36–44.
11 Arbustini E, Dal Bello B, Morbini P, Burke AP, Bocciarelli M, Specchia G, Virmani R: Plaque erosion is a major substrate for coronary thrombosis in acute myocardial infarction. Heart 1999; 82:269–272.
12 Falk E: Stable versus unstable atherosclerosis: clinical aspects. Am Heart J 1999;138:S421–S425.
13 Davies MJ: The pathophysiology of acute coronary syndromes. Heart 2000;83:361–366.
14 Virmani R, Kolodgie FD, Burke AP, Farb A, Schwartz SM: Lessons from sudden coronary death: a comprehensive morphological classification scheme for atherosclerotic lesions. Arterioscler Thromb Vasc Biol 2000;20:1262–1275.
15 Libby P: Current concepts of the pathogenesis of the acute coronary syndromes. Circulation 2001;104:365–372.
16 Burke AP, Kolodgie FD, Farb A, Weber DK, Malcom GT, Smialek J, Virmani R: Healed plaque ruptures and sudden coronary death: evidence that subclinical rupture has a role in plaque progression. Circulation 2001;103:934–940.
17 Mann J, Davies MJ: Mechanisms of progression in native coronary artery disease: role of healed plaque disruption. Heart 1999;82:265–268.
18 Varnava AM, Mills PG, Davies MJ: Relationship between coronary artery remodeling and plaque vulnerability. Circulation 2002;105:939–943.
19 Ambrose JA: Prognostic implications of lesion irregularity on coronary angiography. J Am Coll Cardiol 1991;18:675–566.
20 Vallabhajosula S, Fuster V: Atherosclerosis: imaging techniques and the evolving role of nuclear medicine. J Nucl Med 1997;38:1788–1796.
21 Schaar JA, De Korte CL, Mastik F, Strijder C, Pasterkamp G, Boersma E, Serruys PW, Van Der Steen AFW: Characterizing vulnerable plaque features with intravascular elastography. Circulation 2003;108:2636–2641.
22 Huang H, Virmani R, Younis H, Burke AP, Kamm RD, Lee RT: The impact of calcification on the biomechanical stability of atherosclerotic plaques. Circulation 2001;103:1051–1056.
23 Schmermund A, Erbel R: Unstable coronary plaque and its relation to coronary calcium. Circulation 2001;104:1682–1687.

24   Jang IK, Bouma BE, Kang DH, Park SJ, Park SW, Seung KB, Choi KB, Shishkov M, Schlendorf K, Pomerantsev E, Houser SL, Aretz HT, Tearney GJ: Visualization of coronary atherosclerotic plaques in patients using optical coherence tomography: comparison with intravascular ultrasound. J Am Coll Cardiol 2002;39:604–609.

25   Nair A, Kuban BD, Tuzcu EM, Schoenhagen P, Nissen SE, Vince DG: Coronary plaque classification with intravascular ultrasound radiofrequency data analysis. Circulation 2002;106:2200–2206.

26   Nieman K, van der Lugt A, Pattynama PM, de Feyter PJ: Noninvasive visualization of atherosclerotic plaque with electron beam and multislice spiral computed tomography. J Interv Cardiol 2003;16:123–128.

27   Moreno PR, Muller JE: Detection of high-risk atherosclerotic coronary plaques by intravascular spectroscopy. J Interv Cardiol 2003;16:243–252.

28   Baldewsing RA, Schaar JA, Mastik F, Oomens CWJ, van der Steen AFW: Assessment of vulnerable plaque composition by matching the deformation of a parametric plaque model to measured plaque deformation. IEEE Trans Med Imaging 2005;24:514–528.

29   Baldewsing RA, Mastik F, Schaar JA, van der Steen AFW: A compounding method for reconstructing the heterogeneous Young's modulus distribution of atherosclerotic plaques from their radial strain. Proceedings of the Fourth International Conference on the Ultrasonic Measurement and Imaging of Tissue Elasticity, 2005, p 68.

30   MacNeill BD, Lowe HC, Takano M, Fuster V, Jang IK: Intravascular modalities for detection of vulnerable plaque: current status. Arterioscler Thromb Vasc Biol 2003;23:1333–1342.

31   Prati F, Arbustini E, Labellarte A, Bello BD, Sommariva L, Mallus MT, Pagano A, Boccanelli A: Correlation between high frequency intravascular ultrasound and histomorphology in human coronary arteries. Heart 2001;85:567–570.

32   Komiyama N, Berry G, Kolz M, Oshima A, Metz J, Preuss P, Brisken A, Moore M, Yock P, Fitzgerald P: Tissue characterization of atherosclerotic plaques by intravascular ultrasound radiofrequency signal analysis: an in vitro study of human coronary arteries. Am Heart J 2000;140:565–574.

33   Hiro T, Fujii T, Yasumoto K, Murata T, Murashige A, Matsuzaki M: Detection of fibrous cap in atherosclerotic plaque by intravascular ultrasound by use of color mapping of angle-dependent echo-intensity variation. Circulation 2001;103:1206–1211.

34   Falk E, Shah PK, Fuster V: Coronary plaque disruption. Circulation 1995;92:657–671.

35   Moreno PR, Falk E, Palacios IF, Newell JB, Fuster V, Fallon JT: Macrophage infiltration in acute coronary syndromes. Implications for plaque rupture. Circulation 1994;90:775–778.

36   Loree HM, Tobias BJ, Gibson LJ, Kamm RD, Small DM, Lee RT: Mechanical properties of model atherosclerotic lesion lipid pools. Arterioscler Thromb 1994;14:230–234.

37   Loree HM, Grodzinsky AJ, Park SY, Gibson LJ, Lee RT: Static circumferential tangential modulus of human atherosclerotic tissue. J Biomech 1994;27:195–204.

38   Lee RT, Richardson G, Loree HM, Gordzinsky AJ, Gharib SA, Schoen FJ, Pandian N: Prediction of mechanical properties of human atherosclerotic tissue by high-frequency intravascular ultrasound imaging. Arterioscler Thromb 1992;12:1–5.

39   Lendon CL, Davies MJ, Born GVR, Richardson PD: Atherosclerotic plaque caps are locally weakened when macrophage density is increased. Atherosclerosis 1991;87:87–90.

40   Loree HM, Kamm RD, Stringfellow RG, Lee RT: Effects of fibrous cap thickness on peak circumferential stress in model atherosclerotic vessels. Circ Res 1992;71:850–858.

41   Richardson PD, Davies MJ, Born GVR: Influence of plaque configuration and stress distribution on fissuring of coronary atherosclerotic plaques. Lancet 1989;ii:941–944.

42   Ophir J, Céspedes I, Ponnekanti H, Yazdi Y, Li X: Elastography: a quantitative method for imaging the elasticity of biological tissues. Ultrason Imaging 1991;13:111–134.

43   Céspedes EI, Ophir J, Ponnekanti H, Maklad N: Elastography: elasticity imaging using ultrasound with application to muscle and breast in vivo. Ultrason Imaging 1993;17:73–88.

44   Céspedes EI, Huang Y, Ophir J, Spratt S: Methods for estimation of subsample time delays of digitized echo signals. Ultrason Imaging 1995;17:142–171.

45   Konofagou EE: Quo vadis elasticity imaging? Ultrasonics 2004;42:331–336.

46   Sarvazyan AP, Emelianov SY, Skovorada AR: Intracavity device for elasticity imaging. US patent 5,265,612, November 39. 1993.

47   Doyley M, Mastik F, de Korte CL, Carlier S, Céspedes E, Serruys P, Bom N, van der Steen AFW: Advancing intravascular ultrasonic palpation towards clinical applications. Ultrasound Med Biol 2001;27:1471–1480.

48   Céspedes EI, de Korte CL, van der Steen AFW: Intraluminal ultrasonic palpation: assessment of local and cross-sectional tissue stiffness. Ultrasound Med Biol 2000;26:385–396.

49   Talhami HE, Wilson LS, Neale ML: Spectral tissue strain: a new technique for imaging tissue strain using intravascular ultrasound. Ultrasound Med Biol 1994;20:759–772.

50   Ryan LK, Foster FS: Ultrasonic measurement of differential displacement and strain in a vascular model. Ultrason Imaging 1997;19:19–38.

51   Varghese T, Ophir J: Characterization of elastographic noise using the envelope of echo signals. Ultrasound Med Biol 1998;24:543–555.

52   Shapo BM, Crowe JR, Skovoroda AR, Eberle M, Cohn NA, O'Donnell M: Displacement and strain imaging of coronary arteries with intraluminal ultrasound. IEEE Trans Ultrason Ferroelectr Freq Control 1996;43:234–246.

53   De Korte CL, van der Steen AFW, Céspedes EI, Pasterkamp G: Intravascular ultrasound elastography of human arteries: initial experience in vitro. Ultrasound Med Biol 1998;24:401–408.

54   Doyley MM, de Korte CL, Mastik F, Carlier S, van der Steen AFW: Advancing intravascular palpography towards clinical applications; in Wells PNT, Halliwell M (eds): Acoustical Imaging. New York, Plenum Press, 2000, pp 493–500.

55   De Korte CL, Carlier SG, Mastik F, Doyley MM, van der Steen AFW, Céspedes EI, Serruys PW, Bom N: Intracoronary elastography in the catheterisation laboratory: preliminary patient results; in IEEE Ultrasonics Symposium, Lake Tahoe/CA, 1999, pp 1649–1652.

56   De Korte CL, Pasterkamp G, van der Steen AFW, Woutman HA, Bom N: Characterization of plaque components using intravascular ultrasound elastography in human femoral and coronary arteries in vitro. Circulation 2000;102:617–623.

57   De Korte CL, Sierevogel MJ, Mastik F, Strijder C, Schaar JA, Velema E, Pasterkamp G, Serruys PW, van der Steen AFW: Identification of atherosclerotic plaque components with intravascular ultrasound elastography in vivo: a Yucatan pig study. Circulation 2002;105:1627–1630.

58   De Korte CL, Carlier SG, Mastik F, Doyley MM, van der Steen AF, Serruys PW, Bom N: Morphological and mechanical information of coronary arteries obtained with intravascular elastography; feasibility study in vivo. Eur Heart J 2002;23:405–413.

59   Schaar JA, Regar E, Mastik F, McFadden EP, Saia F, Disco C, de Korte CL, de Feyter PJ, van der Steen AFW, Serruys PW: Incidence of vulnerable plaque patterns in humans: assessment with three-dimensional intravascular palpography and correlation with clinical presentation. Circulation 2004;109:2716–2719.

60   De Korte CL, Céspedes EI, van der Steen AFW: Influence of catheter position on estimated strain in intravascular elastography. IEEE Trans Ultrason Ferroelectr Freq Control 1999;46:616–625.

61   Ophir J, Céspedes EI, Garra B, Ponnekanti H, Huang Y, Maklad N: Elastography: ultrasonic imaging of tissue strain and elastic modulus in vivo. Eur J Ultrasound 1996;3:49–70.

62   Fung YC: Biomechanics: Mechanical Properties of Living Tissues, ed 2. New York, Springer, 1993.

63   Salunke NV, Topoleski LD: Biomechanics of atherosclerotic plaque. Crit Rev Biomed Eng 1997;25:243–285.

64   Raghavan KR, Yagle AE: Forward and inverse problems in elasticity imaging of soft tissues. IEEE Trans Nucl Sci 1994;41:1639–1648.

65   Sumi C, Suzuki A, Nakayama K: Estimation of shear modulus distribution in soft tissue from strain distribution. IEEE Trans Biomed Eng 1995;42:193–202.

66   Skovoroda AR, Emelianov SY, O'Donnell M: Tissue elasticity reconstruction based on ultrasonic displacement and strain images. IEEE Trans Ultrason Ferroelectr Freq Control 1995;42:747–765.

67   Kallel F, Bertrand M: Tissue elasticity reconstruction using linear perturbation method. IEEE Trans Med Imaging 1996;15:299–313.

68   Beattie D, Xu C, Vito R, Glagov S, Whang MC: Mechanical analysis of heterogeneous, atherosclerotic human aorta. J Biomech Eng 1998;120:602–607.

69   Vorp DA, Rajagopal KR, Smolinski PJ, Borovetz HS: Identification of elastic properties of homogeneous, orthotropic vascular segments in distension. J Biomech 1995;28:501–512.

70   Chandran KB, Mun JH, Choi KK, Chen JS, Hamilton A, Nagaraj A, McPherson DD: A method for in-vivo analysis for regional arterial wall material property alterations with atherosclerosis: preliminary results. Med Eng Phys 2003;25:289–298.

71   Soualmi L, Bertrand M, Mongrain R, Tardif JC. Forward and inverse problems in endovascular elastography, in Lees S, Ferrari LA (eds): Acoustical Imaging. New York, Plenum, 1997, pp 203–209.

72   Wan M, Li Y, Li J, Cui Y, Zhou X: Strain imaging and elasticity reconstruction of arteries based on intravascular ultrasound video images. IEEE Trans Biomed Eng 2001;48:116–120.

73   Bank AJ: Intravascular ultrasound studies of arterial elastic mechanics. Pathol Biol (Paris) 1999; 47:731–737.

74   Kanai H, Hasegawa H, Ichiki M, Tezuka F, Koiwa Y: Elasticity imaging of atheroma with transcutaneous ultrasound: preliminary study. Circulation 2003;107:3018–3021.

75   Barbone PE, Bamber JC: Quantitative elasticity imaging: what can and cannot be inferred from strain images. Phys Med Biol 2002;47:2147–2164.

76   Barbone PE, Gokhale NH: Elastic modulus imaging: on the uniqueness and nonuniqueness of the elastography inverse problem in two dimensions. Inverse Probl 2004;20:283–296.

77   Virmani R, Burke AP, Kolodgie FD, Farb A: Pathology of the thin-cap fibroatheroma: a type of vulnerable plaque. J Interv Cardiol 2003;16:267–272.

78   Baldewsing RA, de Korte CL, Schaar JA, Mastik F, van der Steen AFW: A finite element model for performing intravascular ultrasound elastography of human atherosclerotic coronary arteries. Ultrasound Med Biol 2004;30:803–813.

79   Baldewsing RA, De Korte CL, Schaar JA, Mastik F, van der Steen AFW: Finite element modeling and intravascular ultrasound elastography of vulnerable plaques: parameter variation. Ultrasonics 2004;42:723–729.

80   Baldewsing RA, Mastik F, Schaar JA, Serruys PW, van der Steen AFW: Young's modulus reconstruction of vulnerable atherosclerotic plaque components using deformable curves. Ultrasound Med Biol 2006;32:201–210.

81   Van Mieghem CA, Bruining N, Schaar JA, McFadden E, Mollet N, Cademartiri F, Mastik F, Ligthart JM, Granillo GA, Valgimigli M, Sianos G, van der Giessen WJ, Backx B, Morel MA, Van Es GA, Sawyer JD, Kaplow J, Zalewski A, van der Steen AF, de Feyter P, Serruys PW: Rationale and methods of the integrated biomarker and imaging study (IBIS): combining invasive and non-invasive imaging with biomarkers to detect subclinical atherosclerosis and assess coronary lesion biology. Int J Cardiovasc Imaging 2005;21:425–441.

Radj A. Baldewsing, PhD
Biomedical Engineering, Room Ee 23.02
Thorax Center, Erasmus Medical Center Rotterdam, PO Box 1738
NL–3000 DR, Rotterdam (The Netherlands)
Tel. +31 10 4089 363, Fax +31 10 4089 445, E-Mail r.baldewsing@erasmusmc.nl

Safar ME, Frohlich ED (eds): Atherosclerosis, Large Arteries and Cardiovascular Risk.
Adv Cardiol. Basel, Karger, 2007, vol 44, pp 62–75

··························

Endothelial Function, Mechanical Stress and Atherosclerosis

Daniel Hayoz   Lucia Mazzolai

Department of Medicine, Vascular Medicine, CHUV, Lausanne, Switzerland

Abstract

Atherosclerosis and its complications represent the leading cause of morbidity and
mortality in the industrialized as well as in the developing countries. Classical cardiovascular risk factors have been identified over the past decades leading to recommendations
for life style modifications and to the development of efficient and well-tolerated drug
regimens aimed at reducing the occurrence of cardiovascular complications. The endothelium due to its position in the circulation is the first organ being exposed to circulating
noxious elements and solutes as well as to the mechanical aggressions generated by heart-
beats and pulsating blood flow. This review addresses the relevance of the combined effects of the mechanical stress and cardiovascular risk factors on the early phases of
atherosclerosis.

This chapter on endothelium involves four sections: normal endothelial
function; effect of atherosclerosis; role of mechanical stress, and relation between arterial stiffness and endothelial function.

Normal Endothelial Function

The endothelium is a monolayer of endothelial cells lining the vasculature. It lies at the interface of the vessel wall and the circulating blood and con-
stitutes a protective barrier between the two elements. Endothelial cells play a
crucial role in maintaining vascular homeostasis. They function as sensors
and integrators of hemodynamic and hormonal stimuli and they control the

bidirectional transport of macromolecules and blood gases through the vascular wall [1]. As a result, endothelial cells release a number of autocrine and paracrine factors that regulate vascular permeability, vasomotion, coagulation, cell adhesion, inflammation and mitogenesis [2]. Disruption of the balanced release of these bioactive factors can be a critical factor in the pathogenesis of vascular diseases and more specifically of atherogenesis.

It is now well established that endothelial dysfunction is a very early event if not the earliest in the process of atherogenesis and therefore, testing endothelial function may serve as a biomarker of lesion formation [3]. For this reason it became manifest that evaluation of endothelial function integrity was of utmost importance in vascular biology both in clinical as well as in experimental conditions. Impairment in endothelial function has been related to all known atherogenic risk factors (dyslipidemia, hypertension, smoking, diabetes mellitus, aging, menopause…). Several studies have now recognized the prognostic value of endothelial dysfunction for atherothrombotic complications [4–8]. Although endothelial dysfunction may not homogeneously affect the vascular bed, strong evidence suggests that a close relationship exists between human peripheral artery and coronary vasomotor abnormalities leading to the concept of systemic endothelial dysfunction [9]. As a consequence, endothelial function testing is no longer restricted to patients undergoing invasive cardiac catheterization. Originally, endothelial function was assessed during quantitative angiography by measuring the vasomotor response of epicardial arteries to increasing concentrations of muscarinic receptor agonists (acetylcholine, metacholine) [10]. Nowadays, it can be tested in the upper limb by measuring forearm blood flow using strain gauge plethysmography during intra-arterial infusion of muscarinic receptor agonists [11]. The brachial artery is the most frequent peripheral artery tested for this purpose. However, the test remains invasive and therefore limited to research centers. With the advent of high-resolution ultrasound technology, a totally non-invasive method was proposed to evaluate endothelial function [12, 13]. Reactive hyperemia following a localized ischemic stimulus, distal to the measuring site, generates an increased shear stress that induces nitric oxide (NO) release. This test, known as the endothelial-dependent flow-mediated dilation (FMD) of the conduit artery, is now widely used to test the integrity of endothelial function [14]. As demonstrated years ago it is less sensitive than the muscarinic receptor challenge but much more practical and it can be applied to asymptomatic populations as well as to patients [10]. Indeed, subjects with cardiovascular risk factors and smooth coronary arteries show paradoxical vasoconstriction upon intracoronary acetylcholine infusion [10]. In patients with significant coronary artery disease, diagnosed at angiography, preserved although reduced FMD could still be observed despite significant vasoconstriction during ace-

Table 1. Current methods to assess in vivo endothelial function in human subjects

Method	Vascular bed	Convenience	Risk	Accuracy
Venous occlusion plethysmography	Forearm resistance vessels	Invasive	Arterial cannulation Critical vasoconstriction	Highly accurate
Laser Doppler flowmetry (reactive hyperemia, iontophoresis)	Skin microvessels	Non-invasive	None	High accuracy for acute pharmacological or physical challenges Needs further validation
Flow-mediated dilation	Conduit arteries	Non-invasive (echo-Doppler) Invasive (flow-wire)	None Critical vasoconstriction Arterial cannulation and dissection	Equipment-dependent (hardware, software)
PET scan	Resistance vessels	Non-invasive Very expensive	Irradiation	Highly accurate Needs further validation
Pulse wave analysis	Large and small arteries	Non-invasive Ease of use	None	Further characterization needed to establish association between arterial stiffness and endothelial function

tylcholine challenge. In the latter case, blood flow was increased by peripheral arteriolar dilation following papaverine infusion distally from the arterial segment under investigation.

Brachial artery FMD was shown to be predictive of clinical complications associated with atherosclerosis [9]. Although more easily available than the invasive techniques, brachial FMD assessment performed by high-resolution ultrasound remains quite a challenging test and requires appropriate qualification and training. In this respect, guidelines have been published to try to standardize the methods and protocols between centers in order to be able to compare results among investigators [14].

Recently, more practical and simpler devices have been designed to measure endothelial function (table 1). One such device uses a digital plethysmography technique based on an observation that was made earlier in hypercholesterolemic patients demonstrating reduced flow reserve and elevated resistance during hyperemia [15]. This system allows to assess endothelial function in a very simple way. Using this device, it has been demonstrated that digital reactive hyperemia response can identify patients with early coronary microvascular endothelial dysfunction [16]. Further studies will be needed to fully assess the potential of this simple and non-invasive endothelial function test.

Laser Doppler iontophoresis is another attractive technique requiring specific tools to assess skin microvascular endothelial function [17, 18]. The test is quite reproducible but several problems still need to be overcome such as variability in skin conductivity and current-induced vasodilation. As for the previously mentioned plethysmography method, further studies will be necessary to evaluate the prognostic value of skin microvascular dysfunction in detecting individuals at increased coronary heart disease (CHD) [19].

A number of circulating factors have been considered for their potential predictive value of endothelial function and atherothrombotic complications. Among them, highly sensitive CRP, which is closely related to systemic and vascular low-grade inflammation, has been identified as one of the most valuable factors. Elevated levels of circulating CRP have been shown to be closely associated with the increased 10-year risk of CHD, regardless of the presence or absence of known cardiac risk factors. A single CRP measurement provided information beyond conventional risk assessment, especially in intermediate-Framingham-risk men and high-Framingham-risk women [20]. Can CRP measurements replace the predictive value of the cumbersome FMD assessment in determining the quality of endothelial function? Apparently not, as demonstrated in a large healthy cohort of subjects in whom the predictive value of CRP was shown to be largely independent of abnormalities in endothelial function assessed by FMD testing [21].

Microalbuminuria is another laboratory parameter which is considered to be a marker of endothelial dysfunction. Whether microalbuminuria is associated with FMD has recently been investigated in an elderly population. Microalbuminuria is linearly associated with impaired endothelium-dependent flow-mediated vasodilation in elderly individuals without and with diabetes [22]. Unfortunately, microalbuminuria, which is easy to measure, appears to be a rather late marker of endothelial dysfunction. Indeed, endothelial dysfunction, as estimated by plasma von Willebrand factor concentration, precedes and may predict the development of microalbuminuria in insulin-dependent diabetes mellitus [23].

In conclusion, up to now, no circulating factor has been convincingly shown to yield earlier and more sensitive information on endothelial function as a prognostic factor of cardiovascular events than muscarinic receptor stimulation or FMD.

Endothelial Function and Atherosclerosis

As mentioned in the previous section, endothelial dysfunction represents the primary event in atherogenesis. We have described above the different methods currently used for the in vivo assessment of endothelial function. In this section we present some of the main mechanisms linking endothelial dysfunction to atherosclerosis. Endothelial cells are the target of local and systemic injuries. Among the systemic factors that affect endothelium homeostasis, hyperlipidemia, diabetes mellitus, hypertension and smoking represent the most prevalent conditions in clinical settings. The initial description of the endothelium-derived vasodilator agent by Furchgott and Zawadski [24] later identified as NO occupies a key position in the pathogenesis of atherosclerosis. NO was first described as a vasodilator whose production can be controlled by different physiological agonists as well as by pharmacological agents acting on the endothelial isoform of the NO synthase (eNOS or NOSIII) gene. NO not only regulates vascular tone by directly acting on smooth muscle cells, but it also counterbalances the action of other vasoconstrictors such as endothelin-1 (ET-1) [25] and angiotensin II (Ang II) [26]. In addition, NO limits recruitment of leukocytes, inhibits platelet adhesion and aggregation, inhibits smooth muscle cells proliferation and tissue factor production [27]. Although not limited to NO metabolism, endothelium homeostasis is greatly dependent on the NO-balanced release because of the pleiotropic actions NO exerts in controlling most of the other endothelial factors. Reduced NO bioavailability is the common denominator of endothelial dysfunction associated with cardiovascular risk factors.

Most of these cardiovascular risk factors are associated with an increased production of reactive oxygen species (ROS), such as the superoxide radicals which in turn reduce vascular NO bioavailability [28]. Superoxide radicals can react with NO released by endothelial nitric oxide synthase (eNOS), thereby generating peroxynitrite. A vicious circle can then be initiated where the anti-atherosclerotic NO-producing enzyme is converted into an enzyme (uncoupling) that may trigger or even accelerate the atherosclerotic process by producing superoxide rather than NO. Therefore, reducing ROS and improving eNOS activity to increase NO bioavailability represents the mainstay of the management of cardiovascular risk factors in primary and secondary prevention.

Low-grade inflammation has been shown to contribute to atherogenesis. Leukocyte recruitment and monocyte adhesion on the activated endothelium represent one of the earliest responses in the inflammatory process associated with atherosclerosis [29]. Complex interactions exist between cytokines, chemokines, and inflammation in the development of atherosclerosis. However, cardiovascular hormones directly involved in the control of hemodynamics and volume homeostasis may also play a crucial role in the initiation and the development of atherosclerotic plaques. We have recently demonstrated the pressure independent role of an activated renin-angiotensin-aldosterone system on atherosclerotic plaque development and vulnerability [30]. To study the contribution of Ang II in plaque vulnerability, hypertensive hypercholesterol-

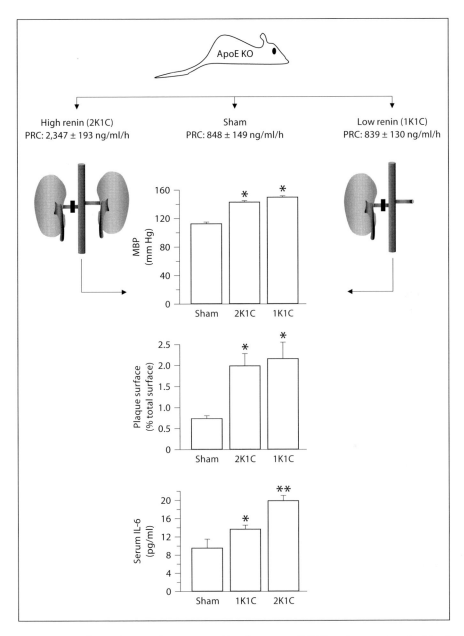

Fig. 1. Atherosclerotic plaque, mean blood pressure (MBP) and serum interleukin-6 (IL-6) in ApoE knockout (ApoE KO) mice: sham is compared to high-renin and low-renin animals. K = Kidney; C = clip; PRC = plasma renin concentration. * p < 0.05 versus sham; ** p < 0.05 versus 1K1C.

emic ApoE$^{-/-}$ mice were generated with either normal or endogenously increased Ang II production (renovascular hypertension models) (fig. 1). Hypertensive high Ang II ApoE$^{-/-}$ mice developed unstable plaques, whereas in hypertensive normal Ang II ApoE$^{-/-}$ mice, plaques showed a stable phenotype. Vulnerable plaques from high Ang II ApoE$^{-/-}$ mice had a thinner fibrous cap, larger lipid core, and increased macrophage content than even more hypertensive but normal Ang II ApoE$^{-/-}$ mice. Our findings suggest that Ang II via the AT1 receptor, within the context of hypertension and hypercholesterolemia, independently from its hemodynamic effect behaves as a local modulator of atherosclerotic plaque phenotype probably via a T-helper cells switch. The exact role of the AT2 receptor in the proatherogenic process remains to be further clarified since recent data have demonstrated contradictory results [31, 32].

Mechanical Stress and Endothelial Function

It is well established that endothelial dysfunction can be demonstrated quite early in the setting of cardiovascular risk factors such as hypercholesterolemia, hypertension, diabetes mellitus, and chronic smoking. However, despite the systemic effects of these cardiovascular risk factors, atherosclerosis is a focal disease which clearly shows a non-random distribution within the arterial vasculature [33]. Plaques persistently occur at definite sites such as branch points and curved areas of conduit arteries [34]. The clinical manifestations of atherothrombotic complications are determined by the non-random localization of atherosclerotic plaques. Strong evidence suggests that fluid dynamics and mechanical forces play a critical role in the initiation and the focal distribution of atherosclerotic lesions [35, 36].

Mechanical forces affecting the endothelial cells during the cardiac cycle can be distinguished in two types. The first is parallel to the flow direction. It is due to the frictional forces generated by the viscous fluid on the luminal surface of blood vessels, we therefore talk about shear stress. The second force is due to the cyclic strain and is known as circumferential stretch. It is perpendicular to the vessel wall. Circumferential stretch is a critical parameter for smooth muscle cells while it has been shown to play a minor role on the endothelium when combined with near physiological flow conditions (mean shear stress of 10 dyn/cm^2) [37]. Conversely, several reports have demonstrated that cyclic strain mediates a significant endothelial response in the absence of flow and/or when supraphysiological strain conditions (10–20% strain) are applied [38]. Similarly, endothelial cell activation can be observed when cells are acutely submitted to cyclic strain from resting culture conditions.

Therefore, in this section we will mainly focus on shear stress, the tangential drag force which appears to be the predominant mechanical stimulus inducing changes in structure and function of endothelial cells. Early experiments were performed in in vitro flow models to study fluid dynamics along the different carotid bulb sections and revealed that low shear stress zones matched arterial surface alterations observed in cadaveric arteries. Regions exposed to low mean and oscillatory (bidirectional) shear stress were found to be prone to develop atherosclerotic lesions. These observations are somehow in opposition with those made in animal models where endothelial lesions were demonstrated in regions exposed to high shear stress induced by lumen reduction [39] but corroborate data obtained in more physiological atherosclerosis animal models [40]. The latter confirmed that low shear stress zones with cyclic reversal flow direction are prone to develop early atherosclerotic transformations. Therefore, it became manifest that disturbed blood flow plays a critical role in determining plaque location. Because it is quite difficult to study individual hemodynamic effects on endothelial functions in animal models, owing to the redundant biofeedback systems, several in vitro models mimicking physiological blood flow conditions were developed. Our laboratory has played a seminal role in this development by proposing to study the effect of combined and controlled hemodynamic parameters on different endothelial cells seeded on tubular structures with biomechanical properties similar to those of native arteries. Primary as well as endothelial cell lines have been studied to better appreciate the mechanisms by which endothelial cells sense and respond to changes in shear stress, cyclic strain, and hydrostatic pressure [37, 41, 42].

Like other laboratories, we were able to show that shear stress has a profound effect on endothelial cell cytoskeletal proteins. Endothelial cells respond in a dose-dependent manner to the increase in shear stress by reorganizing their stress fibers and by releasing atheroprotective factors or by reducing atherogenic mediators. Stress fibers are aligned in parallel to the flow direction and perpendicular to the circumferential strain and the Rho-ROCK pathway plays a critical role in the flow-induced rearrangement of the stress fibers [43]. The effects observed using the in vitro flow modulation were in total accordance with the observations made by Nerem et al. [44] using animal models of flow disturbances.

For a given mean shear stress value, we showed that pulsatile shear stress exerts a greater influence on endothelial cells than a constant shear stress [42]. Because endothelial cells in vivo are subjected to concomitant shear stress and cyclic strain, acting in perpendicular directions, a time lag between flow and pressure waves generated by wave reflection may influence cell function. Indeed, asynchronous shear stress and circumferential strain were demonstrated to induce an atherogenic profile of eNOS, ET-1 and COX-2 [45]. These results emphasize the importance of local hemodynamic conditions on the localization and initiation of atherosclerosis.

As mentioned earlier, increased production of ROS, such as the superoxide radicals, leads to decreased NO vascular bioavailability, thus promoting atherosclerosis. Shear stress modulates the redox state of the endothelial cells [46]. We demonstrated that the pulsatility of flow, but not cyclic stretch, was a critical determinant of flow-induced superoxide anion production [42]. p22phox mRNA levels increased in cells exposed to both unidirectional and oscillatory shear stress, suggesting that p22phox gene expression upregulation contributes to flow-induced increase in superoxide anion production in endothelial cells. Different results were obtained in absence of pulsatility but do not correspond to the in vivo situation and therefore should be interpreted with limitation [47]. Agents that block the renin-angiotensin system (ACE-I and ARBs) [48, 49] and statins [50] have been shown to favorably influence oxidative stress by reducing or suppressing NADPH oxidase activity independently from their primary therapeutic effect.

Shear stress does appear to have a favorable effect on inflammation. Indeed, endothelial cells release a number of factors that prevent atherogenesis such as NO, prostacyclin and SOD, to name a few that counteract inflammatory stimuli. Physiologic flow conditions have a positive impact by turning on atheroprotective genes and by turning off genes that contribute to atherosclerosis initiation or progression (adhesion molecules). Recently, Berk and colleagues [51] demonstrated that preconditioning of endothelial cells by steady laminar flow decreased apoptosis and reduced TNF-mediated endothelial cell activation by inactivation of the MAPK cascade. All these in vitro results must be interpreted bearing in mind that cells are not exposed to the full physiopathological array of conditions such as hyperlipidemia and increased oxidative stress that are normally found in the in vivo situation.

Nitric Oxide and Age-Related Changes in Stiffness

Arterial stiffness is frequently considered to result mainly from the distending pressure and from the quality/quantity of elastic and collagen fibers arterial media content. However, the media is rich in smooth muscle cells that respond actively to sympathetic activation and to the paracrine release of vasomediators such as NO, ET-1 and prostacyclin to name a few. Therefore, it is not surprising that alterations in NO bioavailability influences arterial stiffness [52]. There are different ways to assess arterial elasticity. Pulse pressure which is a surrogate of large artery stiffness has been shown to be a strong independent predictor of the endothelial response to muscarinic receptor agonists in normotensive subjects [53]. Similar results have been obtained in healthy subjects and in patients with coronary artery disease in whom an inverse correlation was observed between the degree of arterial stiffness and impaired endothelial function [54].

Recently, it has become evident that for any given mean blood pressure level, aging is accompanied by vascular wall stiffening which induces opposite hemodynamic effects on blood pressure [55]. Systolic blood pressure tends to steadily increase with aging whereas diastolic blood pressure reaches a plateau around age 55–60 years before declining [56]. This trend which has been observed in most of the studied populations so far clearly shows that pulse pressure, thus arterial stiffness, increases with age.

Pulse wave velocity is another measure of arterial stiffness which is a good predictor of cardiovascular outcome in various clinical settings such as hypertension, diabetes and end-stage renal disease [57, 58]. In the latter case, accumulation of asymmetrical dimethylarginine, a potent inhibitor of eNOS, may play a critical role in the development of severe arterial stiffening in combination with media calcification due to hyperphosphatemia [59]. With aging of the population, new problems are emerging. It has been observed in the general population that low bone mass is associated with a higher mortality rate due to atherosclerotic cardiovascular disease. The degree of aortic calcification is strongly related with a lower bone mineral density. Therefore, one may speculate that low bone mineral density is a predictor of increased arterial stiffness [60, 61]. Patients with chronic renal failure also present with renal osteodystrophy. Preliminary data tend to support that pulse wave velocity is related to the severity of osteodystrophy in ESRD patients and with osteoporosis in the general elderly population [62]. To which extent endothelial dysfunction contributes to large artery stiffening with time remains to be fully addressed. Studies have looked at the acute effect of NO blockade in healthy volunteers showing an increased arterial stiffness [52]. To discriminate the effect of blood pressure increase from that of the inhibition of NO release vasoconstricting agents such as noradrenaline and dobutamine were compared to L-NMMA measuring carotido-femoral PVW as a marker of elastic artery stiffness in healthy volunteers. No apparent effect of NO blockade other than the pressure effect could be detected. This observation may not be true for muscular arteries where other factors than NO may play a role in modulating vascular tone. Chronic inhibition of NO synthase or clinical conditions associated with endothelial dysfunction may induce vascular remodeling which in the long run may favor development of atherosclerosis and increased left ventricular afterload.

Endothelial function is impaired with increasing age and may therefore contribute to the steady increase in arterial stiffness observed in epidemiological studies. Measures aimed at controlling cardiovascular risk factors which improve endothelial function may reverse some of the age-related stiffening of the conduit arteries by influencing both on the active component of the vessel wall via smooth muscle tone and on the passive elements such as the elastic and collagen fibers and the matrix proteins.

There is now a very large body of evidence showing that endothelial dysfunction is an early marker of atherosclerotic changes. Several mechanisms are implicated in the progression of endothelial dysfunction. Some of them are modifiable and measures to limit atherosclerosis development via endothelial alteration have proven successful. Although interesting, the demonstration of an improvement in endothelial function should be taken with great caution before being considered as a valid surrogate of clinical improvement. Indeed, recent clinical trials have demonstrated a discrepancy between improved endothelial function following estrogen, COX-2 inhibitors or vitamin treatment and increased cardiovascular events [63, 64].

References

1   Vanhoutte PM: Endothelium and control of vascular function. State of the art lecture. Hypertension 1989;13:658–667.
2   Rubanyi GM: The role of endothelium in cardiovascular homeostasis and diseases. J Cardiovasc Pharmacol 1993;4:S1–S14.
3   Ganz P, Vita JA: Testing endothelial vasomotor function. Circulation 2003;108:2049–2053.
4   Schachinger V, Britten MB, Zeiher AM: Prognostic impact of coronary vasodilator dysfunction on adverse long-term outcome of coronary heart disease. Circulation 2000;101:1899–1906.
5   Vita JA, Keaney JF Jr: Endothelial function: a barometer for cardiovascular risk? Circulation 2002;106:640–642.
6   Suwaidi JA, Hamasaki S, Higano ST, et al: Long-term follow-up of patients with mild coronary artery disease and endothelial dysfunction. Circulation 2000;101:948–954.
7   Halcox JP, Schenke WH, Zalos G, et al: Prognostic value of coronary vascular endothelial dysfunction. Circulation 2002;106:653–658.
8   Lerman A, Zeiher AM: Endothelial function: cardiac events. Circulation 2005;111:363–368.
9   Kuvin JT, Patel AR, Sliney KA, Pandian NG, Rand WM, Udelson JE, Karas RH: Peripheral vascular endothelial function testing as a noninvasive indicator of coronary artery disease. J Am Coll Cardiol 2001;38:1843–1849.
10   Zeiher AM, Drexler H, Wollschlager H, Just H: Modulation of coronary vasomotor tone in humans. Progressive endothelial dysfunction with different early stages of coronary atherosclerosis. Circulation 1991;83:391–401.
11   Panza JA, Quyyumi AA, Callahan TS, Epstein SE: Effect of antihypertensive treatment on endothelium-dependent vascular relaxation in patients with essential hypertension. J Am Coll Cardiol 1993;21:1145–1151.
12   Sinoway LI, Hendrickson C, Davidson WR Jr, Prophet S, Zelis R: Characteristics of flow-mediated brachial artery vasodilation in human subjects. Circ Res 1989;64:32–42.
13   Hayoz D, Drexler H, Münzel T, Hornig B, Zeiher AM, Just H, Brunner HR, Zelis R: Flow mediated arterial dilation is abnormal in congestive failure. Circulation 1993;87(suppl VII):VII-92–VII-96.
14   Corretti MC, Anderson TJ, Benjamin EJ, et al: Guidelines for the ultrasound assessment of endothelial-dependent flow-mediated vasodilation of the brachial artery: a report of the International Brachial Artery Reactivity Task Force. J Am Coll Cardiol 2002;39:257–265.

15   Hayoz D, Weber R, Rutschmann B, Darioli R, Burnier M, Waeber B, Brunner HR: Post-ischemic blood flow response in hypercholesterolemic patients. Hypertension 1995;26:497–502.

16   Bonetti PO, Pumper GM, Higano ST, Holmes DR Jr, Kuvin JT, Lerman A: Noninvasive identification of patients with early coronary atherosclerosis by assessment of digital reactive hyperemia. J Am Coll Cardiol 2004;44:2137–2141.

17   Morris SJ, Shore AC: Skin blood flow responses to the iontophoresis of acetylcholine and sodium nitroprusside in man: possible mechanisms. J Physiol 1996;496:531–542.

18   De Jongh RT, Serne EH, Ijzerman RG, de Vries G, Stehouwer CD: Impaired microvascular function in obesity: implications for obesity-associated microangiopathy, hypertension, and insulin resistance. Circulation 2004;109:2529–2535.

19   Ijzerman RG, de Jongh RT, Beijk MA, van Weissenbruch MM, Delemarre-van de Waal HA, Serne EH, Stehouwer CD: Individuals at increased coronary heart disease risk are characterized by an impaired microvascular function in skin. Eur J Clin Invest 2003;33:536–542.

20   Cushman M, Arnold AM, Psaty BM, Manolio TA, Kuller LH, Burke GL, Polak JF, Tracy RP: C-reactive protein and the 10-year incidence of coronary heart disease in older men and women: the cardiovascular health study. Circulation 2005;112:25–31.

21   Verma S, Wang CH, Lonn E, Charbonneau F, Buithieu J, Title LM, Fung M, Edworthy S, Robertson AC, Anderson TJ, FATE Investigators: Cross-sectional evaluation of brachial artery flow-mediated vasodilation and C-reactive protein in healthy individuals. Eur Heart J 2004;25:1754–1760.

22   Stehouwer CD, Henry RM, Dekker JM, Nijpels G, Heine RJ, Bouter LM: Microalbuminuria is associated with impaired brachial artery, flow-mediated vasodilation in elderly individuals without and with diabetes: further evidence for a link between microalbuminuria and endothelial dysfunction – the Hoorn Study. Kidney Int Suppl 2004;92:S42–44.

23   Stehouwer CD, Fischer HR, van Kuijk AW, Polak BC, Donker AJ: Endothelial dysfunction precedes development of microalbuminuria in insulin-dependent diabetes mellitus. Diabetes 1995; 44:561–564.

24   Furchgott RF, Zawadski JV: The obligatory role of endothelial cells in the relaxation of arterial smooth muscle by acetylcholine. Nature 1980;288:373–376.

25   Schiffrin EL, Touyz RM: Vascular biology of endothelin. J Cardiovasc Pharmacol 1998;32(suppl 3):S2–S13.

26   Dimmeler S, Rippmann V, Weiland U, Haendeler J, Zeiher AM: Angiotensin II induces apoptosis of human endothelial cells. Protective effect of nitric oxide. Circ Res 1997;81:970–976.

27   Chen XL, Tummala PE, Olbrych MT, Alexander RW, Medford RM: Angiotensin II induces monocyte chemoattractant protein-1 gene expression in rat vascular smooth muscle cells. Circ Res 1998;83:952–959.

28   Munzel T, Daiber A, Ullrich V, Mulsch A: Vascular consequences of endothelial nitric oxide synthase uncoupling for the activity and expression of the soluble guanylyl cyclase and the cGMP-dependent protein kinase. Arterioscler Thromb Vasc Biol 2005;25:1551–1557.

29   Libby P, Theroux P: Pathophysiology of coronary artery disease. Circulation 2005;111:3481–3488.

30   Mazzolai L, Duchosal MA, Korber M, Bouzourene K, Aubert JF, Hao H, Vallet V, Brunner HR, Nussberger J, Gabbiani G, Hayoz D: Endogenous angiotensin II induces atherosclerotic plaque vulnerability and elicits a Th1 response in ApoE$^{-/-}$ mice. Hypertension 2004;44:277–282.

31   Johansson ME, Wickman A, Fitzgerald SM, Gan LM, Bergstrom G: Angiotensin II, type 2 receptor is not involved in the angiotensin II-mediated pro-atherogenic process in ApoE$^{-/-}$ mice. J Hypertens 2005;23:1541–1549.

32   Iwai M, Chen R, Li Z, Shiuchi T, Suzuki J, Ide A, Tsuda M, Okumura M, Min LJ, Mogi M, Horiuchi M: Deletion of angiotensin II type 2 receptor exaggerated atherosclerosis in apolipoprotein E-null mice. Circulation 2005;112:1636–1643.

33   Cornhill JF, Herderick EE, Stary HC: Topography of human aortic sudanophilic lesions. Monogr Atheroscler 1990;15:13–19.

34   DeBakey ME, Lawrie GM, Gleaser DH: Patterns of atherosclerosis and their surgical significance. Ann Surg 1985;201:115–131.

35   Pohl U, Holtz J, Busse R, Bassenge E: Crucial role of endothelium in the vasodilator response to increased flow in vivo. Hypertension 1986;8:37–47.

36   Langille BL, O'Donnell F: Reduction in arterial diameter produced by chronic decreases in blood flow are endothelium-dependent. Science 1986;231:405–407.

37   Ziegler T, Silacci P, Harrison VJ, Hayoz D: Nitric oxide synthase expression in endothelial cells exposed to mechanical forces. Hypertension 1998;32:351–355.

38   Okada M, Matsumori A, Ono K, Furukawa Y, Shioi T, Iwasaki A, Matsushima K, Sasayama S: Cyclic stretch upregulates production of interleukin-8 and monocyte chemotactic and activating factor/monocyte chemoattractant protein-1 in human endothelial cells. Arterioscler Thromb Vasc Biol 1998;18:894–901.

39   Fry DL: Acute vascular endothelial changes associated with increased blood velocity gradients. Circ Res 1968;22:165–192.

40   Bassiouny HS, Zarins CK, Kadowaki MH, Glagov S: Hemodynamic stress and experimental aortoiliac atherosclerosis. J Vasc Surg 1994;19:426–434.

41   Zhao S, Suciu A, Ziegler T, Moore JE Jr, Burki E, Meister JJ, Brunner HR: Synergistic effects of fluid shear stress and cyclic circumferential stretch on vascular endothelial cell morphology and cytoskeleton. Arterioscler Thromb Vasc Biol 1995;15:1781–1786.

42   Silacci P, Desgeorges A, Mazzolai L, Chambaz C, Hayoz D: Flow pulsatility is a critical determinant of oxidative stress in endothelial cells. Hypertension 2001;38:1162–1166.

43   Lin T, Zeng L, Liu Y, DeFea K, Schwartz MA, Chien S, Shyy JY: Rho-ROCK-LIMK-cofilin pathway regulates shear stress activation of sterol regulatory element binding proteins. Circ Res 2003; 92:1296–304.

44   Nerem RM, Levesque MJ, Cornhill JF: Vascular endothelial morphology as an indicator of the pattern of blood flow. J Biomech Eng 1981;103:172–176.

45   Dancu MB, Berardi DE, Vanden Heuvel JP, Tarbell JM: Asynchronous shear stress and circumferential strain reduces endothelial NO synthase and cyclooxygenase-2 but induces endothelin-1 gene expression in endothelial cells. Arterioscler Thromb Vasc Biol 2004;24:2088–2094.

46   Hojo Y, Saito Y, Tanimoto T, Hoefen RJ, Baines CP, Yamamoto K, Haendeler J, Asmis R, Berk BC: Fluid shear stress attenuates hydrogen peroxide-induced c-Jun NH2-terminal kinase activation via a glutathione reductase-mediated mechanism. Circ Res 2002;91:712–718.

47   De Keulenaer GW, Chappell DC, Ishizaka N, Nerem RM, Alexander RW, Griendling KK: Oscillatory and steady laminar shear stress differentially affect human endothelial redox state: role of a superoxide-producing NADH oxidase. Circ Res 1998;82:1094–1101.

48   Tsuda M, Iwai M, Li JM, Li HS, Min LJ, Ide A, Okumura M, Suzuki J, Mogi M, Suzuki H, Horiuchi M: Inhibitory effects of AT1 receptor blocker, olmesartan, and estrogen on atherosclerosis via anti-oxidative stress. Hypertension 2005;45:545–551.

49   Hornig B, Landmesser U, Kohler C, Ahlersmann D, Spiekermann S, Christoph A, Tatge H, Drexler H: Comparative effect of ace inhibition and angiotensin II type 1 receptor antagonism on bioavailability of nitric oxide in patients with coronary artery disease: role of superoxide dismutase. Circulation 2001;103:799–805.

50   Pizzi C, Manfrini O, Fontana F, Bugiardini R: Angiotensin-converting enzyme inhibitors and 3-hydroxy-3-methylglutaryl coenzyme A reductase in cardiac syndrome X: role of superoxide dismutase activity. Circulation 2004;109:53–58.

51   Yamawaki H, Lehoux S, Berk BC: Chronic physiological shear stress inhibits tumor necrosis factor-induced proinflammatory responses in rabbit aorta perfused ex vivo. Circulation 2003;108: 1619–1625.

52   Stewart AD, Millasseau SC, Kearney MT, Ritter JM, Chowienczyk PJ: Effects of inhibition of basal nitric oxide synthesis on carotid-femoral pulse wave velocity and augmentation index in humans. Hypertension 2003;42:915–918.

53   Ceravolo R, Maio R, Pujia A, Sciacqua A, Ventura G, Costa MC, Sesti G, Perticone F: Pulse pressure and endothelial dysfunction in never-treated hypertensive patients. J Am Coll Cardiol 2003; 41:1753–1758.

54   Ichigi Y, Takano H, Umetani K, Kawabata K, Obata JE, Kitta Y, Kodama Y, Mende A, Nakamura T, Fujioka D, Saito Y, Kugiyama K: Increased ambulatory pulse pressure is a strong risk factor for coronary endothelial vasomotor dysfunction. J Am Coll Cardiol 2005;45:1461–1466.

55 Sutton-Tyrrell K, Najjar SS, Boudreau RM, Venkitachalam L, Kupelian V, Simonsick EM, Havlik R, Lakatta EG, Spurgeon H, Kritchevsky S, Pahor M, Bauer D, Newman A, Health ABC Study: Elevated aortic pulse wave velocity, a marker of arterial stiffness, predicts cardiovascular events in well-functioning older adults. Circulation 2005;111:3384–3390.

56 Franklin SS, Gustin W 4th, Wong ND, Larson MG, Weber MA, Kannel WB, Levy D: Hemodynamic patterns of age-related changes in blood pressure. The Framingham Heart Study. Circulation 1997;96:308–315.

57 Benetos A, Adamopoulos C, Bureau JM, Temmar M, Labat C, Bean K, Thomas F, Pannier B, Asmar R, Zureik M, Safar M, Guize L: Determinants of accelerated progression of arterial stiffness in normotensive subjects and in treated hypertensive subjects over a 6-year period. Circulation 2002;105:1202–1207.

58 Blacher J, Guerin AP, Pannier B, Marchais SJ, Safar ME, London GM: Impact of aortic stiffness on survival in end-stage renal disease. Circulation 1999;99:2434–2439.

59 Shinohara K, Shoji T, Kimoto E, Yokoyama H, Fujiwara S, Hatsuda S, Maeno T, Shoji T, Fukumoto S, Emoto M, Koyama H, Nishizawa Y: Effect of atorvastatin on regional arterial stiffness in patients with type 2 diabetes mellitus. J Atheroscler Thromb 2005;12:205–210.

60 Hirose K, Tomiyama H, Okazaki R, Arai T, Koji Y, Zaydun G, Hori S, Yamashina A: Increased pulse wave velocity associated with reduced calcaneal quantitative osteo-sono index: possible relationship between atherosclerosis and osteopenia. J Clin Endocrinol Metab 2003;88:2573–2578.

61 Joki N, Hase H, Shiratake M, Kishi N, Tochigi S, Imamura Y: Calcaneal osteopenia is a new marker for arterial stiffness in chronic hemodialysis patients. Am J Nephrol 2005;25:196–202.

62 Yamada S, Inaba M, Goto H, Nagata-Sakurai M, Kumeda Y, Imanishi Y, Emoto M, Ishimura E, Nishizawa Y: Associations between physical activity, peripheral atherosclerosis and bone status in healthy Japanese women. Atherosclerosis 2006;188:196–202.

63 Grady D, Herrington D, Bittner V, Blumenthal R, Davidson M, Hlatky M, Hsia J, Hulley S, Herd A, Khan S, Newby LK, Waters D, Vittinghoff E, Wenger N, HERS Research Group: Cardiovascular disease outcomes during 6.8 years of hormone therapy: Heart and Estrogen/progestin Replacement Study follow-up (HERS II). JAMA 2002;288:49–57.

64 Bresalier RS, Sandler RS, Quan H, Bolognese JA, Oxenius B, Horgan K, Lines C, Riddell R, Morton D, Lanas A, Konstam MA, Baron JA, Adenomatous Polyp Prevention on Vioxx (APPROVe) Trial Investigators: Cardiovascular events associated with rofecoxib in a colorectal adenoma chemoprevention trial. N Engl J Med 2005;352:1092–1102.

Daniel Hayoz
Department of Medicine, Vascular Medicine, CHUV
CH–1011 Lausanne (Switzerland)
Tel. +41 21 3140 750/52, Fax +41 21 3140 761
E-Mail daniel.hayoz@chuv.hospvd.ch

Safar ME, Frohlich ED (eds): Atherosclerosis, Large Arteries and Cardiovascular Risk.
Adv Cardiol. Basel, Karger, 2007, vol 44, pp 76–95

······················

Arterial Stiffness and Extracellular Matrix

Javier Díez

Division of Cardiovascular Sciences, Centre for Applied Medical Research and
University Clinic, School of Medicine, University of Navarra, Pamplona, Spain

Abstract

The growing prevalence and associated risk of arterial stiffness provide a major challenge to better understand the underlying causes and the resultant physiological impact of this condition. Structural components within the arterial wall, mainly collagen and elastin, are considered to be major determinants of arterial stiffness. Thus, quantitative and qualitative alterations of collagen and elastin fibers are involved in arterial stiffening that is associated with the aging process and disease states such as hypertension, diabetes, atherosclerosis, and chronic renal failure. Elucidation of mechanisms leading to the above alterations will aid in more specifically targeted therapeutic interventions because currently available cardiovascular medications fall short at reducing the stiffness of the large arteries. Reduction of arterial stiffness will likely have a significant impact on morbidity and mortality of older adults, as well as subjects suffering from cardiovascular and renal diseases.

Copyright © 2007 S. Karger AG, Basel

Introduction

Increased arterial stiffness is a hallmark of the aging process and the consequence of many disease states such as hypertension, diabetes, atherosclerosis, and chronic renal failure. Accordingly, there is a marked increase in the incidence and prevalence of clinical surrogate markers of arterial stiffness, such as pulse pressure and isolated systolic hypertension, with age and these associated conditions [1–5]. Arterial stiffness is also a marker for increased

Table 1. Collagen types present in vascular tissue classified in accordance with their structural properties

Fibrillar	Sheet-forming	Fibril-associated	Microfibrillar
Type I	Type IV	Type XV	Type VI
Type III	Type VIII	Type XVIII	
Type V		Type XIX	

cardiovascular risk, including myocardial infarction, heart failure, and total mortality, as well as stroke, dementia, and renal disease [6–14].

Although arterial stiffness is a dynamic parameter, which can be modulated by changes in smooth muscle tone [15], endothelial function [16], and the vasa vasorum microcirculation network [17], it is classically recognized that structural components within the arterial wall, mainly extracellular (ECM) macromolecules, together with transmural pressure are the major determinants of arterial stiffness [18]. This chapter reviews the contribution of ECM macromolecules to arterial stiffness, including the roles of collagen, elastin, and other ECM proteins. In addition, the potential role of vascular integrins that act as a link between the ECM and the intracellular environment will also be considered.

Vascular Collagen

By definition, a collagen is a structural protein of the ECM that contains at least one domain in the characteristic triple helical conformation [19]. The triple helix is formed by three polypeptide chains (α chains). All collagen molecules are characterized by a central collagen domain composed of repeating Gly-Xaa-Yaa triplets, a high concentration of proline, alanine, and lysine residues and non-collagenous domains at their terminal ends [20, 21]. To date, 20 different collagen types have been identified [22]. Collagen types I, III, IV, V, VI, VIII, XV, XVIII, and XIX have all been detected in normal adult vascular tissue [23–27]. Based on their structural properties, these collagens can be described as fibrillar and non-fibrillar (table 1). Fibrillar collagen types I and III are the major collagens detectable in vessels, representing 60 and 30% of vascular collagens, respectively [28, 29]. These molecules contain triple helical domains of about 1,000 amino acids, highly conserved carboxy-terminal non-collagenous domains of about 250 amino acids, and variable amino-terminal non-collagenous domains of 50–520 amino acids [20] (fig. 1).

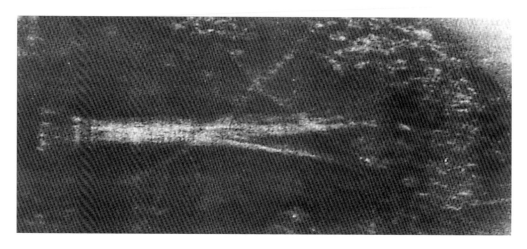

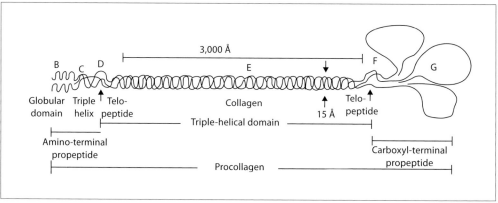

3,000 Å

B C D   E   F   G

Globular Triple Telo-   Collagen   Telo-
domain   helix   peptide   15 Å peptide

                              Triple-helical domain

Amino-terminal
propeptide   Carboxyl-terminal
                                                    propeptide

                              Procollagen

Fig. 1. Electron micrograph of segment-long-spacing aggregates of procollagen type I (top) and a model of procollagen type I molecule (bottom). B = Amino-terminal propeptide extension; C = minor triple helix of the amino-terminal protease cleavage site; D = amino-terminal telopeptide; E = triple helix; F = carboxy-terminal telopeptide; G = carboxy-terminal propeptide extension.

The regulation of collagen deposition and turnover in tissue is complex (fig. 2). Firstly, the amount of procollagen precursors secreted by the cells is controlled at the level of transcription [30] and by regulating intracellular degradation [31]. Secondly, extracellular conversion in collagen molecules and deposition are controlled by proteolytic processing and is counteracted by degradation via collagenolytic enzymes.

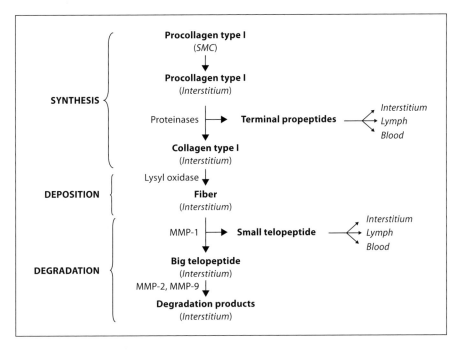

Fig. 2. Diagrammatic representation of fibrillar collagen turnover in the vascular wall. SMC = Smooth muscle cell; MMP = matrix metalloproteinase.

Synthesis and Secretion

While most of the collagens in the vascular intima and media are synthesized by smooth muscle cells (SMCs), fibroblasts are responsible for collagen synthesis in the adventitia. Contractile SMCs in the arterial media are responsible for the gross muscular changes that occur in the vessel in response to nervous and paracrine stimuli. These are quiescent cells which in the adult show little division, migration, or matrix production. SMCs are, however, phenotypically plastic and can modulate to the so-called synthetic phenotype. These cells resemble the more immature fetal or neonatal cells and are commonly found in secondary culture and in the arterial intima; they migrate, divide, and produce ECM, namely collagen. Thus, a number of chemical and physical factors influence collagen production by SMCs through their phenotypic modulation (table 2) [32].

After secretion of procollagen molecules in the extracellular compartment, the amino- and carboxy-terminal non-collagenous domains are removed by specific proteinases. The resulting collagen triple helices aggregate in quarter-staggered fibrils. Newly formed collagen fibrils are soluble in salt solutions and

Table 2. Factors influencing collagen synthesis and secretion by vascular smooth muscle cells

Stimulating factors	Inhibiting factors
Transforming growth factor-β	Basic fibroblast growth factor
Platelet-derived growth factor	Interferon-γ
Angiotensin II	Tumor necrosis factor-α
Periodic stretching	Prostaglandin E_2
Insulin?	Cell-matrix contact
Aldosterone?	Nitric oxide?

dilute acid, and have no tensile strength. During the formation of intermolecular cross-linking, collagen fibers become increasingly insoluble, more refractory to the action of enzymes and show a progressive increase in tensile strength. The cross-linking process is initiated by the enzyme lysyl oxidase, through the oxidation of specific lysine or hydroxylysine residues in the telopeptide regions. The resulting aldehydes undergo a series of reactions with adjacent reactive residues to give both inter- and intramolecular cross-links [33].

Degradation and Turnover

The metabolic turnover of mature collagen in adult animals is relatively slow [34]. Although only small amounts of these proteins are degraded normally, increased degradation and fragmentation of collagen fibers are observed in vascular diseases. Collagenolytic enzymes are found in a number of mammalian cells and tissues including polymorphonuclear neutrophils and monocytes/macrophages. Collagenolytic enzymes are mainly matrix metalloproteinases (MMPs) and have been described extensively in previous reviews [35, 36]. Vascular MMPs include collagenases (MMP-1 and MMP-8), gelatinases (MMP-2 and MMP-9), elastases (MMP-7 and MMP-12), stromelysins (MMP-3) and membrane-type metalloproteinases (MT1-MMP) (table 3). The substrate specificity differs for the various MMPs present in the vascular wall. Whereas MMP-1 degrades collagen types I and III, gelatinases act on gelatin and collagen type IV, and MMP-3 degrades proteoglycans, fibronectin, and laminin [37].

The proteolytic activity of each MMP is tightly regulated at three levels: first, gene expression and protein secretion levels; second, activation of the inactive pro-enzyme, and, third, inhibition by the tissue inhibitors of MMPs (TIMPs) or other inhibitors (α_2-macroglobulin). The activation of secreted pro-MMPs requires the disruption of the Cys-Zn^{2+} (cysteine switch) interaction and the removal of the propeptide. In vivo, pro-MMPs are activated

Table 3. Metalloproteinases active on extracellular macromolecules present within the vascular wall and cellular origin

Detectable in vascular cells	Detectable in inflammatory cells
MMP-1 (ECs)[1]	MMP-1 (monocytes)
MMP-2 (ECs, SMCs, fibroblasts)	MMP-2 (macrophages, PMNs)
MMP-3 (SMCs) [1]	MMP-7 (monocytes)
MMP-7 (SMCs)	MMP-8 (PMNs)
MMP-9 (ECs, SMCs, fibroblasts) [1]	MMP-9 (macrophages, PMNs)
MT1-MMP (SMCs)	MMP-12 (macrophages)
	MT1-MMP (macrophages)

[1] Enzymes not expressed in basal conditions.
MMP = Matrix metalloproteinase; MT-MMP = membrane-type MMP; ECs = endothelial cells; PMNs = polymorphonuclear neutrophils; SMCs = smooth muscle cells.

by tissue or plasma proteinases – plasmin, thrombin, other MMPs or MT-MMPs – and reactive oxygen species. The activation of MMPs and their inhibition by TIMPs are the main regulatory mechanisms of MMP activities in the vascular wall [35, 36]. The very well controlled balance between active proteinases and inhibitors is perturbed during pathological processes, particularly when polymorphonuclear neutrophils or macrophages are present. However, through their capacity to synthesize enzyme inhibitors, SMCs have an extremely high capacity to respond to these increased enzyme levels.

Functions in the Vascular Wall

The biomechanical properties of vessels, particularly of the major arteries, are largely dependent on the absolute and relative quantities of fibrillar collagens (and elastin) [38]. Collagen fibers run longitudinally in the intima and adventitia, and run spirally between muscle layers in the media [39]. These fibers are often crimped or 'wavy' in order to both allow and resist distension of the vessel [40]. The larger diameter type I fibers are believed to confer high tensile strength while the thinner, type III fibers are associated with increased tissue flexibility [41]. Molecules of fibrillar collagen type V can either form fine type V filaments or can copolymerize with type I and III molecules in larger fibers. It is believed that inclusion of type V molecules may regulate assembly and structure of the vascular collagen fiber network [42].

Vascular collagens may also interact with SMCs resulting in changes of their phenotype and activity. In fact, type I collagen promotes change to the synthetic phenotypic while type IV collagen inhibits, or even reverses, this change [43, 44]. In addition, interactions with the surrounding collagen matrix may control collagen production in phenotypically modified SMCs by posttranslational mechanisms. For instance, SMCs grown inside type I collagen lattices, unlike cells grown on plastic, do not dramatically increase fibrillar collagen secretion in response to serum and growth factors [45]. Serum increases transcription and translation of collagen mRNA in lattice cells, but intracellular degradation of the newly translated collagen prevents it from being secreted [46].

Finally, the possibility exists that collagen and other ECM molecules participate in the regulation of vascular tone. Recently, Davis et al. [47] defined matricryptic sites as biologically active sites that are not exposed in the mature secreted form of ECM molecules, but which become exposed following conformational or structural changes in these molecules (e.g., the Arg-Gly-Asp peptide or RGD sequence). The same authors hypothesized that exposure of matricryptic sites in altered ECM molecules is a critical component of a coordinated vascular response to tissue injury. In support of this notion, they showed that proteolytic fragments of collagen type I (which contain the RGD sequence) induce vasoconstriction [48, 49]. Furthermore, it has been shown that these molecules induce integrin-dependent vasoconstrictor effects that are regulated through calcium signaling and which are mediated in some cases by the L-type calcium channel of SMCs [48].

Vascular Elastin and Other ECM Molecules

Elastin is the most abundant protein of the large arteries that are subjected to a large pulsatile pressure generated by cardiac contraction [50–52]. However, elastin is also detectable in resistance arteries – mainly in the internal and external elastic lamina – and veins. Elastin represents 90% of the elastic fibers, the other constituents being microfibrillar glycoproteins such as fibrillins and microfibrillar-associated glycoproteins [53–55]. The precursor of elastin, tropoelastin, is a highly hydrophobic protein which is soluble in salt solution like the collagen triple helix. In contrast, elastin is an insoluble protein. This insolubility results from the cross-linking process between lysine residues. Cross-linking of tropoelastin molecules begins with the oxidative deamination of some lysine residues by lysyl oxidase, as previously described for collagen cross-linking. The spontaneous condensation reaction between four lysine/allysine residues leads to the formation of the specific cross-links for elastin, desmosine and isodesmosine. Cross-links resulting from the condensation of two or three lysine/allysine residues are also detectable in elastin [33]. This cross-linking process confers to elastin its function, i.e. elasticity, essential in large arteries which distend during systole and recoil during diastole. Another property of elastin has been recently demonstrated by the study of patients suffering from supravalvular aortic stenosis and of knockout mice for elastin: elastin controls, directly or indirectly, the proliferation and phenotype of SMCs [56–58].

Other structural glycoproteins play an essential role in the structure and function of the ECM in the arterial wall, including fibronectin, vitronectin, laminin, entactin/nidogen, tenascin and thrombospondin. These glycoproteins have a multidomain structure, potentially enabling simultaneous interactions between cells and other ECM components [59, 60].

The proteoglycans contained in the vascular wall are the large aggregating proteoglycans aggrecan and versican, the small non-aggregating interstitial proteoglycans biglycan, decorin and fibromodulin and the cell-associated proteoglycans syndecan, fibroglycan and glypican. Proteoglycans are proteins that have one or more attached glycosaminoglycan chains [61, 62]. They contain distinct protein and carbohydrate domain structures, which interact with other ECM molecules. They participate in ECM assembly and confer specific properties to the tissues (hydration, filtration, etc.). Proteoglycans also regulate various cellular activities (proliferation, differentiation, adhesion, migration) and control cytokine biodisponibility and stability (basic fibroblast growth factor, transforming growth factor-β or TGF-β, etc.) [63].

Vascular Integrins

Integrins are a large family of cell surface receptors that provide for adhesion of cells to both the ECM and neighboring cells. In addition, integrins act as a membrane coupling and assembly point for a growing list of cytoskeletal and cell signaling components. Of the approximately 24 known integrins, 16 have been reported to have involvement in some aspect of vascular biology (table 4), including the processes involved in the synthesis, degradation, and structural modification of the ECM [64].

As early as 1976, Leung et al. [65] had shown that SMCs grown on elastic sheets and stimulated by cyclic strain upregulate their synthesis of collagen I and III. Integrins are the best candidates for being the mechanosensors capable of detecting changes in stress and strain. In addition to their role in regulating ECM production, integrins also participate in controlling the production of several MMPs. Type VIII collagen binding of $\alpha_1\beta_1$ and $\alpha_2\beta_1$ integrins stimulates MMP-2 and MMP-9 expression and activity in SMCs [66], while osteopontin and tenascin-C do so through ligation of the $\alpha_v\beta_3$ integrin [67, 68].

Table 4. Integrin heterodimers present in vascular cells

Endothelial cells	Smooth muscle cells
$\alpha_1\beta_1$	$\alpha_1\beta_1$
$\alpha_2\beta_1$	$\alpha_2\beta_1$
$\alpha_3\beta_1$	$\alpha_3\beta_1$
$\alpha_5\beta_1$	$\alpha_4\beta_1$
$\alpha_6\beta_1$	$\alpha_5\beta_1$
$\alpha_6\beta_4$	$\alpha_6\beta_1$
$\alpha_V\beta_3$	$\alpha_7\beta_1$
$\alpha_V\beta_5$	$\alpha_8\beta_1$
	$\alpha_9\beta_1$
	$\alpha_V\beta_1$
	$\alpha_V\beta_3$
	$\alpha_V\beta_5$
	$\alpha_6\beta_4$

SMCs transformation from a contractile to a synthetic/proliferative phenotype is, in part, modulated by integrin $\alpha_5\beta_1$ [69]. Interestingly, integrins $\alpha_1\beta_1$, $\alpha_2\beta_1$, and $\alpha_V\beta_3$ are upregulated during the phenotypic transformation [70–72]. As mentioned before, contact with the surrounding collagen matrix may control ECM production in phenotypically modified SMCs. In this regard, cell adhesion studies in SMCs indicate that the $\alpha_1\beta_1$ and $\alpha_2\beta_1$ integrins may be the dominant receptors for triple helical domains in collagen types I and III [73, 74].

Integrins have been also implicated in the conformational and structural rearrangement of ECM proteins. ECM proteins synthesized and secreted by cells of the vascular wall need to be in an ordered arrangement for best performing their structural support role. Recent evidence suggests that integrins may be, in part, responsible for this process. For example, experiments carried on in primary human foreskin fibroblasts show that soluble fibronectin molecules are converted into elaborate fibrillar matrices in a process that requires the participation of integrins [75]. Soluble fibronectin molecules bind $\alpha_5\beta_1$ integrins in complex cellular contacts that run parallel to actin bundles of the cytoskeleton. Once ligated to $\alpha_5\beta_1$, fibronectin can be actively translocated along stress fibers.

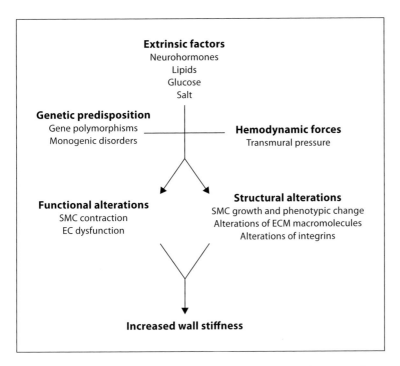

Fig. 3. Schematic view of the multiple causes and mechanisms of arterial stiffness. SMC = Smooth muscle cell; EC = endothelial cell; ECM = extracellular matrix.

ECM Molecules, Integrins and Arterial Stiffness

Arterial stiffening develops from a complex process of interactions between stable and dynamic factors determining structural and functional changes of the vessel wall (fig. 3). This process is influenced by hemodynamic forces [76] as well as by genetic determinants [77] and extrinsic factors such as vasoactive substances, hormones, salt, lipids and glucose regulation [78] (fig. 3).

The structural changes involved in arterial stiffness include cellular changes (i.e., SMC hypertrophy and/or hyperplasia), and non-cellular changes (i.e., increased collagen deposition, reduction in the elastin/collagen ratio, alterations in the organization of collagen and elastin fibers, and alteration in the glycosaminoglycan contents and metabolism) [76]. These changes are not uniformly disseminated throughout the vascular tree but are often patchy [79–81] occurring in central and conduit arteries while sparing more peripheral arteries [82, 83]. On the other hand, since SMC and ECM volume in large ar-

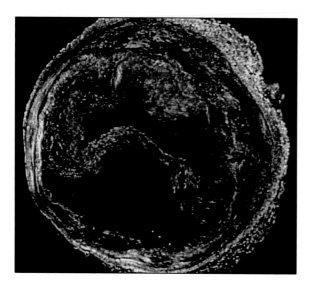

Fig. 4. Section of a human aorta stained with sirius red and photographed under polarized light. Whereas deposition of collagen type I fibers (red/yellow) is predominantly seen within the intima, collagen type III fibers (green) are mostly accumulated in the media and the adventitia.

teries is roughly 50–50%, whereas in resistance arteries more than 70% of the tissue volume is occupied by SMC, cellular changes are likely to have more impact on stiffness of resistance arteries [76]. In contrast, stiffness of large arteries is more likely influenced by non-cellular changes [76].

On gross pathologic vascular specimens, structural changes related to arterial stiffness manifest as a doubling to tripling of intima-medial thickness between ages 20 and 90 [84, 85]. Histological examination of the intima of stiffened vessels reveals abnormal and disarrayed endothelial cells, increased collagen (fig. 4), frayed and broken elastin molecules, infiltration of SMCs, macrophages and mononuclear cells, and increased MMPs, cell adhesion molecules and cytokines, namely TGF-β [86].

Role of ECM Macromolecules

In order to explain the respective role of collagen and elastin on the stiffness of the vessel wall, Burton [87] assessed the Young's modulus (wall tension per centimeter wall thickness for 100% diameter increase) of isolated elastic and collagen tissues and showed that the latter made the major contribution to the stiffness of the vessel wall. These data were expanded in the experiments of Dobrin et al. [88] in which human isolated arterial vessels were studied in the presence of elastase and collagenase. With elastase, the pressure-volume relationship of the arterial vessel was shifted towards higher values of arterial diameter and volume, indicating that the loss of elastin greatly influenced the geometry of the vessel without changing its mechanical properties (i.e. the slope of the curve). On the other hand, with collagenase the slope of the curve increased greatly, indicating a decreased stiffness of the vessel wall, without substantial change in its geometry.

The relative content of ECM macromolecules is normally held stable by a slow, but dynamic, process of production and degradation. Dysregulation of this balance, mainly by stimulation of an inflammatory milieu, leads to over-production of abnormal collagen and diminished quantities of normal elastin, which contribute to vascular stiffness [89]. Increased luminal pressure, or hypertension, also stimulates excessive collagen production and facilitates disruption and fracture of elastin [90]. In addition, several neurohumoral factors, particularly those related to the renin-angiotensin-aldosterone system, may induce collagen accumulation and reduce elastin deposition, thus leading to increased arterial stiffness [91–93]. In this regard, it is of interest to mention that some studies have shown positive associations between aortic stiffness and polymorphisms of genes encoding for angiotensinogen [94], angiotensin-converting enzyme [95, 96], the angiotensin II type 1 receptor [95, 97], and the aldosterone synthase [98].

Collagen molecules provide the tensile strength of the vessel wall and are enzymatically cross-linked soon after their formation to render them insoluble to hydrolytic enzymes [99]. Breaks in the integrity of these intermolecular bonds cause unraveling of the collagen matrix. Moreover, because of their slow hydrolytic turnover rate, collagen is particularly susceptible to non-enzymatic glycation cross-linking. This leads to increased collagen content, often with a more unorganized and dysfunctional fiber distribution resulting in increased stiffness. Elastin molecules are also stabilized by cross-linking to form desmosine and isodesmosine. Disruption of these cross-links contributes to weakening of the elastin array with predisposition to mineralization by calcium and phosphorous, together increasing arterial stiffness [100–102]. In addition, activation of various serine proteases and MMPs generate broken and frayed elastin molecules [103]. In this regard, it has been reported recently that aortic stiffness is related to serum MMP-9 levels and serum elastase activity in patients with isolated systolic hypertension and apparently healthy individuals [104]. Furthermore, it has been reported that aortic stiffness is greater in aged subjects homozygous for the 5A promoter polymorphism of MMP-3 than aged subjects homozygous for the 6A promoter polymorphism [105]. Interestingly, both MMP-3 gene and protein expression were higher in 6A subjects than in 5A subjects [105].

Arterial stiffness is also caused by advanced glycation end products (AGEs), which result from non-enzymatic protein glycation to form irreversible cross-links between long-lived proteins such as collagen [106, 107]. AGE-linked collagen is stiffer and less susceptible to hydrolytic turnover. This results in an accumulation of structurally inadequate collagen molecules [108]. Similarly, elastin molecules are susceptible to AGE cross-linking reducing the elasticity of the wall [109, 110].

Increased deposition of chondroitin sulfate, heparin sulfate, proteoglycans, and fibronectin can also contribute to stiffening of the arterial wall [111]. Of interest, recent studies by Et-Taouil et al. [112], performed in spontaneously hypertensive rats, indicate that the aortic wall glycosaminoglycans contents play a more important role than the collagen and elastin contents, in terms of wall rigidity or compliance.

Potential Role of Integrins

In addition to changes in ECM protein components, alterations in vascular expression of integrins have been reported in clinical conditions that are associated with increased arterial stiffness (i.e., diabetes and hypertension) [113–116]. Recently, Durier et al. [117] determined the expression profiles of the human aorta and identified several genes that were differently expressed between patients with increased aortic stiffness and patients with distensible aorta. In particular, integrins α_{2b}, α_6, β_3, and β_5 transcript levels were different between stiff and distensible aortas. The α_{2b} and α_6 integrin transcripts were present in all samples from stiff aortas, and absent in all samples from distensible aortas. Integrin α_6 forms heterodimers with β_1 or a β_4 integrin subunit, binds to laminin, and plays a role in the regulation of SMC phenotype [118]. The β_5 integrin transcript was less abundant in stiff aortas than in distensible aortas. The β_5 subunit of the integrin receptor, generally coupled with the α_V subunit, forms a heterodimer involved in cell adhesion to vitronectin and osteopontin [118]. It has been shown that osteopontin interacts with collagen and fibronectin, which suggests a possible role in ECM organization and stability [119, 120].

On the other hand, the possibility exists that collagen glycation affects integrin binding sequences through alterations in protein structure, possibly by either exposing or making less accessible integrin binding sites. For instance, it has been shown that modification of RGD sequences in collagen by AGEs inhibits cell-matrix interactions, most likely via the loss of specific residues involved in integrin-mediated cell attachment [121]. Therefore, to determine the exact role of integrins in arterial stiffness, there is a need for studies involving use of specific anti-integrin agents and of transgenic animal models.

Conclusions and Perspectives

Arterial stiffness is an important, independent predictor of cardiovascular risk. Alterations in structural components within the arterial wall, namely ECM macromolecules, are major determinants of increased arterial stiffness. Importantly, direct pharmacological manipulation of ECM macromolecules seems to be possible and therapeutic strategies that specifically target collagen and elastin in large arteries to reduce stiffness may be helpful, particularly in those individuals with increased arterial stiffening. For instance, recent data suggest that a thialozium derivative (ALT-711), which breaks down established AGE cross-links between collagen and elastin proteins, can reduce arterial stiffness in diabetic rats [122], older monkeys [123] and older humans with increased arterial stiffness [124]. The time has come to perform therapeutic trials designed to test whether an improvement in morbidity and mortality is produced on the basis of influencing arterial stiffness in elderly people and patients suffering from cardiovascular diseases and/or chronic renal failure [125].

References

1   Chobanian AV, Bakris GL, Black HR, Cushman WC, Green LA, Izzo JL Jr, Jones DW, Materson BJ, Oparil S, Wright JT Jr, Roccella EJ: The Seventh Report of the Joint National Committee on Prevention, Detection, Evaluation, and Treatment of High Blood Pressure: the JNC 7 report. JAMA 2003;289:2560–2572.

2   Scuteri A, Najjar SS, Muller DC, Andres R, Hougaku H, Metter EJ, Lakatta EG: Metabolic syndrome amplifies the age-associated increases in vascular thickness and stiffness. J Am Coll Cardiol 2004;43:1388–1395.

3   Dart A, Kingwell B: Pulse pressure – a review of mechanisms and clinical relevance. J Am Coll Cardiol 2001;37:975–984.

4   Lakatta EG, Levy D: Arterial and cardiac aging: major shareholders in cardiovascular disease enterprises. I. Aging arteries: a 'set up' for vascular disease. Circulation 2003;107:139–146.

5   Collins AJ, Li S, Gilbertson DT, Liu J, Chen SC, Herzog CA: Chronic kidney disease and cardiovascular disease in the Medicare population. Kidney Int 2003;64(suppl 87):S24–S31.

6   Chae CU, Pfeffer MA, Glynn RJ, Mitchell GF, Taylor JO, Hennekens CH: Increased pulse pressure and risk of heart failure in the elderly. JAMA 1999;281:634–639.

7   Franklin SS, Larson MG, Khan SA, Wong ND, Leip FP, Kannel WB, Levy D: Does the relation of blood pressure to coronary heart disease risk change with aging? The Framingham Heart Study. Circulation 2001;103:1245–1249.

8   Mitchell GF, Pfeffer MA, Braunwald E, Rouleau JL, Bernstein V, Geltman EM, Flaker GC: Sphygmomanometrically determined pulse pressure is a powerful independent predictor of recurrent events after myocardial infarction in patients with impaired left ventricular function. Circulation 1997;96:4254–4260.

9   Vaccarino V, Berger A, Abramson J, Black H, Setaro J, Davey J, Krumholz H: Pulse pressure and risk of cardiovascular events in the systolic hypertension in the elderly program. Am J Cardiol 2001;88:980–986.

10   Kostis J, Lawrence-Nelson J, Ranjan R, Wilson A, Kostis W, Lacy C: Association of increased pulse pressure with the development of heart failure in SHEP. Systolic Hypertension in the Elderly (SHEP) Cooperative Research Group. Am J Hypertens 2001;14:798–803.

11   Blacher J, Guerin AP, Pannier B, Marchais SJ, Safar ME, London GM: Impact of aortic stiffness on survival in end-stage renal disease. Circulation 1999;99:2434–2439.

12   Forette F, Seux ML, Staessen JA, Thijs L, Birkenhager WH, Babarskiene MR, Babeanu S, Bossini A, Gil-Extremera B, Girerd X, Laks T, Lilov E, Moisseyev V, Tuomilehto J, Vanhanen H, Webster J, Yodfat Y, Fagard R: Prevention of dementia in randomised double-blind placebo-controlled Systolic Hypertension in Europe (Syst-Eur) trial. Lancet 1998;352:1347–1351.

13   Benetos A, Safar M, Rudnichi A, Smulyan H, Richard JL, Ducimetière P, Guize L: Pulse pressure: a predictor of long-term cardiovascular mortality in a French male population. Hypertension 1997;30:1410–1415.

14   Cohn JN, Quyyumi AA, Hollenberg NK, Jamerson KA: Surrogate markers for cardiovascular disease. Functional markers. Circulation 2004;109(suppl IV):IV-31–IV-46.

15   Gow BS: The influence of vascular smooth muscle on the viscoelastic properties of blood vessels; in Bergel DH (ed): Cardiovascular Fluid Dynamics. London, Academic Press, 1972, pp 66–97.

16   Wilkinson IB, McEniery CM: Arterial stiffness, endothelial function and novel pharmacological approaches. Clin Exp Pharmacol Physiol 2004;31:795–799.

17   Angouras D, Sokoli DP, Dosios T, Kostomitsopoulos N, Boudoulas H, Skalkeas G, Karayannacos PE: Effect of impaired vasa vasorum flow on the structure and mechanics of the thoracic aorta: implications for the pathogenesis of aortic dissection. Eur J Cardiothoracic Surg 2000;17:468–473.

18   Glagov S: Hemodynamic risk factors: mechanical stress, mural architecture, medial nutrition and vulnerability of arteries to atherosclerosis; in Wissler RW, Geer JC (eds): The Pathogenesis of Atherosclerosis. Baltimore, Williams & Wilkins, 1972, pp 164–199.

19   Van der Rest M, Bruckner P: Collagens: diversity at the molecular and supramolecular levels. Curr Opin Struct Biol 1993;3:430–436.

20   Vuorio E, De Crombugghe B: The family of collagen genes. Annu Rev Biochem 1990;59:837–872.

21   Van der Rest M, Garrone R: Collagen family of proteins. FASEB J 1991;5:2814–2823.

22   Koch M, Foley JE, Hahn R, Zhou P, Burgeson RE, Gerecke DR, Gordon MK: Alpha 1 (XX) collagen, a new member of the collagen subfamily, fibril-associated collagens with interrupted triple helices. J Biol Chem 2001;276:23120–23126.

23   Katsuda S, Okada Y, Minamoto T, Oda Y, Matsui Y, Nakanishi I: Collagens in human atherosclerosis. Immunohistochemical analysis using collagen type-specific antibodies. Arterioscler Thromb 1992;12:494–502.

24   Kittleberger R Davis PF, Flynn DW, Greenhill NS: Distribution of type VIII collagen in tissues: an immunohistochemical study. Connect Tissue Res 1990;24:303–318.

25   Myers JC, Dion AS, Abraham V, Amenta PS: Type XV collagen exhibits a widespread distribution in human tissues but a distinct localisation in basement membrane zones. Cell Tissue Res 1996;286:493–505.

26   Autio-Harmainen H, Pihlajaniemi T: The short and long forms of type XVIII collagen show clear tissue specificities in their expression and location in basement membrane zones in humans. Am J Pathol 1998;153:611–626.

27   Myers JC, Li D, Bageris A, Abraham V, Dion AS, Amenta PS: Biochemical and immunohistochemical characterization of human type XIX defines a novel class of basement membrane zone collagens. Am J Pathol 1997;151:1729–1740.

28   Prockop DJ, Kivirikko KI: Collagens: molecular biology, diseases, and potentials for therapy. Annu Rev Biochem 1995;64:403–434.

29   Mayne R. Collagenous proteins of blood vessels. Arteriosclerosis 1986;6:585–593.

30   Slack JL, Liska DJ, Bornstein P: Regulation of expression of type I collagen genes. Am J Med Genet 1993;45:140–151.

31   Laurent J: Dynamic state of collagen: pathways of collagen degradation in vivo and their possible role in regulation of collagen mass. Am J Physiol 1987;252:C1–C9.

32   Fitzsimmons CM, Shanahan CM: Vascular extracellular matrix; in Lanzer P, Topol EJ (eds): Panvascular Medicine. Berlin, Springer, 2002, pp 217–231.

33   Reiser K, McCormick RJ, Rucker RB: Enzymatic and nonenzymatic cross-linking of collagen and elastin. FASEB J 1992;6:2439–2449.

34 Shapiro SD, Endicott SK, Province MA, Pierce JA, Campbell EJ: Marked longevity of human lung parenchymal elastic fibers deduced from prevalence of D-aspartate and nuclear weapons-related radiocarbon. J Clin Invest 1991;87:1828–1834.

35 Bode W, Maskos K: Structural basis of matrix metalloproteinases and their physiological inhibitors, the tissue inhibitors of metalloproteinases. Biol Chem 2003;384:863–872.

36 Visse R, Nagase H: Matrix metalloproteinases and tissue inhibitors of metalloproteinases. Structure, function, and biochemistry. Circ Res 2003;92:827–839.

37 Palombo D, Maione M, Cifiello BI, Udini M, Maggio D, Lupo M: Matrix metalloproteinases. Their role in degenerative chronic diseases of abdominal aorta. J Cardiovasc Surg 1999;40:257–260.

38 Robins SP, Farquharson C: Connective tissue components of the blood vessel wall in health and disease; in Stehbens WE, Lie JT (eds): Vascular Pathology. London, Chapman & Hall Medical, 1995, pp 89–127.

39 Clarke JM, Glagov S: Transmural organisation of the arterial media. Atherosclerosis 1985;5:19–34.

40 Wolinsky H, Glagov S: Structural basis for the static mechanical properties of the aortic media. Circ Res 1967;20:99–111.

41 Barnes MJ, Farndale RW: Collagens in atherosclerosis. Exp Gerontol 1999;34:513–525.

42 Birk DE, Fitch JM, Babiarz J, Linsenmayer TF: Collagen type I and V are present in the same fibril in the avian corneal stroma. J Cell Biol 1988;106:999–1008.

43 Yamamoto M, Yamamoto K, Noumura T: Type I collagen promotes modulation of cultured rabbit arterial smooth muscle cells from a contractile to a synthetic phenotype. Exp Cell Res 1993;204:121–129.

44 Hirose M, Kosugi H, Nakazato K, Hayashi T: Restoration to a quiescent and contractile phenotype from a proliferative phenotype of myofibroblast-like human aortic smooth muscle cells by culture on type IV collagen gels. J Biochem 1999;125:991–1000.

45 Thie M, Harrach B, Schoenherr E, Kresse H, Robenek H, Rauterberg J: Responsiveness of aortic smooth muscle cells to soluble growth mediators is influenced by cell-matrix contact. Arterioscler Thromb 1993;13:994–1004.

46 Redecker-Beuke B, Thie M, Rauterberg J, Robenek H: Aortic smooth muscle cells in a three-dimensional collagen lattice culture. Evidence for posttranslational regulation of collagen synthesis. Arterioscler Thromb 1993;11:1572–1579.

47 Davis GE, Bayless KJ, Davis MJ, Meininger GA: Regulation of tissue injury responses by the exposure of matricryptic sites within extracellular matrix molecules. Am J Pathol 2000;156:1489–1498.

48 Mogford JE, Davies GE, Meininger GA: RGDN peptide interaction with endothelial $\alpha_5\beta_1$ integrin causes sustained endothelin-dependent vasoconstriction of rat skeletal muscle arterioles. J Clin Invest 1997;100:1647–1653.

49 Waitkus-Edwards KR, Martínez-Lemus LA, Wu X, Trzeciakowski JP, Davis MJ, Davis GE, Maininger GA: $\alpha_4\beta_1$ integrin activation of L-type calcium channels in vascular smooth muscle causes arteriole vasoconstriction. Circ Res 2002;90:473–480.

50 Jacob MP: Élastine: préparation, caractérisation, structure, biosynthèse et catabolisme. C R Soc Biol 1993;187:166–180.

51 Rosenbloom J, Abrams WR, Mecham R: Extracellular matrix. 4. The elastic fiber. FASEB J 1993;7:1208–1218.

52 Debelle L, Tamburro AM: Elastin: molecular description and function. Int J Biochem Cell Biol 1999;31:261–272.

53 Handford PA, Downing AK, Reinhardt DP, Sakai LY: Fibrillin: from domain structure to supramolecular assembly. Matrix Biol 2000;1:457–470.

54 Sherratt MJ, Wess TJ, Baldock C, Ashworth J, Purslow PP, Shuttleworth CA, Kielty CM: Fibrillin-rich microfibrils of the extracellular matrix: ultrastructure and assembly. Micron 2001;32:185–200.

55 Gibson MA, Hatzinikolas G, Kumaratilake JS, Sandberg LB, Nicholl JK, Sutherland GR, Cleary EG: Further characterization of proteins associated with elastic fiber microfibrils including the molecular cloning of MAGP-2 (MP25). J Biol Chem 1996;271:1096–1103.

56 Li DY, Brooke B, Davis EC, Mecham RP, Sorensen LK, Boak BB, Eichwald E, Keating MT: Elastin is an essential determinant of arterial morphogenesis. Nature 1998;393:276–280.

57 Li DY, Faury G, Taylor DG, Davis EC, Boyle WA, Mecham RP, Stenzel P, Boak B, Keating MT: Novel arterial pathology in mice and humans hemizygous for elastin. J Clin Invest 1998;102: 1783–1787.

58 Milewicz DM, Urban Z, Boyd C: Genetic disorders of the elastic fiber system. Matrix Biol 2000; 19:4714–4780.

59 Chothia C, Jones EY: The molecular structure of cell adhesion molecules. Annu Rev Biochem 1997;66:823–862.

60 Labat-Robert J: Cell-matrix interactions, alterations with aging, involvement in agiogenesis. Pathol Biol 1998;46:527–533.

61 Iozzo RV: Matrix proteoglycans: from molecular design to cellular function. Annu Rev Biochem 1998;67:609–652.

62 Praillet C, Grimaud JA, Lortat-Jacob H: Les protéoglycannes. I. Molécules aux multiples fonctions… futures molécules thérapeutiques? M/S 1998;14:412–420.

63 Praillet C, Lortat-Jacob H, Grimaud JA: Les protéoglycannes. II. Rôles en pathologie. M/S 1998; 14:421–428.

64 Martínez-Lemus LA, Wu X, Wilson E, Hill MA, Davis GE, Davis MJ, Meininger GA: Integrins as unique receptors for vascular control. J Vasc Res 2003;40:211–223.

65 Leung DY, Glagov S, Mathews MB: Cyclic stretching stimulates synthesis of matrix components by arterial smooth muscle cells in vitro. Science 1976;191:475–477.

66 Hou G, Mulholland D, Gronska MA, Bendeck MP: Type VIII collagen stimulates smooth muscle cell migration and matrix metalloproteinase synthesis after arterial injury. Am J Pathol 2000; 156:467–476.

67 Bendeck MP, Irvin C, Reidy M, Smith L, Mulholland D, Horton M, Giachelli CM: Smooth muscle cell matrix metalloproteinase production is stimulated via $\alpha_v\beta_3$ integrin. Arterioscler Thromb Vasc Biol 2000;20:1467–1472.

68 Jian B, Jones PL, Li Q, Mohler ER 3rd, Shoen FJ, Levy RJ: Matrix metalloproteinase-2 is associated with tenascin-C in calcific aortic stenosis. Am J Pathol 2001;159:321–327.

69 Pankov R, Cukierman E, Katz BZ, Matsumoto K, Lin DC, Lin S, Hahn C, Yamada KM: Integrin dynamics and matrix assembly: tensin-dependent translocation of $\alpha_5\beta_1$ integrins promotes early fibronectin fibrillogenesis. J Cell Biol 2000;148:1075–1090.

70 Barillari G, Albonici L, Incerpi S, Bogetto L, Pistritto G, Volpi A, Ensoli B, Manzari V: Inflammatory cytokines stimulate vascular smooth muscle cells locomotion and growth by enhancing $\alpha_5\beta_1$ integrin expression and function. Atherosclerosis 2001;154:377–385.

71 Byzova TV, Rabbani R, D'Souza SE, Plow EF: Role of integrin $\alpha_v\beta_3$ in vascular biology. Thromb Haemost 1998;80:726–734.

72 Doi M, Shichiri M, Yoshida M, Marumo F, Hirata Y: Suppression of integrin α_v expression by endothelin-1 in vascular smooth muscle cells. Hypertens Res 2000;23:643–649.

73 Wayner EA, Carter WG: Identification of multiple cell adhesion receptors for collagen and fibronectin in human fibrosarcoma cells possessing unique α- and common β-subunits. J Cell Biol 1987;105:1873–1884.

74 Gullberg D, Gehlsen KR, Turner DC, Ahlen K, Zijenah LS, Barnes MJ, Rubin K: Analysis of $\alpha_1\beta_1$, $\alpha_2\beta_1$ and $\alpha_3\beta_1$ integrins in cell-collagen interactions: identification of conformation dependent $\alpha_1\beta_1$ binding sites in collagen type I. EMBO J 1992;11:3865–3873.

75 Pankov R, Cukierman E, Katz BZ, Matsumoto K, Lin DC, Lin S, Hahn C, Yamada KM: Integrin dynamics and matrix assembly: tensin-dependent translocation of $\alpha_5\beta_1$ integrins promotes early fibronectin fibrillogenesis. J Cell Biol 2000;148:1075–1090.

76 Et-Taouil K, Safar M, Plante GE: Mechanisms and consequences of large artery rigidity. Can J Physiol Pharmacol 2003;81:205–211.

77 Laurent A, Boutouyrie P, Lacolley P: Structural and genetic bases of arterial stiffness. Hypertension 2005;45:1050–1055.

78 Zieman SJ; Melenovsky V, Kass DA: Mechanisms, pathophysiology, and therapy of arterial stiffness. Arterioscler Thromb Vasc Biol 2005;25:932–943.

79 Galis ZS, Khatri JJ: Matrix metalloproteinases in vascular remodeling and atherogenesis: the good, the bad, and the ugly. Circ Res 2002;90:251–262.

80 Beattie D, Xu C, Vito R, Glagov S, Whang MC: Mechanical analysis of heterogeneous, atherosclerotic human aorta. J Biomech Eng 1998;120:602–607.

81 Bassiouny HS, Zarins CK, Kadowaki MH, Glagov S: Hemodynamic stress and experimental aortoiliac atherosclerosis. J Vasc Surg 1994;19:426–434.

82 Benetos A, Laurent S, Hoeks AP, Boutouyrie PH, Safar ME: Arterial alterations with aging and high blood pressure. A noninvasive study of carotid and femoral arteries. Arterioscler Thromb 1993;13:90–97.

83 Gillessen T, Gillessen F, Sieberth H, Hanrath P, Heintz B: Age-related changes in the elastic properties of the aortic tree in normotensive patients: investigation by intravascular ultrasound. Eur J Med Res 1995;1:144–148.

84 Nagai Y, Metter EJ, Earley CJ, Kemper MK, Becker LC, Lakatta EG, Fleg JL: Increased carotid artery intimal-medial thickness in asymptomatic older subjects with exercise-induced myocardial ischemia. Circulation 1998;98:1504–1509.

85 O'Leary DH, Polak JF, Kronmal RA, Manolio TA, Burke GL, Wolfson SK Jr: Carotid-artery intima and media thickness as a risk factor for myocardial infarction and stroke in older adults. Cardiovascular Health Study Collaborative Research Group. N Engl J Med 1999;340:14–22.

86 Lakatta EG: Arterial and cardiac aging: major shareholders in cardiovascular disease enterprises. III. Cellular and molecular clues to heart and arterial aging. Circulation 2003;107:490–497.

87 Burton AC: Relation of structure to function of tissues of the wall of blood vessels. Physiol Rev 1954;34:619–624.

88 Dobrin PB, Baker WH, Gley WC: Elastolytic and collagenolytic studies of arteries: implications for the mechanical properties of aneurysms. Arch Surg 1984;119:406–409.

89 Johnson CP, Baugh R, Wilson CA, Burns J: Age related changes in the tunica media of the vertebral artery: implications for the assessment of vessels injured by trauma. J Clin Pathol 2001;54: 139–145.

90 Xu C, Zarins CK, Pannaraj PS, Bassiouny HS, Glagov S: Hypercholesterolemia superimposed by experimental hypertension induces differential distribution of collagen and elastin. Arterioscler Thromb Vasc Biol 2000;20:2566–2572.

91 Ahimastos AA, Natoli AK, Lawler A, Blombery PA, Kingwell PA: Ramipril reduces large-artery stiffness in peripheral arterial disease and promotes elastogenic remodeling in cell culture. Hypertension 2005;45:1194–1199.

92 Nehme JA; Lacolley P, Labat C, Challande P, Robidel E, Perret C, Leenhardt A, Safar ME, Delcayre C, Milliez P: Spironolactone improves carotid artery fibrosis and distensibility in rat postischaemic heart failure. J Mol Cell Cardiol 2005;39:511–519.

93 Tokimitsu I, Kato H, Wachi H, Tajima S: Elastin synthesis is inhibited by angiotensin II but not by platelet-derived growth factor in arterial smooth muscle cells. Biochim Biophys Acta 1994; 1207:68–73.

94 Bozec E, Lacolley P, Bergaya S, Boutouyrie P, Meneton P, Herisse-Legrand M, Boulanger CM, Alhenc-Gelas F, Kim HS, Laurent S, Dabire H: Arterial stiffness and angiotensinogen gene in hypertensive patients and mutant mice. J Hypertens 2004;22:1299–1307.

95 Benetos A, Topouchian J, Ricard S, Gautier S, Bonnardeaux A, Asmar R, Poirier O, Soubrier F, Safar M, Cambien F: Influence of angiotensin II type 1 receptor polymorphism on aortic stiffness in never-treated hypertensive patients. Hypertension 1995;26:44–47.

96 Balkestein EJ, Wang JG, Struijker-Boudier HA, Barlassina C, Bianchi G, Birkenhager WH, Brand E, Den Hond E, Fagard R, Hermann SM, Van Bortel LM, Staessen JA: Carotid and femoral intima-media thickness in relation to three candidate genes in a Caucasian population. J Hypertens 2002;20:1551–1561.

97 Lajemi M, Labat C, Gautier S, Lacolley P, Safar M, Asmar R, Cambien F, Benetos A: Angiotensin II type 1 receptor-153 A/G and 1166 A/C gene polymorphisms and increase in aortic stiffness with age in hypertensive subjects. J Hypertens 2001;19:407–413.

98 Pojoga L, Gautier S, Blanc H, Guyene TT, Poirier O, Cambien F, Benetos A: Genetic determination of plasma aldosterone levels in essential hypertension. Am J Hypertens 1998;11:856–860.

99 Reiser K, McCormick RJ, Rucker RB: Enzymatic and nonenzymatic cross-linking of collagen and elastin. FASEB J 1992;6:2439–2449.

100 Watanabe M, Sawai T, Nagura H, Suyama K: Age-related alteration of cross-linking amino acids of elastin in human aorta. Tohoku J Exp Med 1996;180:115–130.

101   Spina M, Garbin G: Age-related chemical changes in human elastins from non-atherosclerotic areas of thoracic aorta. Atherosclerosis 1976;24:267–279.
102   Cattell MA, Anderson JC, Hasleton PS: Age-related changes in amounts and concentrations of collagen and elastin in normotensive human thoracic aorta. Clin Chim Acta 1996;245:73–84.
103   Avolio A, Jones D, Tafazzoli-Shadpour M: Quantification of alterations in structure and function of elastin in the arterial media. Hypertension 1998;32:170–175.
104   Yasmin, Wallace S, McEniery CM, Dakham Z, Pusalkar P, Maki-Petaja K, Ashby MJ, Cockcroft JR, Wilkinson IB: Matrix metalloproteinase-9 (MMP-9), MMP-2, and serum elastase activity are associated with systolic hypertension and arterial stiffness. Arterioscler Thromb Vasc Biol 2005;25:372–378.
105   Medley TL, Kingwell BA, Gatzka CD, Pillay P, Cole TJ: Matrix metalloproteinase-3 genotype contributes to age-related aortic stiffening through modulation of gene and protein expression. Circ Res 2003;92:1254–1261.
106   Lee A, Cerami A: Role of glycation in aging. Ann NY Acad Sci 1992;663:63–70.
107   Bailey AJ: Molecular mechanisms of ageing in connective tissues. Mech Ageing Dev 2001;122:735–755.
108   Verzijil N, DeGroot J, Thorpe SR, Bank RA, Shaw JN, Lyons TJ, Bijlsma JW, Lafeber FP, Baynes JW, TeKoppele J: Effect of collagen turnover on the accumulation of advanced glycation end products. J Biol Chem 2000;275:39027–39031.
109   Winlove CP, Parker KH, Avery NC, Bailey AJ: Interactions of elastin and aorta with sugars in vitro and their effects on biochemical and physical properties. Diabetologia 1996;39:1131–1139.
110   Konova E, Baydanoff S, Atanasova M, Velkova A: Age-related changes in the glycaton of human aortic elastin. Exp Gerontol 2004;39:249–254.
111   Lakatta EG: Cardiovascular regulatory mechanisms in advanced age. Physiol Rev 1993;73:413–467.
112   Et-Taouil K, Schiavi P, Levy BI, Plante GE: Sodium intake, large artery stiffness, and proteoglycans in the spontaneously hypertensive rat. Hypertension 2001;38:1172–1176.
113   Roth T, Podesta F, Stepp MA, Boeri D, Lorenzi M: Integrin overexpression induced by high glucose and by human diabetes: potential pathway to cell dysfunction in diabetic microangiopathy. Proc Natl Acad Sci USA 1993;90:9640–9644.
114   Regoli M, Bendayan M: Alterations in the expression of the $\alpha_3\beta_1$ integrin in certain membrane domains of the glomerular epithelial cells (podocytes) in diabetes mellitus. Diabetologia 1997;40:15–22.
115   Bezie Y, Lamaziere JM, Laurent S, Challande P, Cunha RS, Bonnet J, Lacolley P: Fibronectin expression and aortic wall elastic modulus in spontaneously hypertensive rats. Arterioscler Thromb Vasc Biol 1998;18:1027–1034.
116   Intengan HD, Thibault G, Li JS, Schiffrin EL: Resistance artery mechanics, structure, and extracellular components in spontaneously hypertensive rats: effects of angiotensin receptor antagonism and converting enzyme inhibition. Circulation 1999;100:2267–2275.
117   Durier S, Fassot C, Laurent S, Boutouyrie P, Couetil JP, Fine E, Lacolley P, Dzau VJ, Pratt RE: Physiologic genomics of human arteries. Quantitative relationship between gene expression and arterial stiffness. Circulation 2003;108:1845–1851.
118   Moiseeva EP: Adhesion receptors of vascular smooth muscle cells and their functions. Cardiovasc Res 2001;52:372–386.
119   Mukherjee BB, Nemir M, Beninati S, Cordella-Miele E, Singh K, Chackalaparampil I, Shanmugam V, DeVougue MW, Mukherjee AB: Interaction of osteopontin with fibronectin and other extracellular matrix molecules. Ann NY Acad Sci 1995;760:201–212.
120   Kaartinen MT, Pirhonen A, Linnala-Kankhunen A, Maenpaa PH: Cross-linking of osteopontin by tissue transglutaminase increases its collagen binding properties. J Biol Chem 1999;274:1729–1735.
121   Paul RG, Bailey AJ: The effect of advanced glycation end-product formation upon cell-matrix interactions. Int J Biochem Cell Biol 1999;31:653–660.
122   Wolffenbutel BH, Boulanger CM, Crijns FR, Huijberts MS, Poitevin P, Swennen GN, Vasan S, Egan JJ, Ulrich P, Cerami A, Levy BI: Breakers of advanced glycation end products restore large artery properties in experimental diabetes. Proc Natl Acad Sci USA 1998;95:4630–4634.

123 Vaitkevicius PV, Lane M, Spurgeon H, Ingram DK, Roth GS, Egan JJ, Vasan S, Wagle DR, Ulrich P, Brines M, Wuerth JP, Cerami A, Lakatta EG: A cross-link breaker has sustained effects on arterial and ventricular properties in older rhesus monkeys. Proc Natl Acad Sci USA 2001;98: 1171–1175.
124 Kass DA, Shapiro EP, Kawaguchi M, Capriotti AR, Scuteri A, deGroof RC, Lakatta EG: Impaired arterial compliance by a novel advanced glycation end-product cross-link breaker. Circulation 2001;104:1464–1470.
125 Safar ME, Lavy BI, Struijker-Boudier H: Current perspectives on arterial stiffness and pulse pressure in hypertension and cardiovascular diseases. Circulation 2003;107:2864–2869.

Dr. Javier Díez
Area de Ciencias Cardiovasculares, Edificio CIMA, Avda. Pío XII, 55
ES–31008 Pamplona (Spain)
Tel. +34 948 194 700, Fax +34 948 194 716
E-Mail jadimar@unav.es

Safar ME, Frohlich ED (eds): Atherosclerosis, Large Arteries and Cardiovascular Risk.
Adv Cardiol. Basel, Karger, 2007, vol 44, pp 96–116

· ·

Animal Models of Arterial Stiffness

Jeffrey Atkinson

Pharmacology Laboratory, Pharmacy Faculty, UHP-Nancy, Nancy, France

Abstract

Animal models of large artery wall stiffness fall into two categories: firstly those that slowly develop multifactorial vascular dysfunction spontaneously, such as the ageing rat. The second type of model consists of those in which a specific pathology is induced by surgical, chemical, or genetic means. Such models are based on a short-term, highly traumatic insult to the arterial wall of a young animal and its acute reaction to such insult. This is very different from the human situation in which changes in wall stiffness arise from the long-term accumulation of relatively minor episodes of vascular insult in the vulnerable elderly.

In this chapter, I will discuss animal models of human, age-linked arterial wall damage leading to increased wall stiffness. Such animal models generally exhibit diffuse, dilatory, medial arteriosclerotic deterioration, essentially following non-enzymatic, post-transcriptional modification of extracellular matrix proteins rather than focalized obstructive intimal atheroma. In man the two processes – arteriosclerosis and atheroma – often develop simultaneously with age such that a temporal relationship may mask any causal relationship (see later). The pathophysiology and clinical consequences of increased large artery wall stiffness are shown in figure 1.

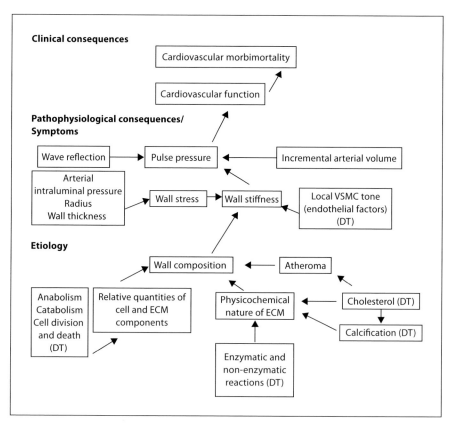

Fig. 1. Etiology, pathophysiology and clinical consequences of increase large artery stiffness. VSMC = Vascular smooth muscle cells; ECM = extracellular matrix; DT = drug target. Enzymatic and non-enzymatic post-transcriptional modifications of ECM include proteolysis, racemation, cross-linking, glycation, nitration.

Within this scheme, animal models are used in preclinical research regarding: (1) proof of concept for a supposed etiological factor or pathophysiological consequence, and (2) evaluation of efficacy of a new drug candidate, generally in terms of some surrogate change in cardiovascular function (e.g. decreased wall stiffness, systolic or pulse pressure) but almost never in terms of cardiovascular morbimortality (potential drug targets are indicated DT).

Animal models generally involve a single massive insult to one supposedly rate-limiting system over a short period in a young, short-lived mammal, in most cases the rat. They supposedly mimic the changes following the slow accumulation over a long period of millions of minor insults to multiple sys-

Table 1. Animal models for preclinical proof of concept and evaluation of candidate drug activity in the area of large artery stiffness

---

1. Natural occurrence of arterial stiffness in mammals and its impact on cardiovascular function; relationship to hypertension and atheroma

2. Induction of arterial stiffness
   a. Surgery
      i. Induction of arterial stiffness by ischemia
      ii. Replacement of the aorta by a stiff tube
   b. Chemical
      i. Neurohormonal factors
      ii. Imbalance between salt handling and the renin-angiotensin-aldosterone system
      iii. Cross-linking of collagen and elastin
      iv. Calcification
      v. Treatment with enzymes
   c. Genetic modification

---

tems culminating in pathological change in an elderly, long-lived mammal (man). It is possible that the rat and other laboratory mammals do not live long enough to develop the same cardiovascular changes seen in man, cardiovascular pathology being essentially seen in the elderly. It is possible that animals such as the rat die from cancer [1] and nephropathy [2] before reaching an age at which they start to develop cardiovascular disease. Whilst lifespans may be very different, there is no reason to suspect that the time courses of key biochemical events such as scleroprotein turnover and post-transcriptional modification of extracellular matrix proteins is different between man and other mammals. Finally, it should be noted that although pronounced changes in salt intake, body weight or aerobic capacity may modify some aspects of cardiovascular aging, few – if any – efficacious drugs or drug candidates with a direct, specific effect on large artery stiffness are available. Thus there is no standard treatment to which a new treatment could be compared.

Interest in animal models of arterial wall stiffness arose at an early date [e.g. 3]. The latter author expressed his hope '...to be enabled to obtain trustworthy data from experiments on the blood vessels of living animals': the problem still exists. Models for the study of large artery stiffness are given in table 1. This subject has been reviewed previously [4–8].

Natural Occurrence of Increased Arterial Stiffness in Mammals and Its Impact on Cardiovascular Function, Relationship to Hypertension and Atheroma

As seen above, aging can be considered as an accumulation of deteriorative changes over time during post-maturational life that underlie an ever increasing vulnerability to external insults thereby decreasing the capacity of the organism to survive [9]. In this respect, animals share with man some of the external challenges, i.e. cardiovascular risk factors such as obesity or lack of exercise, but not others such as smoking or hypertension. Furthermore, it is uncertain whether age-linked increasing vulnerability of the cardiovascular system decreases the survival capacity of animals other than man. For instance, chronically lowering blood pressure in spontaneously hypertensive rats increased lifespan by 43% [10], but chronically lowering blood pressure in normotensive rats with the same treatment (ACE inhibition), and by the same percentage amount, did not modify survival [2], although carotid artery compliance was chronically increased by the hypotensive treatment [11].

Changes in the properties of large arteries with age have been extensively studied by Michel et al. [11], our group [12, 13] and others. Large artery wall stiffness increases progressively with age in rats. This is not due to an increase in wall stress, which in fact may fall by up to 30% between the ages of 3–6 and 30 months. Mean arterial pressure does not increase with age and although aortic diameter increases, the wall thickens (fig. 2). However, the elastic modulus/wall stress ratio increases, suggesting that there is some change in wall composition. Although there is some variability in published reports, changes in the absolute amounts of wall components – important determinants in aging and other (patho)physiological states of changes in wall stiffness [14] – do not appear to be pronounced. Thus, processes such as non-enzymatic post-transcriptional modification of extracellular matrix proteins may be involved (glycation [13], calcification [11]).

As stroke volume does not change significantly with age in the normotensive rat (thus cardiac function appears to be maintained [11]), yet compliance decreases (in parallel with the increase in EM/WS), it is to be expected that pulse and systolic pressures increase. Michel et al. [11] found a small (26%) increase in pulse pressure that we did not find. Neither group found any increase in systolic pressure. Thus, old rats do not suffer from isolated systolic hypertension. It should be noted that in both studies, as is often the case in animal studies, blood pressure was measured under anesthesia with low-frequency, fluid-filled cannula and this could lead to an underestimation of peak systolic pressure.

In the rare studies on the evolution of blood pressure with age in other animals, there is no report to our knowledge of isolated systolic hypertension

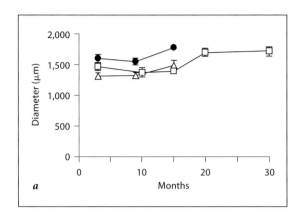

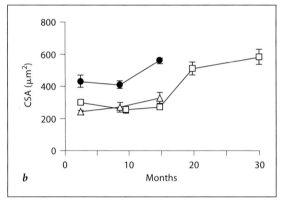

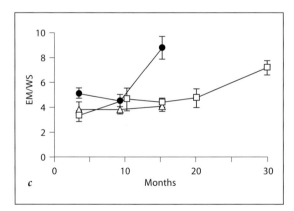

Fig. 2. Changes with age in spontaneously hypertensive (●) and normotensive rats (WKY △, WAG □) in (***a***) thoracic aorta diameter, (***b***) wall cross-sectional area (CSA) and (***c***) elastic modulus/wall stress (EM/WS) [data from 12, 13].

developing with age (e.g. dog [15], fox: Atkinson, Barrat and Lartaud, unpubl. results).

In the rat, left ventricular hypertrophy develops with age and Michel et al. [11] attributed this to an increase in cardiac afterload with an increase in impedance. In summary, there is evidence in the normotensive rat that large artery wall stiffness increases with age following non-enzymatic post-transcriptional modification of extracellular matrix proteins [13], and that although isolated systolic hypertension does not develop, increased wall stiffness has an impact on cardiac structure, if not function. Increased large artery stiffness may have an impact on downstream tissue perfusion as, for instance, cerebral blood flow autoregulation is perturbed with age in the same rat strain [16]. These changes in cardiac and arterial structure and function occur in the absence of atheroma and hypertension (as defined by an increase in mean arterial pressure).

Two provisos should be noted. As mortality increases rapidly in the normotensive rat beyond the median lifespan (approx. 27 months in most strains), 30-month-old rats may be 'survivors' which have a different phenotype and genotype from those who do not survive: increased large artery stiffness may be one of the factors involved in their survival.

Secondly, as can be seen in figure 2, chronic hypertension appears to 'prematurely age' the wall as 15-month-old SHR have elastic modulus/wall stress ratios equivalent to those of 30-month-old normotensive rats. This may be related to an increase in wall stress that is augmented by 10–15% in SHR [12] or in pulse pressure (increased by 30%) and thus in cyclic wall shock. Amplification of age-linked changes by chronic hypertension also suggests that whilst antihypertensive treatment may correct wall stiffness in young hypertensives [17], in old hypertensives an additional 'vasculoprotective' action may be required (fig. 3). The etiology of the increased aortic wall stiffness in old SHR is not clearly defined, although calcification or an increase in the collagen/elastin ratio do not seem to be of prime importance [12]. Other changes such as a change in the type of collagen [18, 19] or in fibronectin [20] may be involved. The SHR remains hypertensive up to 15 months of age but it does not develop isolated systolic hypertension [12]. Concerning the cardiac consequences, with advancing age, left ventricular pumping activity decreases and this is accompanied by ventricular hypertrophy and fibrosis [21]. Finally, the median lifespan in SHR is 18 months (rather than 27 months in normotensive rat strains [22]) and when comparing hypertensive and normotensive strains it may be more appropriate to use indicators of biological aging such as telomerase activity [23].

A distinction has to be made between atheroma (a localized, intimal (at least initially) event), and arteriosclerosis (a diffuse medial change), although

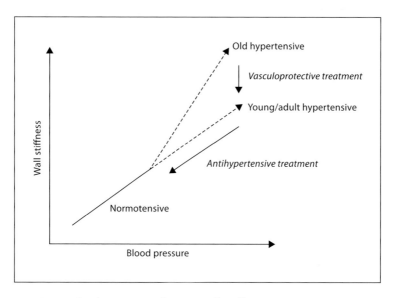

Fig. 3. Blood pressure and aortic wall stiffness.

this theoretical separation of the two probably does not reflect clinical reality in which vascular pathology involves both processes.

Whilst some authors suggest a close association between atheroma and wall stiffness [24], others have provided evidence that local plaque formation does not modify diffuse wall stiffness [25].

As plaque formation frequently occurs in the context of vascular aging, hypertension, diabetes, smoking, etc., it is possible that atheroma and wall stiffness occur concomitantly without there being a causal relationship between the two. Furthermore, as pointed out by Dobrin [26], early atheroma lesions are soft, occupy only a small portion of the wall and so probably have little effect on wall stiffness. As it enlarges, the lesion involves medial degeneration and plaque calcification and this will increase wall stiffness. Thus, contradiction in the reports on the link between atheroma and wall stiffness may reflect the stage of the disease which is being studied.

This latter point is confirmed by studies in animals fed a high cholesterol, atherogenic diet (rabbits: Dalessandri et al. [27], Hayashi et al. [28], Sato et al. [29]; minipigs: Augier et al. [30]; monkeys: Farrar et al. [31, 32]). In these models, marked changes in wall stiffness took several months to develop and were not observed until widespread plaque formation involving changes such as a loss of medial elastin and calcification.

Induction of Arterial Stiffness by Ischemia

Many animal models of human cardiovascular pathology are based on the induction of ischemia, which indeed is an important element in the etiology of many age-linked cardiovascular diseases such as myocardial infarction and stroke. The smooth muscle cells of the media of the aortic wall are irrigated with blood from the lumen and from the adventitia (via the vasa vasorum). A variety of procedures exist for the interruption of the vasa vasorum circulation [33]. Wilens et al. [34] showed that ligation of the intercostal arteries in the dog produced adventitial degeneration several days later, the media showing only minor changes. There were no functional studies in this paper. Heistad et al. [35] showed that intercostal ligation reduced medial conductance in the dog and Angouras et al. [36] showed increased wall stiffness in the pig aorta. These models merit further investigation given their possible pertinence to the importance of ischemia in the age-linked increase in wall stiffness in man and the relative roles of the adventitia and the media in wall stiffness [37].

Replacement of the Aorta by a Stiff Tube

It has been argued that stiffening of the aorta and an increase in impedance will increase telesystolic heart work and decrease diastolic coronary perfusion – these effects having a negative impact on cardiac performance. Thus, cardiac coupling with a stiff aorta should produce an imbalance between myocardial flow and metabolic demand leading to hypertrophy and maybe ultimately, failure. This theory has proven difficult to refute or confirm in animal models. In an acute study in dogs in which the aorta was surgically bypassed by a stiff tube, although peak systolic pressure and wall stress increased as predicted, coronary flow in fact rose due to compensatory enhanced systolic perfusion [38]. In chronic studies such as in the vitamin D + nicotine rat model (VDN, see below), baseline stroke volume, cardiac output and the cardiac response to venous overload were maintained for 1 month following induction of aortic stiffness [39]. This could be due to left ventricular hypertrophy, fibrosis (changes also observed in the old SHR, see above) and a change in ventricular myosin isoform [40], and a compensatory increase in aortic compliance following dilatation [41]. At a later stage of 14 months, cardiac output did decrease but only slightly (–17% [42]). Cardiac insult linked to aortic stiffening could be amplified by phenomena such as induced reduction in coronary flow. In this respect, it would be interesting to study the impact of changes in aortic wall stiffening on cardiac performance following induction myocardial ischemia in the VDN. This may provide a 'double' animal model of the cardiac impact of aortic wall stiffening post-infarct.

Another aspect to be studied in this area is the impact of cyclic stress on wall structure. Nichols and O'Rourke [43] suggested that one of the major events occurring during aging is represented by the changes in arterial wall structure induced by exposure to the cyclic stress of each pressure (and flow) wave and the concomitant wall deformation of each systole. This may produce an initial, adaptive response, as it has been known for many years that, in vitro at least [44], cyclic stretching of arterial cells stimulated the formation of matrix components. Similar phenomena may occur in vivo [45, 46]. Mulvany [47] and others have suggested that the (small diameter?) arterial wall becomes less stiff when exposed to increased pressure due to remodeling, with a shift from the elements with a high elastic modulus to those with lower modulus. Results are sometimes equivocal, however, as in a non-pulsatile left-heart bypass model in the goat a reduction in aortic pulse pressure from 43 to 17 mm Hg produced an increase in aortic wall elastin content with no significant change in wall stiffness [48].

Ultimately, cumulative exposure to cyclic stress leads to fatigue of the wall materials (scleroproteins and others) leading to rupture with dilatation and an increase in wall stiffness. This two-stage response to increased cyclic stress may explain the results obtained with adult and old SHR rats (see above). How cumulative cyclic stress affects chemical processes such as non-enzymatic post-transcriptional modification of scleroproteins [49] could be investigated in the future in animal models.

Neurohormonal Factors

Neurohormonal factors circulating in the blood, liberated from the endothelium or from autonomic nerves in the wall, could modify wall stiffness by a downstream change in resistance and hence in upstream distending pressure, or by a local vasomotor action. Concerning the latter, isobaric changes in wall stiffness, independent of changes in arterial diameter, are difficult to interpret: norepinephrine (α-adrenoceptor agonist) lowers the elastic modulus of the dog carotid artery [50] whereas urapridil (α-adrenoceptor antagonist) increases rat carotid artery compliance [51]. It is also possible that neurohormonal factors modify wall structure via a trophic action. Different animal models are available to study the latter. Neurotoxic agents given to young animals produce more or less specific destruction of one or more neurohormonal systems. Results are sometimes equivocal: guanethidine-induced sympathectomy lowers aortic distensibility [52] whereas 6-hydroxydopamine-induced sympathectomy increases carotid distensibility [53]. Another approach is to use genetically modified mice. In α_2A-adrenoceptor KO mice, whilst there was a hyperadrenergic state with hypertension, no intrinsic changes in wall stiffness were observed [54].

The involvement of endothelial factors is also equivocal. Certain authors have suggested that in man the age-linked increase in wall stiffness and progressive endothelium dysfunction are causally related [55]. Proof of concept in animals is more difficult. Increasing endothelial prostanoid activity, for example with fish oils [56], apparently increases arterial distensibility. Inhibition of the action of nitric oxide with arginine analogues that are inhibitors of nitric oxide synthase is another possibility. Several weeks of such inhibition produces hypertension and a decrease in carotid artery distensibility that was lower than in SHR rats of the same blood pressure, suggesting that the effect of nitric oxide inhibition on wall structure was not simply related to distending pressure [57].

Imbalance between Salt Handling and the Renin-Angiotensin-Aldosterone System

It is interesting to note that whatever the maneuver – high or low renin, aldosterone, salt balance, etc. – the changes in arterial mechanics are often similar. Thus the arterial wall becomes stiffer with conditions of high renin/normal-low salt or low renin/high salt (see table 2). This discrepancy may be explained by differences in genetic sensitivity in various rat strains used (SHR, SHR-SP, Dahl). There may be a pressure and time factor involved. For example, in the two-kidney, one-clip model, the intrinsic properties of the carotid artery wall were similar to those of normotensive controls up to 5 weeks following clipping [58], but at 9 weeks the wall became thicker and yet stiffer. Thus in this model as in others (aging in SHR or normotensive rats) at an early stage the main determinant of stiffness appears to be wall stress, but at a later stage intrinsic changes in wall composition occurs. Whether such changes are similar in the wide-ranging models involving salt and the renin-angiotensin-aldosterone system is unlikely. Comparisons between different models at different time intervals have received scant attention. For example, Cox [59] reported that carotid artery wall thickness to lumen diameter was greater in deoxycorticosterone + saline (DOCA) hypertension than in two-kidney, one-clip hypertension in the rat, but wall stiffness was similar. These equivocal results could also be explained by the multifactorial nature of increased wall stiffness. Factors such as salt and intracellular calcium overload followed by smooth

Table 2. Changes in the balance between renal handling of salt and the renin-angtiotensin-aldosterone system [95–100]

	Species	Effects	Ref.
High plasma renin level			
Renal artery stenosis	rat	↑ impedance ↓ compliance	97
Renal artery stenosis	dog	↓ compliance	96
Low plasma renin level Aldosterone			
Uninephrectomy + aldosterone analogue	rat	↑ impedance ↓ compliance	98
Uninephrectomy + aldosterone analogue + salt	rat	↑ impedance ↓ compliance	100
Genetic salt-sensitive			
SHR	rat	Medial necrosis	60
Dahl	rat	↓ compliance	95
SHR-SP	rat	↓ distensibility	99

muscle cell death and medionecrosis may characterize high salt models [60]. Angiotensin II/aldosterone-induced fibrosis may characterize high renin models [61].

Cross-Linking of Collagen and Elastin

Extracellular matrix scleroprotein function is dependent on optimal interfibrillar cross-linking. Several models are available to investigate the effects of a decrease in cross-linking. In mammals, intoxication with β-aminopropionitrile from *Lathyrus odoratus* inhibits the lysyl oxidase enzyme involved in forming cross-links from lysine and hydroxylysine residues in tropocollagen and tropoelastin, and produces arterial dilatation. In spite of the increase in diameter, β-aminopropionitrile reduces arterial wall stiffness following changes in the secondary characteristics of the connective tissue matrix without affecting connective tissue content [62, 63].

In the blotchy mouse model there is decreased activity of protein copper transporters and thus of lysyl oxidase. Again such mice suffer from aortic aneurysm [64] and it is to be expected that they also suffer from changes in wall stiffness.

Many studies have reported an increase in elastin fiber fluorescence with age in the arterial wall. Brüel and Oxlund [49] reported that the age-related increase in aortic stiffness in rats was associated with an accumulation of fluorescent material in elastin (and collagen). They suggested that this was due to the formation of advanced glycation end-products (advanced Maillard products of the terminal phase of non-enzymatic browning). Others have reported that elastin can incorporate glucose and ribose and form AGEs [65]. The relative importance of glycation of elastin compared to glycation of collagen (see below) remains to be explored.

The nitrite ion, a by-product of nitrogen oxides, reacts with tyrosine in elastin and such non-enzymatic nitration produces marked structural disruption [66]. The in vivo physiological and pathological importance of this for increased vascular wall stiffness is unknown.

It should be noted that elastin fluorescence could be caused by many factors including dityrosine, products of lipid peroxidation and reactive carbonyl compounds and quinones. Fluorescence can also be caused by the extraction procedure used. Thus, caution should be used in the interpretation of the results of fluorescence studies [67].

There may be a link between chemical modification of elastin and calcification. Cross-linking may be involved in calcification; for instance, in the streptozotocin-induced diabetes rat model, glycation of elastin accelerates calcification [68]. Pentosidine, an advanced glycation end-product, colocates with both elastic fibers and calcium deposits in the aortic media of patients with end-stage renal disease [69]. The authors concluded that modification of elastin by the Maillard reaction was involved in calcification.

An increase in cross-linking associated with aging and diabetes is thought to be linked to glycation of collagen with an increase in arterial stiffness [13, 70–74]. Such glycation can be modified with cross-link inhibitors or breakers, and this may form one type of treatment of vascular aging with vasculoprotective drugs (fig. 3).

Changes in wall stiffness are also to be expected in mice with differing semicarbazide-sensitive amine oxidase expression. Semicarbazide-sensitive amine oxidases constitute a diverse group of copper-dependent enzymes that amongst other functions are capable of deaminating amines with the production of formaldehyde, ammonia, hydrogen peroxide, etc. This leads to modification of scleroproteins via highly reactive aldehydes and formation of cross-links or exacerbation of the formation of advance glycation end-products. In a transgenic model for overexpression of human semicarbazide-sensitive amine oxidase in mice, elastic lamina were markedly abnormal and there was an increase in pulse pressure (with a decrease in mean arterial pressure) [75]. This model merits further investigation.

Finally, as several of the above models depend on copper deficiency, it would be interesting to study the effects of copper deficiency in the diet on arterial wall stiffness [76].

Calcification

Calcification of arteries is a common phenomenon especially in the elderly. The calcification of elastin can produce an increase in elastic fiber elastic modulus per se or cause a transfer of strain onto stiffer components such as collagen.

It was suggested 60 years ago that elastocalcinosis is implicated in the age-related decrease in arterial elasticity [77]; the time course of the increase in aortic wall stiffness [78] closely parallels the rise in medial calcification with age [77]. Other observations suggest a link between wall calcification and increased wall stiffness. Asymptomatic hypertensive patients with high aortic pulse wave velocity values show abdominal aortic calcifications [79]. In end-stage renal failure, aortic pulse wave velocity is related to aortic calcification [80].

Proof of the concept that elastocalcinosis is an important etiological factor in the development of fiber fragmentation followed by increased arterial wall stiffness can be obtained in animal models. Arteries contain up to 5 times more calcium than other soft tissues and calcify with age (2- to 3-fold), whereas the other soft tissues do not [81]. In the aorta of the normotensive rat, calcium bound to elastin increases with age [11] and elastocalcinosis and wall stiffness increase in parallel with age [11, 13].

Pronounced arterial calcification can be obtained with different experimental maneuvers. Periadventitial application of calcium chloride to the rat abdominal aorta produces calcification and chronic degeneration of elastic lamellae [82].

Elastocalcinosis of an order of magnitude similar to that observed in man can be produced by hypervitaminosis D, alone or in combination with nicotine or cholesterol. In the rat hypervitaminosis D + nicotine (VDN) model (fig. 4 [6]), there are no changes in aortic wall thickness, wall thickness to lumen ratio or wall stress. There is an increase in elastic modulus/wall stress ratio (following fragmentation of the medial elastic network) with an increase in aortic impedance and a decrease in systemic arterial and in situ and in vitro carotid artery compliance. Mean blood pressure remains at a normotensive level, and VDN animals suffer from isolated systolic hypertension following increased wall rigidity but no change in stroke volume.

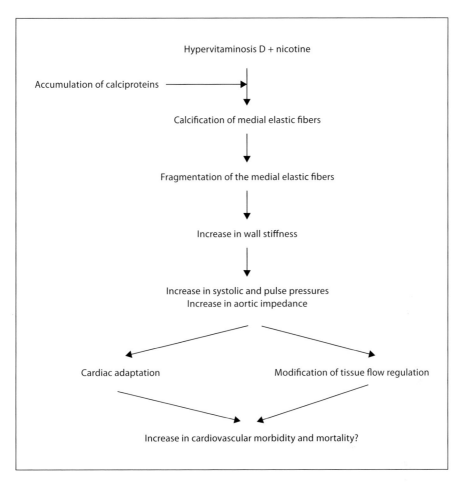

Fig. 4. Elastocalcinosis and wall mechanics in the hypervitaminosis D + nicotine rat model [6].

Other animal models of isolated systolic hypertension following calcification and elastic fiber fragmentation can be produced by inhibiting the maturation of Gla protein by treatment of rats with warfarin (and vitamin K) [83]. Matrix Gla protein inhibits elastocalcinosis; thus in the warfarin model the aortic media is calcified, elastin content decreases, and pulse wave velocity and pressure pulsatility are increased.

Treatment with Enzymes

Preferential destruction of elastin or collagen with enzymes (or acid) show that the main load-bearing element of the wall is elastin and that destruction of collagen produces dilatation rather then increased stiffness [84, 85]. However, results with elastase treatment are equivocal. Elastase treatment damages elastic fibers [86] and produces aneurysm [87]. However, in the cholesterol-fed rabbit, elastase treatment reduced wall stiffness [88]. The use of such chemical or enzymatic methods to produce chronic changes in wall stiffness merits further attention.

Genetic Modification

In animal models and in man the extent to which changes in long-lived tissues – such as scleroproteins – account for age-related pathology is extremely difficult to determine. Although the cumulative damage to long-lived proteins is similar across a given population, the magnitude of the degenerative changes varies between different individuals, suggesting that such changes may predispose to, rather than cause, age-related diseases [67]. Except in cases with a clear-cut genetic predisposition (Marfan and others), diseases such as arterial dilatation and increased wall stiffness do not occur in the young, presumably because the tissue is not vulnerable. Developmental adaptation to a genetic deficiency early in development may produce a cardiovascular system adapted to the change in the wall mechanics with a very different pathology to the one expected [89]. Mice lacking elastin die of obstructive arterial disease following cell proliferation and reorganization of smooth muscle [90]. Elastin haploinsufficiency in mice produces an increase in elastic lamellae [89, 91]. Thus, elastin has also a regulatory effect during arterial development and wall stiffening is not the hallmark of these models. Furthermore, the results of the studies cited above suggest that genetically modified mammals often do not develop the expected phenotype.

Microfibrillar fibrillin is a large macromolecular non-collagenous glycoprotein which forms, together with amorphous elastin (and other components), the elastic fiber. Evidence for the importance of fibrillin in aortic mechanics has come from the identification of the gene for fibrillin (FBN1) as the gene causing Marfan. The latter is a dominantly inherited disorder characterized by skeletal, ocular and cardiovascular abnormalities, including aortic root dilatation and dissection with rupture of the wall and premature death [92]. In the mgR/mgR mouse model of Marfan, which is characterized by a hypomorphic mutation of FBN1, aortic dilatation is due to the failure of the adventitial microfibrillar array to sustain wall integrity in the face of hemo-dynamic stress. The resulting increase in wall stress is accompanied by local-ized calcium deposition, macrophage infiltration and metalloproteinase acti-vation [93]. In adult mgR/mgR mice the wall desmosine content is not modi-fied, yet elastic fibers show severe fragmentation [94], suggesting that fragmentation of the medial elastic network and not a defect in early elasto-genesis is the determinant of aortic dilatation in Marfan (as in the VDN mod-el, see above).

Conclusion

A multitude of animal models are available for the study of large artery stiffness. They basically fall into two categories: firstly, those models which develop vascular dysfunction spontaneously, such as the aging rat. This mod-el presents several advantages, such as small size (quantity of drug candidate available for testing may be limited) and a relatively short lifespan. However, like the majority of mammals, the rat does not show pronounced age-linked cardiovascular pathology, possibly because it is not exposed to cardiovascular risk factors such as smoking or hypertension. One cardiovascular risk fac-tor – male sex – is nearly always present, as few experiments are performed on female animals.

The etiology of human vascular pathology, such as that involved in iso-lated systolic hypertension, depends on a complex mosaic of interacting fac-tors, one of which can be isolated in the second broad type of animal model: those in which pathology is induced by surgical, chemical, or genetic means. Such models are based on a short-term, highly traumatic insult to the arterial wall and the processes studied are those involved in the acute reaction to such insult. The insult may be more or less specific and problems of specificity can be partially solved by the use of genetically modified mammals. However, here again, insult is produced in a young animal. This is very different from the hu-man situation in which changes in wall stiffness arise from the long-term ac-cumulation of relatively minor episodes of vascular insult in the vulnerable elderly.

References

1   Sager R: Tumor expression in genes: the puzzle and the promise. Science 1989;246:1406–1412.
2   Heudes D, Chevalier MJ, Scalbert E, Ezan E, Bariety J, Zimmerman A, Corman B: Effect of chronic ANG I-converting enzyme inhibition on aging processes. I. Kidney structure and function. Am J Physiol 1994;266:R1038–R1051.
3   Roy CS: The elastic properties of the arterial wall. J Physiol (Lond) 1880;3:125–159.
4   Atkinson J: Aging of arterial extracellular matrix elastin: causes and consequences (in French). Pathol Biol 1998;46:555–559.
5   Atkinson J: Arterial calcification: mechanisms, consequences and animal models. Pathol Biol 1999;47:677–684.
6   Atkinson J: Elastin and the arterial wall in large arteries and end-organ damage; in Safar M, O'Rourke MF (eds): Hypertension. Amsterdam, Elsevier, 2006, pp 161–174.
7   Wolf YG, Gertz D, Banai S: Animal models in syndromes of accelerated sclerosis. Ann Vasc Surg 1999;13:328–388.
8   Zieman SJ, Melenovsky V, Kass DA: Mechanisms, pathophysiology and therapy of arterial stiffness. Arterioscler Thromb Vasc Biol 2005;25:932–943.
9   Masoro EJ: Handbook of Physiology, chapt 11: Ageing. New York, Oxford University Press, 1995, pp 3–25.
10 Linz W, Wohlfart PW, Schoelkens BA, Becker RHA, Malinski T, Wiemer G: Late treatment with ramipril increases survival in old spontaneously hypertensive rats. Hypertension 1999;34:291–295.
11 Michel JB, Heudes D, Michel O, Poitevin P, Philippe M, Scalbert E, Corman B, Levy BI: Effect of chronic ANG I-converting enzyme inhibition on aging processes. II. Large arteries. Am J Physiol 1994;267:R124–R135.
12 Marque V, Kieffer P, Atkinson J, Lartaud-Idjouadiene I: Elastic properties and composition of the aortic wall in old spontaneously hypertensive rats. Hypertension 1999;34:415–422.
13 Cantini C, Kieffer P, Corman B, Liminana P, Atkinson J, Lartaud-Idjouadiene I: Aminoguanidine and aortic wall mechanics, structure, and composition in aged rats. Hypertension 2001;38:943–948.
14 Wolinsky H: Response of the rat aortic media to hypertension: importance of comparing absolute amounts of wall components. Atherosclerosis 1970;11:251–255.
15 Bodey AR, Mitchell AR: Epidemiological study of blood pressure in domestic dogs. J Small Anim Pract 1996;37:116–125.
16 Lartaud I, Makki T, Bray-des-Boscs L, Niederhoffer N, Atkinson J, Corman B, Capdeville-Atkinson C: Effect of chronic ANG I-converting enzyme inhibition on aging processes. IV. Cerebral blood flow autoregulation. Am J Physiol 1994;267:R687–R694.
17 Zanchi A, Brunner HR, Hayoz D: Age-related changes of the mechanical properties of the carotid artery in spontaneously hypertensive rats. J Hypertens 1997;15:1415–1422.
18 Deyl Z, Jelinek L, Macek K, Chaldakov G, Vaukor VN: Collagen and elastin syntheses in the aorta of spontaneously hypertensive rats. Blood Vessels 1987;24:313–320.
19 Chamiot CP, Renaud JF, Blacher J, Legrand M, Samuel ML, Levy BI, Sassard J, Safar ME: Collagen I and III and mechanical properties of conduit arteries in rats with genetic hypertension. J Vasc Res 1999;36:139–146.
20 Mamuya W, Chobanian A, Brecher P: Age-related changes in fibronectin expression in spontaneously hypertensive, Wistar-Kyoto, and Wistar rat hearts. Circ Res 1992;71:1341–1350.
21 Pfeffer JM, Pfeffer MA, Fishbein MC, Frohlich ED: Cardiac function and morphology with aging in the spontaneously hypertensive rat. Am J Physiol 1979;237:H461–H468.
22 Yamori Y: Development of the spontaneously hypertensive rat and of various spontaneous rat models and their implications; in De Jong W (ed): Handbook of Hypertension, vol 4: Experimental and Genetic Models of Hypertension. Amsterdam, Elsevier, 1984, pp 224–239.
23 Cao Y, Li H, Mu FT, Ebisui O, Funder JW, Liu JP: Telomerase activation causes vascular smooth muscle cell proliferation in genetic hypertension. FASEB J 2002;16:96–98.
24 Wilkinson IB, Cockroft JR, Webb DJ: Pulse wave analysis and arterial stiffness. J Cardiovasc Pharmacol 1998;32(suppl 3):S33–S37.

25 Avolio AP, Chen SG, Wang RP, Zhang CL, Li MF, O'Rourke MF: Effects of aging on changing arterial compliance and left ventricular load in a Northern Chinese urban community. Circulation 1983;68:50–58.

26 Dobrin PB: Physiology and pathophysiology of blood vessels; in Sidaway AN, Sumpio BE, De-Palma RG (eds): The Basic Science of Vascular Disease. Armonk, Futura, 1997, pp 69–105.

27 Dalessandri KM, Bogren H, Lantz BM, Tsukamoto H, Bjorkerud S, Brock J: Aortic compliance in hypercholesterolemic Watanabe rabbits compared to normal New Zealand controls. J Invest Surg 1990;3:245–251.

28 Hayashi K, Ide K, Matsumoto T: Aortic walls in atherosclerotic rabbits – mechanical study. J Biomech Eng 1994;116:284–293.

29 Sato M, Katsuki Y, Kanehiro H, Iimura M, Akada Y, Mizota M, Kunihiro Y: Effects of ethyl all-cis-5,8,11,14,17-icosapentaenoate on the physical properties of arterial walls in high cholesterol diet-fed rabbits. J Cardiovasc Pharmacol 1993;22:1–9.

30 Augier T, Bertolotti C, Friggi A, Charpiot P, Barlatier A, Bodard H, Chareyre C, Guillou J, Luccioni R, Garcon D, Rolland PH: Therapeutic effects of nitric oxide-donor isosorbide dinitrate on atherosclerosis-induced alterations in hemodynamics and arterial viscoelasticity are independent of the wall elastic component. J Cardiovasc Pharmacol 1996;27:752–759.

31 Farrar DJ, Green HD, Bond MG, Wagner WD, Gobbee RA: Aortic pulse wave velocity, elasticity, and composition in a non-human primate model of atherosclerosis. Circ Res 1978;43:52–62.

32 Farrar DJ, Bond MG, Riley WA, Sawyer JK: Anatomic correlates of aortic pulse wave velocity and carotid artery elasticity during atherosclerosis progression and regression in monkeys. Circulation 1991;83:1754–1763.

33 Schichter JG: Experimental medionecrosis of the aorta. Arch Path 1946;42:182–192.

34 Wilens SL: The post-mortem elasticity of the adult aorta. Its relation to age and to distribution of intimal atheromas. Am J Pathol 1937;13:811–834.

35 Heistad DD, Marcus ML, Larsen GE, Armstrong ML: Role of the vasa vasorum in nourishment of the aortic wall. Am J Physiol 1981;240:H781–H787.

36 Angouras D, Sokolis DP, Dosios T, Kostomitsopoulos N, Boudoulas H, Skalkeas G, Karayannacos PE: Effect of impaired vasa vasorum flow on the structure and mechanics of the thoracic aorta: implications for the pathogenesis of aortic dissection. Eur J Cardiothorac Surg 2000;17:468–473.

37 Fung YC: Mechanical properties and active remodeling of blood vessels; in Biomechanics. Mechanical Properties of Living Tissues. New York, Springer, 1993, pp 321–391.

38 Saeki A, Recchia F, Kass DA: Systolic flow augmentation in hearts ejecting into a model of stiff aging vasculature. Circ Res 1995;76:132–141.

39 Lartaud-Idjouadiene I, Niederhoffer N, Debets JJ, Struyker-Boudier HA, Atkinson J, Smits JF: Cardiac function in a rat model of chronic aortic stiffness. Am J Physiol 1997;272:H2211–H2218.

40 Lartaud-Idjouadiene I, Lompré AM, Kieffer P, Colas T, Atkinson J: Cardiac consequences of prolonged exposure to an isolated increase in aortic stiffness. Hypertension 1999;34:63–69.

41 Tatchum-Talom R, Niederhoffer N, Amin F, Makki T, Tankosic P, Atkinson J: Aortic stiffness and left ventricular mass in a rat model of isolated systolic hypertension. Hypertension 1995;26:963–970.

42 Atkinson J, Poitevin P, Chillon JM, Lartaud I, Levy B: Vascular Ca overload produced by vitamin D_3 + nicotine diminishes arterial distensibility in rats. Am J Physiol 1994;266:H540–547.

43 Nichols WW, O'Rourke MF: Aging; in McDonald's Blood Flow in Arteries, ed 4. London, Arnold 1998, pp 347–376.

44 Leung DY, Glagov S, Mathews MB: Cyclic stretching stimulates synthesis of matrix components by arterial smooth muscle cells in vitro. Science 1976;191:475–477.

45 Baumbach GL, Dobrin PB, Hart MN, Heistad DD: Mechanics of cerebral arterioles in hypertensive rats. Circ Res 1988;62:56–64.

46 Baumbach GL: Effects of increased pulse pressure on cerebral arterioles. Hypertension 1996;27:159–167.

47 Mulvany MJ: A reduced elastic modulus of vascular wall components in hypertension? Hypertension 1992;20:7–9.

48 Nishimura T, Tatsumi E, Taenaka Y, Nishinaka T, Nakatani T, Masuzawa T, Nakata M, Nakamura M, Endo S, Takano H: Effects of long-term nonpulsatile heart bypass on the mechanical properties of the aortic wall. ASAIO J 1999;45:455–459.

49 Brüel A, Oxlund H: Changes in biomechanical properties, composition of collagen and elastin, and advanced glycation end products of the aorta in relation to age? Atherosclerosis 1996;127: 155–165.

50 Dobrin PB, Rovick SA: Influence of vascular smooth muscle on contractile mechanics and elasticity of arteries. Am J Physiol 1969;217:1644–1651.

51 Levy BI, Poitevin P, Safar ME: Effects of α_1-blockade on arterial compliance in normotensive and hypertensive rats. Hypertension 1991;17:534–540.

52 Lacolley P, Glaser E, Challande P, Boutouyrie D, Mignot JP, Duriez M, Levy B, Safar ME, Laurent S: Structural changes and in situ aortic pressure-diameter relationship in long-term chemical-sympathectomized rats. Am J Physiol 1995;269:H407–H416.

53 Mangoni AA, Mircoli L, Giannattasio C, Mancia G, Ferrari AU: Effect of sympathectomy on mechanical properties of common carotid and femoral arteries. Hypertension 1997;30:1085–1088.

54 Marque V, Hein L, Atkinson J, Lartaud-Idjouadiene I, Niederhoffer N: Aortic elasticity in α_2A-adrenoceptor knockout mice (abstract). FASEB J 2000;14:A1316.

55 Cockcroft JR, Wilkinson IB, Webb DJ: Age, arterial stiffness and the endothelium. Age Ageing 1997;26:53–60.

56 Chin-Dusting JP, Jovanovska V, Kingwell BA, Du XJ, Dart AM: Effect of fish oil supplementation on aortic compliance in rats: role of the endothelium. Prostaglandins Leukotr Essent Fatty Acids 1998;59:335–340.

57 Delacretaz E, Hayoz D, Osterheld MC, Genton CY, Brunner HR, Waeber B: Long-term nitric oxide synthase inhibition and distensibility of carotid artery in intact rats. Hypertension 1994; 23:967–970.

58 Zanchi A, Wiesel P, Aubert JF, Brunner HR Hayos D: Time course of changes of the mechanical properties of the carotid artery in renal hypertensive rats. Hypertension 1997;29:1199–1203.

59 Cox RH: Alterations in active and passive mechanics of rat carotid artery with experimental hypertension. Am J Physiol 1979;237:H597–H605.

60 Limas C, Westrum B, Limas CJ, Cohn JN: Effect of salt on the vascular lesions of the spontaneously hypertensive rat. Hypertension 1980;2:477–489.

61 Benetos A, Lacolley P, Safar ME: Prevention of aortic fibrosis by spironolactone in spontaneously hypertensive rats. Arterioscler Thromb Vasc Biol 1997;17:1152–1156.

62 Cox RH, Bashey R, Jimenez S: Effects of chronic β-aminoproprionitrile treatment on rat carotid artery. Blood Vessels 1988;25:53–62.

63 Brüel A, Ortoft G, Oxlund H: Inhibition of cross-links in collagen is associated with reduced stiffness of the aorta in young rats. Atherosclerosis 1998;140:135–145.

64 Moursi MM, Beebe HG, Messina LM, Welling TH, Stanley JC: Inhibition of aortic aneurysm development in blotchy mice by β-adrenergic blockade independent of altered lysyl oxidase activity. J Vasc Res 1995;21:792–800.

65 Winlove CP, Parker KH, Avery NC, Bailey AJ: Interactions of elastin and aorta with sugars in vitro and their effects on biochemical and physical properties. Diabetologia 1996;39:1131–1139.

66 Paik DC, Ramey WG, Dillon J, Tilson MD: The nitrite/elastin reaction: implications for in vivo degenerative effects. Connect Tissue Res 1997;36:241–251.

67 Sell DR, Monnier VM: Aging of long-lived proteins: extracellular matrix (collagens, elastin and proteoglycans) and lens crystallin; in Masoro EJ (ed): American Physiological Society Handbook of Physiology, Section 11: Aging. New York, Oxford University Press, 1995, pp 235–305.

68 Tomizawa H, Yamazaki M, Kunika K Itakura M, Yamashita K: Association of elastin glycation and calcium deposit in diabetic rat aorta. Diabetes Res Clin Pract 1993;19:1–8.

69 Sakata N, Norma A, Yamamoto Y, Okamoto K, Meng J, Takebayashi S, Nagai R, Horiuchi S: Modification of elastin by pentosidine is associated with calcification of aortic media in patients with end-stage renal disease. Nephrol Dial Transpl 2003;18:1601–1609.

70 Huijberts MSP, Woffenbuttel BHR, Struijker-Bondier HAJ, Crijns FRL, Nieuwenhuijzen-Kruseman AC, Poitevin P, Levy BI: Aminoguanidine treatment increases elasticity and decreases fluid filtration of large arteries from diabetic rats. J Clin Invest 1993;92:1407–1411.

71 Wolffenbuttel BHR, Boulanger CM, Crijns FRL, Huijberts MSP, Poitevin P, Swenney RNM, Vasan S, Egan JJ, Ulrich P, Cerami A, Levy BI: Breakers of advanced glycation end products restore large artery properties in experimental diabetes. Proc Natl Acad Sci USA 1998;95:4630–4634.

72 Corman B, Duriez M, Poitevin P, Mendes P, Bruneval P, Tedgui A, Levy BI: Aminoguanidine prevents age-related arterial stiffening and cardiac hypertrophy. Proc Natl Acad Sci USA 1998; 95:1301–1306.

73 Vaitkevicius PV, Lane M, Ebersold C, Ingram D, Roth G, Cerami A, Egan J, Lakatta E: Reduction of arterial stiffness in old primates by a novel compound which distributes vascular collagen cross-links. Circulation 1998;98:I-8.

74 Mizutani K, Ikeda K, Kawai Y, Yamori Y: Biomechanical properties and chemical composition of the aorta in genetic hypertensive rats. J Hypertens 1999;17:481–487.

75 Göktürk C, Nilsson J, Nordquist J, Kristensson M, Svensson K, Söderberg C, Israelson M, Garpenstrand H, Sjöquist M, Oreland L, Forsberg-Nilsson K: Overexpression of semicarbazide-sensitive amine oxidase in smooth muscle cells leads to abnormal structure of the aortic elastic laminas. Am J Pathol 2003;163:1921–1928.

76 Klevay LM: Cardiovascular disease from copper deficiency – a history. J Nutr 2000;130:489S–492S.

77 Blumenthal HT, Lansing AI, Wheeler PA: Calcification of the media of the human aorta and its relation to intimal arteriosclerosis, ageing and disease. Am J Pathol 1944;20:665–679.

78 Wilens SL, Macolm JA, Vazquez JM: Experimental infarction (medial necrosis) of the dog's aorta. Am J Pathol 1965;47:695–711.

79 Simon A, Levenson J: Early detection of subclinical atherosclerosis in asymptomatic subjects at high risk for cardiovascular disease. Clin Exp Hypertens 1993;15:1069–1076.

80 London GM, Marchais SJ, Safar ME, Genest AF, Guerin AP, Metivier F, Chedid K, London AM: Aortic and large artery compliance in end-stage renal failure. Kidney Int 1990;37:137–142.

81 Kieffer P, Robert A, Capdeville-Atkinson C, Atkinson J, Lartaud-Idjouadiene I: Age-related calcification in rats. Life Sci 2000;16:2371–2381.

82 Basalyga SM, Simionescu DT, Xiong W, Baxter BT, Starcher BC, Vyavahare NR: Elastin degradation and calcification in an abdominal aorta injury model: role of matrix metalloproteinases. Circulation 2004;11:3480–3487.

83 Essalihi R, Dao HH, Yamaguchi N, Moreau P: A new model of isolated systolic hypertension induced by chronic warfarin and vitamin K treatment. Am J Hypertension 2003;16:103–110.

84 Roach MR, Burton AC: The reason for the slope of the distensibility curve of arteries. Can J Biochem Physiol 1957;35:681–690.

85 Dobrin PB, Baker WH, Gley WC: Elastolytic and collagenolytic studies of arteries. Implications for the mechanical properties of aneurysms. Arch Surg 1984;119:405–409.

86 Anidjar S, Salzmann JL, Gentric D, Lagneau P, Camilleri JP, Michel JB: Elastase-induced experimental aneurysms in rats. Circulation 1990;82:973–981.

87 Boudghene F, Anidjar S, Allaire E, Osborne-Pellegrin M, Bigot JM, Michel JB: Endovascular grafting in elastase-induced experimental aortic aneurysms in dogs: feasibility and preliminary results. J Vasc Interv Radiol 1993;4:497–504.

88 Hayashi K, Takamizawa K, Nakamura T, Kato T, Tsushima N: Effects of elastase on the stiffness and elastic properties of arterial walls in cholesterol-fed rabbits. Atherosclerosis 1987;66:259–267.

89 Faury G: Function-structure relationship in elastic arteries in evolution: from microfibrils to elastin and elastic fibres. Pathol Biol 2001;49:310–325.

90 Li DY, Brooke B, Davis EC Mecham RP, Sorensen LK, Boak BB, Eichwald E, Keating MT: Elastin is an essential determinant of arterial morphogenesis. Nature 1998;393:276–280.

91 Li DY, Faury G, Taylor DG, Davis EC, Boyle WA, Mecham RP, Stenzel P, Boak B, Keating MT: Novel arterial pathology in mice and humans hemizygous for elastin. J Clin Invest 1998;102:1783–1787.

92 Dietz HC, McIntosh I, Sakai LY, Corson GM, Chalberg SC, Pyeritz RE, Francomano CA: Four novel FBN1 mutations: significance for mutant transcript level and EGF-like domain calcium binding in the pathogenesis of Marfan syndrome. Genomics 1993;17:468–475.

93 Pereira L, Lee SY, Gayraud B, Andrikopoulos K, Shapiro SD, Bunton T, Biery NJ, Dietz HC, Sakai LY, Ramirez F: Pathogenetic sequence for aneurysm revealed in mice under-expressing fibrillin-1. Proc Natl Acad Sci USA 1999;96:3819–3823.

94 Marque V, Kieffer P, Gayraud B, Lartaud-Idjouadiene L, Ramirez, F, Atkinson, J: Aortic wall mechanics and composition in a mouse model of Marfan syndrome. Arterioscler Thromb Vasc Biol 2001;21:1184–1189.

95 Benetos A, Bouaziz H, Albaladejo P, Guez D, Safar ME: Carotid artery mechanical properties of Dahl salt-sensitive rats. Hypertension 1995;25:272–277.

96 Brunner MJ, Bishop GG, Shigemi K: Arterial compliance and its control by the baroreflex in hypertensive dogs. Am J Physiol 1993;265:H616–H620.

97 Levy BI, Michel JB, Saltzmann JL, Azizi M, Poitevin P, Safar M, Camilleri JP: Effects of chronic inhibition of converting enzyme on mechanical and structural properties of arteries in rat renovascular hypertension. Circ Res 1988;63:227–239.

98 Levy BI, Poitevin P, Safar ME: Effects of indapamide on the mechanical properties of the arterial wall in desoxycortisone acetate-salt hypertensive rats. Am J Cardiol 1990;65:28H–32H.

99 Levy BI, Poitevin P, Duriez M, Guez DC, Schiavi PD, Safar ME: Sodium survival and the mechanical properties of the carotid artery in stroke-prone hypertensive rats. J Hypertens 1997;15: 251–258.

100 Zuckerman BD, Yin FC: Aortic impedance and compliance in hypertensive rats. Am J Physiol 1989;257:H553–H562.

Jeffrey Atkinson
Laboratoire de Pharmacodynamie, Faculté des Sciences Pharmaceutiques et Biologiques
Université de Nancy I, 7, rue Albert Lebrun
FR–54001 Nancy (France)
Tel. +33 383 682 262, Fax +33 383 682 301, E-Mail Jeffrey.Atkinson@pharma.uhp-nancy.fr

Safar ME, Frohlich ED (eds): Atherosclerosis, Large Arteries and Cardiovascular Risk.
Adv Cardiol. Basel, Karger, 2007, vol 44, pp 117–124

....

Blood Pressure, Large Arteries and Atherosclerosis

Edward D. Frohlich   *Dink Susic*

Ochsner Clinic Foundation, New Orleans, La., USA

Abstract

It is generally accepted that the increased cardiovascular morbidity and mortality in hypertension are related to target organ damage. Classically, the target organs are heart, brain, and kidneys. This brief report examines whether high arterial pressure may also affect other organs, such as aorta and large arteries. An attempt was also made to elucidate the relationship between disorders of the aorta and large arteries and other cardiovascular risk factors to the pathophysiology and treatment of patients with hypertension and its severe comorbid disease, atherosclerosis.

High Blood Pressure and Disorders of the Aorta and Large Arteries

The positive correlation between arterial pressure and adverse cardiovascular events is certainly well documented. It was Sir George Pickering who vigorously opposed the idea of dividing blood pressure into normotension and hypertension stating that '...the various complications, like myocardial infarction and stroke, are also quantitatively related to arterial pressure...' [1]. Furthermore, current therapeutic approaches to cardiovascular disorders are firmly based on this relationship. It thus seems prudent to start the discussion on the relationship between blood pressure and pathophysiology of large arteries by exploring the pressure as a risk factor.

The two most common disorders affecting aorta and large arteries are atherosclerosis, which starts with patchy intimal changes eventually leading to ischemic events distally, and arteriosclerosis, usually consisting of diffuse changes in the media leading to increased vessel stiffness and impairments in conduit and 'windkessel' functions of aorta and large arteries. Both conditions are common in older individuals and often coincide. Still open is the question whether the two diseases may exacerbate one another. Theoretically, there are reasons to believe they do but, since they usually coexist, causality is not easy to prove. Thus, arteriosclerosis increases systolic and pulse pressure, which could intensify endothelial damage and in this way may facilitate the formation of plaques. Similarly, atherosclerosis affects morphology and vascular function, and this may affect arteriolar stiffness. It should be noted, however, that since atherosclerosis may be a patchy disease throughout the aorta and large arteries, and non-invasive techniques are used to estimate and measure stiffness in large segments, all of the plaques probably do not affect actual measurements unless they are very abundant, coalescent, and calcified. On the other hand, the hyperlipidemias adversely affect endothelial function and may therefore increase arterial stiffness. However, in young patients with familial hypercholesterolemia, as well as in the early stages of experimental diet-induced atherosclerosis, aortic distensibility may be actually increased, not decreased [2, 3]. Similarly, arterial wall stiffness has been shown to be reduced around lipid-laden plaques [4]. Yet, later in the course of experimental atherosclerosis [3] as well as in older hypercholesterolemic patients [5], aortic distensibility is decreased. A number of other studies reported controversial results leading to a present conclusion that the interaction between arteriolosclerosis and atherosclerosis still remains to be clarified.

Hypertension and Atherosclerosis

Atherosclerosis is a chronic inflammatory condition that results in formation of an atherosclerotic plaque which, in turn, compromises circulation distally, by vascular occlusion as result of its bulk or by thromboembolic events after rupturing. Hypertension is a known risk factor for atherosclerosis [6]. The compelling link between the two is the vascular endothelium. Atherosclerosis is an extremely complex process that is initiated by endothelial damage facilitated by, among other factors, an increased arterial pressure [7]. The first step in the process is the formation of fatty streaks subendothelially. This pathological derangement starts with lipoprotein (LDL) transport into the arterial wall and its subsequent entrapment in the extracellular matrix. The entrapped LDL is then oxidized and stimulates endothelial cells to secrete various adhesion molecules and chemokines. These attract monocytes that first adhere to the endothelium and then migrate into the subendothelium where they accumulate lipids and transform into foam cells. The activated monocytes release mitogens and chemokines which attract more monocytes and vascular smooth muscle cells. These events lead to formation of atherosclerotic plaques which contain foam cells and activated macrophages and which are structurally unstable due to epithelial injury and the presence of inflammatory cells. Hemodynamic shearing forces, that are even more intense in hypertension and when pulse pressure is increased, can induce plaque rupture, usually at its more proximal point where the shearing forces are intensified. Rupture of the plaque predisposes the flowing blood to the highly thrombogenic constituents of the plaque, thereby leading to thrombus formation and possible embolization. Plaque formation, rupture, and subsequent thrombosis are therefore the major causes of acute cardiovascular events (myocardial infarction, stroke, death).

Hypertension and Stiffness of the Large Arteries

Decreased distensibility of the aorta and large arteries is routinely found in hypertensive patients regardless of the site or method of measurement [8]. Whether this reduction in distensibility is merely due to an increased distending pressure, or is true increased stiffness due to hypertension-induced structural modifications of the arterial wall, remains a matter of considerable debate and investigation [9]. The reasons for the divergent findings are numerous. Apart from the fact that different indexes (pulse pressure, pulse wave velocity, augmentation index, etc.) and different devices are used to estimate arterial stiffness, there are also many other factors that may affect the results. Thus, different vessels may be affected differently by the disparate factors that participate in the two diseases. In one study, a comparison of the properties of common carotid and femoral arteries in normotensive and hypertensive subjects was made [10]. Diameter-pressure curves in carotid and femoral arteries were first determined and, from these measurements, effective compliance and distensibility at the prevailing pressure of each subject and isobaric compliance and distensibility at the same standard pressure in all subjects were calculated. The results demonstrated that, in the carotid artery, hypertensive patients had isobaric compliance and distensibility values that were similar to those of normotensive subjects. However, when determined at actual pressures, the vessels had lower effective compliance and distensibility. On the other hand, hypertensive patients had both effective and isobaric femoral compliance and distensibility values which were lower than normotensive subjects [10]. It is also possible that additional co-existing conditions can affect the distensibility of large arteries in the hypertensive population. Thus, one very recent study indicated that the 'metabolic syndrome' may adversely affect aortic stiffness in hypertensive patients [11]. This study population involved never-treated, non-diabetic, middle-aged patients with essential hypertension who were classified according to the presence or absence of the metabolic syndrome. As an estimate of stiffness, pulse wave velocity was determined in the aorta and upper limb. Aortic pulse wave velocity was found to be higher in a group with metabolic syndrome, whereas upper limb velocity did not differ between the groups. Interestingly, this same study demonstrated that central, but not general, adiposity was an important determinant of aortic stiffness.

It also appears that the effect of high blood pressure on arterial distensibility is not uniform. Thus, some earlier studies [12–14] demonstrated that arterial compliance may be different within different hypertensive populations. Two studies evaluated arterial compliance using three indices: pulse wave velocity, pulse pressure/stroke volume and analysis of diastolic pressure decay [12, 13]. The results demonstrated decreased compliance in hypertensive patients, particularly in the elderly [12]. Moreover, signs of impaired compliance were found even in patients with borderline hypertension [13]. Another study [14] examined pulse wave velocity, compliance, and impedance of brachial artery in normotensive subjects and patients with uncomplicated essential hypertension. Compared to normotensive controls, hypertensive patients were found to have increased pulse wave velocity. However, when the results were related to diastolic pressure and age of the subjects, the data of the majority of hypertensive patients fell within nomograms obtained from normotensive subjects. Yet, a subgroup of hypertensive individuals still demonstrated higher pulse wave velocity, decreased arterial compliance, and increased impedance, suggesting excessive arterial stiffness. This non-uniform change in arterial stiffness in hypertensive individuals may be due to individual differences but it may also reflect differences in the duration of hypertension. Recently, results of the Bogalusa Heart Study clearly indicated that childhood blood pressure predicted arterial stiffness in adulthood [15]. This particular study was conducted in over 800 black and white adults of both sexes who had at least four measurements of traditional risk factors with an average follow-up period of over 26 years. As an estimate of arterial stiffness, brachial-ankle pulse wave velocity was determined. The results further demonstrated that pulse wave velocity was higher in males than in females and in blacks than in whites. When multiple regression analysis was applied, systolic blood pressure in childhood was found to be an independent predictor of increased pulse wave velocity in young adults, in addition to serum cholesterol and triglyceride concentrations and a history of smoking [15]. These findings underscore the importance of the height of arterial pressure over the long term in the evolution of arterial stiffness. Two other earlier studies further support these findings [16, 17]. Data from the Framingham Heart Study showed that untreated hypertension may accelerate the rate of large artery stiffness [16]. Thus, when compared with normotensive subjects, middle-aged and elderly patients with untreated hypertension were more likely to present with an age-related increase in pulse pressure, suggesting increased arterial stiffness [16]. A more recent, longitudinal study compared the progression of aortic stiffness over a 6-year period in treated hypertensive and normotensive subjects and evaluated the determinants of this progression [17]. Carotid-femoral pulse wave velocity was used as an index of aortic stiffness. The results indicated that the annual rates of progression in aortic stiffness were significantly higher in hypertensive than in normotensive subjects. The exceptions were hypertensive subjects with well-controlled arterial pressure levels which were similar to the stiffness progression of normotensives. In addition to high arterial pressure, other determinants of stiffness progression were a faster heart rate and a higher serum creatinine concentration.

In addition to the evidence that hypertension leads to accelerated arterial stiffening, there is also strong evidence that arterial stiffness may affect the development of high blood pressure. Thus, one very recent study [18] demonstrated that aortic stiffness in normotensive individuals was a predictor of future hypertension after correction for risk factors including systolic pressure, age, sex, body mass, heart rate, total serum cholesterol concentration, diabetes, smoking, alcohol consumption, and physical activity. This relationship was noted in younger and older subjects and for both sexes. Thus, elevated arterial pressure and arterial stiffness may apparently aggravate each other, establishing a vicious circle that is ultimately responsible for the adverse age- and pressure-related cardiovascular events.

The observed direct correlation between arterial pressure and stiffness of large arteries later in life provides some important implications. An analysis of the life course in terms of total life expectancy or life expectancy with or without cardiovascular disease was made in over 3,000 Framingham Heart Study participants according to their arterial pressure level at the age of 50 [19]. As compared with hypertensive subjects, total life expectancy was 5.1 and 4.9 years longer for normotensive men and women, respectively. Furthermore, the normotensive men survived 7.2 years longer without cardiovascular disease compared with hypertensive subjects [19]. These findings clearly indicate that increased arterial pressure in adulthood is associated with a large reduction in life expectancy and increased prevalence of cardiovascular disease. As already stated, high blood pressure in adulthood is also associated with greater arterial stiffness later in life. Thus, increased arterial stiffness may be related to lower life expectancy and higher cardiovascular morbidity that was observed in hypertensive subjects [20].

Arterial Stiffness, Target Organ Damage, and Risk of Atherosclerotic Events

Until recently, large artery stiffening with consequent increases in systolic and pulse pressures has been considered as a part of normal aging. However, over time, evidence has accumulated to demonstrate that arterial stiffness is a strong independent predictor of adverse cardiovascular events. Numerous studies in different populations, particularly in the elderly, have shown that it is a major risk factor for stroke, coronary heart disease, cardiovascular and total mortality [21, 22]. Furthermore, in addition to being an established risk factor, increased vascular stiffness is now becoming a potential therapeutic target, particularly in patients at risk of cardiovascular disease. Of course, even before vascular stiffness becomes a legitimate therapeutic target, it should be clearly demonstrated that reduction of arterial stiffness also reduces cardiovascular risk independent of the effects of treatment. Thus far, there have been few large-scale reports that have conclusively demonstrated that reduction of vascular stiffness reduces the adverse cardiovascular events irrespective of other effects. The one exception that indirectly supports this notion is a study that involved 150 patients with end-stage renal disease who were given antihypertensive medication [23]. Pulse wave velocity was measured in all patients before and during treatment. Fifty-nine deaths occurred during the study, 40 related to cardiovascular and 19 to non-cardiovascular causes. There were several predictors of all causes, with cardiovascular mortality with absence of pulse wave decrease in response to arterial pressure lowering being the strongest. These findings clearly indicated that arterial stiffness is a cardiovascular risk factor independent of arterial pressure.

Role of Cardiovascular Drugs and Arterial Stiffness

A number of cardiovascular drugs have been shown to affect arterial stiffness. Many of these agents also lower arterial pressure which, by itself, also increases arterial distensibility. Therefore, this effect must be differentiated from any functional or structural effects of these drugs on arterial wall stiffness. The angiotensin-converting enzyme (ACE) inhibitors, angiotensin (type 1) receptor antagonists, and some of the calcium antagonists have been shown to be effective in improving vascular stiffness, although the ACE inhibitors seem to be more effective than others [24]. On the other hand, the dual ACE and neutral endopeptidase inhibitor omapatrilat was shown to be more effective than enalapril in reducing aortic stiffness [25]. Statins have also demonstrated the ability to reduce arterial stiffness [26]. Most of these drugs also improve endothelial dysfunction and this effect may actually mediate their effect on vascular distensibility. There are also some novel approaches to treating arterial stiffness. Thus, advanced glycation end-product crosslinks are considered significant contributors to increased arterial stiffness in the elderly. A crosslink breaker has been shown to improve arterial distensibility in older patients [27]. In old spontaneously hypertensive rats the same crosslink breaker was shown to increase aortic distensibility and improve survival [28].

In summary, this report examined the relationship between the disorders of the aorta and large arteries and some other cardiovascular risk factors. Evidence was presented to demonstrate that hypertension aggravates age-related stiffening of the aorta and large arteries. Available data also suggest that arterial stiffness is an independent cardiovascular risk factor. Finally, the effects of commonly used cardiovascular drugs were briefly discussed.

References

1   Pickering J: Normotension and hypertension: the mysterious viability of the false. Am J Med 1978;65:561–563.
2   Lehman E, Watts GF, Fatemi-Langroudi B, Gosling R: Aortic compliance in young patients with heterozygous familial hypercholesterolemia. Clin Sci 1992;83:717–721.
3   Newman DL, Gosling RG, Bowden NLR: Changes in aortic distensibility and area ratio with the development of atherosclerosis. Atherosclerosis 1971;14:231–240.
4   Vonesh MJ, Cho CH, Pinto JVJ, Kane BJ, Lee DS, Roth SI, Chandran KB, McPherson DD: Regional vascular mechanical properties by 3-D intravascular ultrasound with finite-element analysis. Am J Physiol 1977;272:H425–H437.
5   Lehman E, Watts GF, Gosling R: Aortic distensibility and hypercholesterolemia. Lancet 1992; 340:1171–1172.
6   Kannel WB: Blood pressure as a cardiovascular risk factor: prevention and treatment. JAMA 1996;275:1571–1576.
7   Berliner JA, Navab M, Fogelman AM, Frank JS, Demer LL, Edwards PA, Watson AD, Lusis AJ: Atherosclerosis: basic mechanisms: oxidation, inflammation, and genetics. Circulation 1995;91: 2488–2496.
8   Simon A, Levenson J: Use of arterial compliance for evaluation of hypertension. Am J Hypertens 1991;4:97–105.
9   McVeigh GE, Hamilton PK, Morgan DR: Evaluation of mechanical arterial properties: clinical, experimental and therapeutic aspects. Clin Sci 2002;102:51–67.
10 Armentano R, Megnien JL, Simon A, Bellenfant F, Barra J, Levenson J: Effects of hypertension on viscoelasticity of carotid and femoral arteries in humans. Hypertension 1995;26:48–54.
11 Schillaci G, Pirro M, Vaudo G, Mannarino MR, Savarese G, Pucci G, Franklin SS, Mannarino E: Metabolic syndrome is associated with aortic stiffness in untreated essential hypertension. Hypertension 2005;45:1078–1082.
12 Messerli FH, Frohlich ED, Ventura HO: Arterial compliance in essential hypertension. J Cardiovasc Pharmacol 1985;7(suppl 2):S33–S35.
13 Ventura H, Messerli FH, Oigman W, Suarez DH, Dreslinski GR, Dunn FG, Reisin E, Frohlich ED: Impaired systemic arterial compliance in borderline hypertension. Am Heart J 1984;108: 132–136.
14 Simon AC, Levenson J, Bouthier J, Safar ME, Avolio AP: Evidence of early degenerative changes in large arteries in human essential hypertension. Hypertension 1985;7:675–680.

15 Li S, Chen W, Srinivasan SR, Berenson GS: Childhood blood pressure as a predictor of arterial stiffness in young adults. The Bogalusa Heart Study. Hypertension 2004;43:541–546.

16 Franklin SS, Gustin W IV, Wong ND, Larson MG, Weber MA, Kannel WB, Levy D: Hemodynamic patterns of age-related changes in blood pressure. The Framingham Heart Study. Circulation 1997;96:308–315.

17 Benetos A, Adamopoulos C, Bureau JM, Temmar M, Labat C, Bean K, Thomas F, Pannier B, Asmar R, Zureik M, Safar M, Guize L: Determinants of accelerated progression of arterial stiffness in normotensive subjects and in treated hypertensive subjects over a 6-year period. Circulation 2002;105:1202–1207.

18 Dernellis J, Panaretou M: Aortic stiffness is an independent predictor of progression to hypertension in nonhypertensive subjects. Hypertension 2005;45:426–431.

19 Franco OH, Peeters A, Bonneux L, deLaet C: Blood pressure in adulthood and life expectancy with cardiovascular disease in men and women: life course analysis. Hypertension 2005;46:280–286.

20 Benetos A: Does blood pressure control contribute to a more successful aging? Hypertension 2005;46:261–262.

21 Nielsen WB, Vestbo J, Jensen GB: Isolated systolic hypertension as a major risk factor for stroke and myocardial infarction and an unexploited source of cardiovascular prevention: a prospective population-based study. J Hum Hypertens 1995;9:175–180.

22 Sutton-Tyrrell K, Najar SS, Boudreau RM, Ventkitachalam L, Kupelian V, Simonsick EM, Havlik R, Lakatt EG, Spurgeon H, Kritchevsky S, Pahor M, Bauer D, Newman A: Elevated aortic pulse wave velocity, a marker of arterial stiffness, predicts cardiovascular events in well-functioning older adults. Circulation 2005;111:3384–3390.

23 Guerin AP, Blacher J, Pannier B, Marchais SJ, Safar ME, London GM: Impact of aortic stiffness attenuation on survival of patients in end-stage renal failure. Circulation 2001;103:987–992.

24 London GM, Pannier B, Guerin AP, Marchais SJ, Safar ME, Cushe JL: Cardiac hypertrophy, aortic compliance, peripheral resistance, and wave reflection in end-stage renal disease: comparative effects of ACE inhibition and calcium channel blockade. Circulation 1994;90:2786–2796.

25 Mitchell GF, Izo JL, Lacourciere Y, Ouellet JP, Neutel J, Quian C, Kerwin LJ, Block AJ, Pfeffer MA: Omapatrilat reduces pulse pressure and proximal aortic stiffness in patients with systolic hypertension: results of the conduit hemodynamics of omapatrilat international research study. Circulation 2002;105:2955–2961.

26 Ferrier KE, Muhlmann MH, Baguet JP, Cameron JD, Jennings GL, Dart AM, Kingwell BA: Intensive cholesterol reduction lowers blood pressure and large artery stiffness in isolated systolic hypertension. J Am Coll Cardiol 2002;39:1020–1025.

27 Kass DA, Shapiro EP, Kawaguchi M, Capriotti AR, Scuteri A, deGroof RC, Lakatta EG: Improved arterial compliance by a novel advanced glycation end-product crosslink breaker. Circulation 2001;104:1464–1470.

28 Susic D, Varagic J, Ahn J, Frohlich ED: Cardiovascular and renal effects of a collagen cross-link breaker (ALT-711) in adult and aged spontaneously hypertensive rats. Am J Hypertens 2004;17:328–333.

Edward D. Frohlich, MD
Ochsner Clinic Foundation
1514 Jefferson Highway
New Orleans, LA 70121 (USA)
Tel. +1 504 842 3700, Fax +1 504 842 3258, E-Mail efrohlich@ochsner.org

Safar ME, Frohlich ED (eds): Atherosclerosis, Large Arteries and Cardiovascular Risk.
Adv Cardiol. Basel, Karger, 2007, vol 44, pp 125–138

....

Arterial Stiffness and Coronary Ischemic Disease

Bronwyn A. Kingwell   Anna A. Ahimastos

Baker Heart Research Institute, Melbourne, Australia

Abstract

Large artery stiffening may be both a cause and a consequence of atherosclerosis and is independently related to coronary outcome. This relationship is likely to be causal given the unfavourable effect of large artery stiffening on coronary hemodynamics. There is clear experimental and clinical evidence that large artery stiffening promotes myocardial ischemia secondary to central pulse pressure elevation. Many agents commonly used to treat ischemic heart disease symptoms also reduce large artery stiffness, through both functional and structural mechanisms. Such effects likely contribute to the anti-ischemic actions of these drugs. However, it remains to be elucidated whether agents specifically targeted to reduce large artery stiffness provide ischemic protection in the setting of coronary disease.

Introduction

Stiff large arteries are associated with coronary artery disease [1–7], myocardial ischemia [8, 9] and coronary mortality [10]. The inter-relationships between large artery stiffness and coronary artery disease are not straightforward and are likely bidirectional (fig. 1). That is, arterial stiffness may be both a cause and a consequence of atherosclerosis. However, regardless of mechanism, it is clear that large artery stiffening exacerbates the ischemic symptoms of coronary disease [9] (fig. 1). The relationship between arterial stiffness and death from coronary artery disease is thus likely to be causal. This chapter will

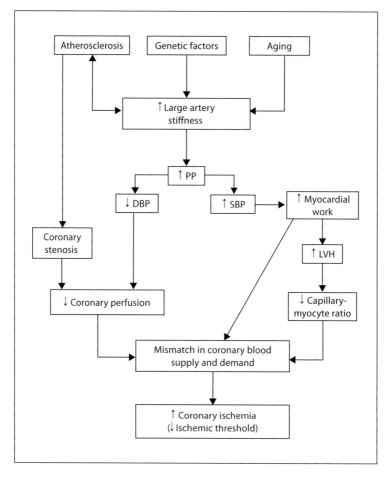

Fig. 1. Schematic diagram showing the proposed links between large artery stiffness, atherosclerosis and coronary ischemic threshold. DBP = Diastolic blood pressure; LVH = left ventricular hypertrophy; PP = pulse pressure; SBP = systolic blood pressure.

discuss the mechanisms linking large artery stiffness and coronary artery disease. It will further examine the consequences for symptoms and outcome. The effect on arterial stiffness of conventional therapies for treatment of coronary disease symptoms will be discussed with regard to mechanisms of benefit. Finally, the therapeutic potential of therapies specifically targeting the large arteries will be discussed with regard to ischemic coronary disease.

Arterial Stiffness as a Risk Factor for Ischemic Heart Disease

Strong relationships between pulse pressure and coronary outcomes provided some of the first definitive evidence that large artery stiffness may be a risk factor for coronary disease [11–13]. In 2002, Boutouyrie et al. [10] published the first study directly relating a measure of large artery stiffness (pulse wave velocity) to coronary outcome during a 15-year follow-up in a hypertensive French cohort. Certainly, indices of arterial stiffness including pulse wave velocity are higher in patients with angiographically determined coronary disease than those without [1–7]. Several studies have also reported a positive correlation between arterial stiffness and the severity of coronary disease. Waddell et al. [6] showed that both systemic arterial compliance and central blood pressure were independently related to the maximum coronary stenosis determined angiographically. Similarly, both augmentation index and augmentation pressure have been associated with an increased risk of angiographically determined coronary disease [14]. Small artery compliance also relates to diffuse, but not focal coronary disease [15]. Interestingly, coronary disease severity and pulse pressure, which is significantly influenced by large artery stiffness, track together in post-menopausal women. In the Estrogen Replacement in Atherosclerosis trial, pulse pressure related closely to standardized measures of minimum angiographically determined coronary lumen diameter during 3.2 years' follow-up [16]. The tight association between stiffness of the large arteries and coronary disease severity suggest that these two phenomena are closely inter-related.

Large artery stiffness may be either a marker or a cause of coronary atherosclerosis or may contribute to coronary ischemia independently of any relationship with coronary atherosclerosis. The first possibility is that atherosclerosis in the coronaries and the aorta develops in parallel, and that large artery stiffness is simply a surrogate measure of atherosclerosis in both regions [17]. That atherosclerosis promotes arterial stiffening is certainly well established. For example in monkeys, development of aortic atherosclerosis on an atherogenic diet has been associated with elevation in pulse wave velocity [18–20]. Of greater interest is the possibility that intrinsic stiffening of the large arteries independently of atherosclerosis, and perhaps related to age or genetic factors, could actually promote atherosclerosis in the coronaries. Certainly large artery stiffness has been shown to be heritable [21] and a number of genes regulating arterial structure have been associated with arterial stiffness in various contexts [21–26]. It would be expected that individuals with intrinsically stiff large vessels would have elevated pulse pressure and that this could contribute to an unfavorable hemodynamic profile promoting atherosclerosis. In vitro studies of rabbit carotid arteries show that elevated pressure pulsatility

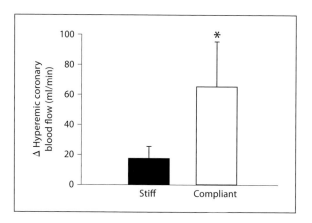

Fig. 2. The change in hyperemic coronary blood flow following percutaneous coronary intervention in patients categorized as having a stiff aorta (central pulse wave velocity ~9 m/s), and as having a compliant aorta (central pulse wave velocity ~6 m/s). Data are presented as mean ± SEM. * p = 0.002 [adapted from 8].

induces endothelial dysfunction as indexed by acetylcholine reactivity [27] and may thus be an antecedent of coronary atherosclerosis.

Regardless of whether large artery stiffness is a marker of coronary atherosclerosis or actually contributes to its development, it would be expected to also have independent detrimental effects on the relationship between myocardial blood supply and demand. Elevated pulse pressure secondary to large artery stiffening could affect coronary outcomes through increased systolic pressure and thus afterload [28]. Chronic afterload elevation would likely lead to development of left ventricular hypertrophy [29–31] and a reduction in capillary to myocyte ratio [32]. Coronary perfusion is also likely to diminish secondary to diastolic pressure reduction. Indeed, it has been elegantly demonstrated in a dog study that ejection into a stiff aortic bypass increases pulse pressure and the energetic cost to the heart to maintain adequate cardiac output [33]. In addition, subendocardial perfusion was particularly compromised when ejection was into a stiff aorta in the setting of an applied coronary stenosis [34]. These data demonstrate that elevation in aortic stiffness tightens the link between cardiac systolic performance and myocardial perfusion [35]. The clinical relevance of this experimental modeling has recently been demonstrated by Leung et al. [8]. In patients undergoing routine percutaneous coronary intervention, those with stiffer aortas had lower coronary blood flow, lower hyperemic coronary blood flow response and a smaller improvement in the hyperemic coronary blood flow after a successful intervention [8]. In this

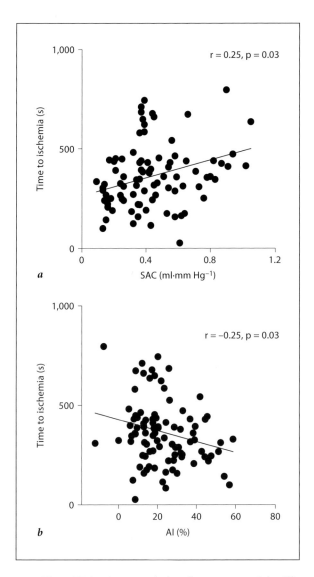

Fig. 3. Univariate correlations between arterial stiffness indices and time to ST segment depression of 1.5 mm (time to ischemia). All data are adjusted to the mean age of the group (62 years) using the slope of the univariate relationship between each variable and age. The full regression equations for SAC (*a*) and AI (*b*) are: Time to ischemia = $-7.47 \cdot age + 179 \cdot SAC + 738$; Time to ischemia = $-7.90 \cdot age - 2.53 \cdot AI + 910$. AI = Augmentation index; SAC = systemic arterial compliance [adapted from 9].

study the patients were dichotomized into those with low (~6 m/s) and high (~9 m/s) pulse wave velocity. Those with lower pulse wave velocity (more compliant arteries) had a dramatic threefold greater coronary hyperemic response after their percutaneous coronary intervention (fig. 2). That this mechanism impacts on physical capacity has been demonstrated by the finding that for any given degree of coronary disease, patients with stiffer large arteries have a lower ischemic threshold during a standard treadmill test [9] (fig. 3). In this study, when the mean systemic arterial compliance of 0.43 was increased to 0.53, the average time to ischemia would increase by 18 s (calculations made for the population mean age of 62 years, fig. 3a), whereas a reduction in the mean augmentation pressure of 23% to 18% increased time to ischemia by 13 s (fig. 3b). Thus the influence of stiffness on ischemic time was modest, but nevertheless measurable. Large artery stiffness is therefore likely to contribute to ischemic risk and be a potential therapeutic target for individuals with coronary disease.

The importance of large artery stiffening as an ischemic mechanism also depends on the prevalence of isolated systolic hypertension and its co-occurrence with coronary artery disease. Isolated systolic hypertension affects 26% of the population over 55 years of age [36], and is a strong predictor of cerebrovascular and cardiac events [28, 37–39]. For males and females aged between 25 and 64 with isolated systolic hypertension, the relative coronary risk is 1.5 and 2.2 respectively, compared to normotensive subjects [28]. The incidence of isolated systolic hypertension amongst those with clinically significant coronary disease is more difficult to quantify. As discussed in the previous section, the close relationship between large artery stiffness and atherosclerotic coronary disease suggests that the majority of coronary patients would have elevated large artery stiffness and therefore pulse pressure. While this elevation will not always fall into the range to be categorized as isolated systolic hypertension, pulse pressure elevation would nevertheless influence ischemic threshold.

Arterial Stiffness as Therapeutic Target in Ischemic Coronary Artery Disease

At present there are no clinically available agents which specifically target the large arteries. However, many conventional cardiovascular therapies, both pharmacological and non-pharmacological, reduce large artery stiffness, and clinical trials of more specific agents are underway. Arterial stiffness can be reduced both via passive (functional) mechanisms and through structural changes to the arterial wall. Functional reduction in arterial stiffness can be achieved through lowering mean arterial pressure or through vasodilation, which alters the relative loading of collagen and elastin in the arterial wall [40]. All antihypertensive and vasodilator agents reduce arterial stiffness via this mechanism. Many agents in these classes and others also influence arterial wall structure and thus biomechanical properties directly. The following section will briefly discuss the interactions of drugs commonly prescribed for treatment of the symptoms of ischemic coronary disease with respect to large artery stiffness and the implications for ischemia and outcome. In addition to their more direct actions, those agents which reduce large artery stiffness are likely to have additional benefit with regard to raising ischemic threshold. This would relate to reduction in pulse pressure and afterload and elevation in coronary perfusion. In the long term this hemodynamic profile might also be favorable with respect to limiting atherosclerotic progression and reducing risk of coronary plaque destabilization and rupture. The effect of drugs used to treat risk factors to improve cardiovascular outcomes are discussed in Section IV of this book.

Nitrates

Nitrates are an important anti-ischemic therapy which are thought to act, at least in part, through release of nitric oxide, although there is currently some controversy surrounding this issue [41, 42]. There is good evidence that under basal conditions, nitric oxide acts to lower both pulse wave velocity and arterial wave reflection [43]. Nitrate drugs would therefore be expected to reduce large artery stiffness and wave reflection. Acute administration of isosorbide dinitrate to untreated hypertensive individuals increased systemic arterial compliance and reduced peripheral wave reflection [44]. This effect was likely secondary to a reduction in mean arterial blood pressure [44]. Similarly, glyceryl trinitrate reduces arterial stiffness acutely in hypertensive patients [45]. In a double-blind randomized placebo-controlled study, isosorbide dinitrate resulted in a reduction in office and ambulatory pulse pressure following 8 weeks of treatment, without a reduction in diastolic blood pressure [46] in patients with isolated systolic hypertension. Similar hemodynamic findings have also been observed with the use of nitroglycerin or molsidomine (a glycosidase-activated nitric oxide donor) in hypertensive patients [47]. The fact that nitrates decrease pulse pressure whilst having no effect on diastolic blood pressure suggests that these agents act mainly on large arteries rather than on small resistance vessels. The blood pressure-lowering effects of chronic nitrate therapy would certainly be expected to mediate reduction in large artery stiffness [48]. In addition, studies in minipigs suggest that chronic nitrate therapy may also improve the viscoelastic properties of the arterial wall [49].

Potassium Channel Openers

Like nitrates, the ATP-sensitive K^+ channel opener, nicorandil, causes vasodilation with subsequent reduction in preload and afterload, and an increase in coronary blood flow. Only a single study has examined the effect of nicorandil on biomechanical artery properties and this was in the periphery. Acute administration of nicorandil reduced brachial artery stiffness as demonstrated by a decrease in brachioradial pulse wave velocity [50]. This was likely mediated by a reduction in mean arterial blood pressure.

β-Blockers

β-Blockers improve symptoms of angina and are commonly prescribed for the treatment of ischemic heart disease. It is generally accepted that β-blockers with vasodilator actions including pindolol, dilevalol, celiprolol and nebivolol have greater efficacy in reducing large artery stiffness than non-vasodilating β-blockers (e.g., atenolol) [51–55]. It is likely that blood pressure reduction may provide benefit, including ischemic protection through reduction in arterial stiffness [53]. Chronic therapy with dilevalol or atenolol for 12 weeks reduced arterial stiffness, while the vasodilator actions of dilevalol had the added benefit of reduction in wave reflection [53]. The selective β_1-blocking agent, bisoprolol, has also been shown to reduce both blood pressure and artery stiffness with chronic treatment [56]. Vasodilating (highly-selective β_1-adrenoceptor antagonist) β-blockers such as nebivolol, but not atenolol which is non-vasodilating, reduce arterial stiffness in sheep [57]. β-Blockers are also commonly prescribed in Marfan syndrome to limit aortic dilation. However, the effect of β blockade on arterial stiffness in this population is somewhat controversial. In both acute [58] and long-term studies of aortic stiffness [59] in Marfan syndrome, β-blockers reduce wall stiffness only in those patients with normal or mildly increased aortic dimensions. In patients with significant aortic dilatation, an increase in wall stiffness is seen with β-blockade. Such an effect could be potentially detrimental in these patients [58]. Thus from the perspective of arterial stiffness, β-blockers with vasodilating activity are likely to be most effective in patients with normal or only mildly elevated aortic dimensions.

Calcium Antagonists

Calcium antagonists cause dilation of epicardial conduit vessels (thus relieving vasospastic angina) and of arterial resistance vessels. They also reduce systemic vascular resistance and arterial pressure and thereby myocardial oxygen demand. Chronic calcium antagonist therapy is generally accepted to reduce arterial stiffness on par with other antihypertensive agents including angiotensin-converting enzyme inhibitors and diuretics [39, 60, 61]. However, there is some evidence that calcium channel blockers may have structural effects on the arterial wall and reduce stiffness by mechanisms additional to blood pressure reduction. In a study comparing 12 weeks of treatment with the calcium channel blocker felodipine or the diuretic hydrochlorothiazide in hypertensive patients, felodipine reduced central and peripheral pulse wave velocity, whereas hydrochlorothiazide did not [62]. Both drugs had similar effects on blood pressure, suggesting that calcium channel blockers may exert direct arterial wall effects. Similarly, peripheral compliance was improved by the calcium channel blocker nicardipine but not by the β-blocker atenolol in hypertensive patients following 8 months of treatment eliciting similar blood pressure effects [63].

Antiplatelet Therapy

Few studies have examined the effects of chronic aspirin therapy on arterial properties. While aspirin treatment at 325 mg/day for 1 week has been associated with a detrimental effect on wave reflection [64], chronic low dose aspirin (100 mg/day) had no significant effect on augmentation index and wave reflection patterns in two studies [64, 65]. On the other hand, low-dose aspirin has slight antihypertensive effects when administered in the evening [66]. Such an effect would be expected to contribute to a reduction in large artery stiffness. It is possible that aspirin could mediate effects on arterial stiffness via its anti-inflammatory actions which decrease arterial tone [67]. It has recently been shown that inflammation caused by *Salmonella typhi* vaccination increases pulse wave velocity [68]. In reducing acute inflammation, aspirin may therefore reduce arterial stiffness [68]. Whether other antiplatelet agents affect arterial properties is unknown.

Experimental Therapies Which May More Directly Target the Large Arteries

Compliance of the arterial wall is dependent on two primary scaffolding proteins, collagen and elastin. Dysregulation in the production and degradation of these two molecules can lead to overproduction of abnormal collagen and reduced quantities of normal elastin, contributing to increased arterial stiffness. In addition, irreversible non-enzymatic cross-linking of arterial matrix components can be caused by advanced glycation end products (AGEs) [69]. Drugs which prevent cross-link formation or break existing cross-links are in development. Aminoguanidine, which inhibits cross-link formation, improves arterial compliance and reduces pulse wave velocity; however, high doses can result in glomerulonephritis [70]. Alagebrium or ALT-711 is an AGE cross-link breaker and reverses arterial stiffening without influencing blood pressure in animal models [71]. Furthermore, in a randomized, clinical trial in patients with elevated pulse pressure, ALT-711 significantly reduced pulse pressure and pulse wave velocity and increased arterial compliance [72]. AGE breakers would be expected to have particular efficacy in patients with diabetes. However, non-diabetic individuals with coronary disease are known to have elevated AGE levels proportional to the number of diseased vessels [73] and these individuals may also benefit. Clinical trials are currently underway to examine the effect of ALT-711 on large artery stiffness in patients with coronary artery disease, diabetes and isolated systolic hypertension [74]. Finally, since genetic modulation of extracellular matrix components and matrix metalloproteinases contribute to atherosclerotic differences in large artery mechanical properties, these proteins may be important targets for therapy [23, 24, 75].

To summarize: Large artery stiffening is closely related to coronary atherosclerosis and outcome. Parallels in atherosclerotic burden between these beds likely explain part of this relationship. In addition, large artery stiffness per se promotes an unfavorable hemodynamic profile which may cause endothelial disruption, which further promotes the atherosclerotic process. Furthermore, studies in both animals and man indicate that large artery stiffening promotes a mismatch in cardiac blood supply and demand through pulse pressure elevation. Many agents commonly used to treat ischemic heart disease symptoms including nitrates, aspirin, vasodilating adrenergic antagonists, calcium antagonists and potassium channel openers, reduce large artery stiffness, at least in part, through reduction in mean arterial pressure. Some of these agents may also have structural effects on the arterial wall which influence arterial biomechanical properties. AGE breakers such as ALT-711 have shown promise in directly reducing large artery stiffness via structural effects. It remains to be determined whether agents specifically targeted to reduce large artery stiffness provide ischemic protection in the setting of coronary disease.

References

1   Hirai T, Sasayama S, Kawasaki T, Yagi S: Stiffness of systemic arteries in patients with myocardial infarction. A noninvasive method to predict severity of coronary atherosclerosis. Circulation 1989;80:78–86.
2   Triposkiadis F, Kallikazaros I, Trikas A, Stefanadis C, Stratos C, Tsekoura D, et al: A comparative study of the effect of coronary artery disease on ascending and abdominal aorta distensibility and pulse wave velocity. Acta Cardiol 1993;48:221–233.
3   Barenbrock M, Spieker C, Kerber S, Vielhauer C, Hoeks AP, Zidek W, et al: Different effects of hypertension, atherosclerosis and hyperlipidaemia on arterial distensibility. J Hypertens 1995; 13:1712–1717.
4   Cameron JD, Jennings GL, Dart AM: Systemic arterial compliance is decreased in newly-diagnosed patients with coronary heart disease: implications for prediction of risk. J Cardiovasc Risk 1996;3:495–500.

5   Gatzka CD, Cameron JD, Kingwell BA, Dart AM: Relation between coronary artery disease, aortic stiffness, and left ventricular structure in a population sample. Hypertension 1998;32: 575–578.

6   Waddell TK, Dart AM, Medley TL, Cameron JD, Kingwell BA: Carotid pressure is a better predictor of coronary artery disease severity than brachial pressure. Hypertension 2001;38:927–931.

7   Lim HE, Park CG, Shin SH, Ahn JC, Seo HS, Oh DJ: Aortic pulse wave velocity as an independent marker of coronary artery disease. Blood Press 2004;13:369–375.

8   Leung MC, Meredith IT, Cameron JD: Aortic stiffness affects the coronary blood flow response to percutaneous coronary intervention. Am J Physiol Heart Circ Physiol 2005;290:H624–H630.

9   Kingwell BA, Waddell TK, Medley TL, Cameron JD, Dart AM: Large artery stiffness predicts ischemic threshold in patients with coronary artery disease. J Am Coll Cardiol 2002;40:773–779.

10 Boutouyrie P, Tropeano AI, Asmar R, Gautier I, Benetos A, Lacolley P, et al: Aortic stiffness is an independent predictor of primary coronary events in hypertensive patients: a longitudinal study. Hypertension 2002;39:10–15.

11 Darne B, Girerd X, Safar M, Cambien F, Guize L: Pulsatile versus steady component of blood pressure: a cross-sectional analysis and a prospective analysis on cardiovascular mortality. Hypertension 1989;13:392–400.

12 Benetos A, Safar M, Rudnichi A, Smulyan H, Richard JL, Ducimetiere P, et al: Pulse pressure: a predictor of long-term cardiovascular mortality in a French male population. Hypertension 1997;30:1410–1415.

13 Domanski MJ, Mitchell GF, Norman JE, Exner DV, Pitt B, Pfeffer MA: Independent prognostic information provided by sphygmomanometrically determined pulse pressure and mean arterial pressure in patients with left ventricular dysfunction. J Am Coll Cardiol 1999;33:951–958.

14 Weber T, Auer J, O'Rourke MF, Kvas E, Lassnig E, Berent R, et al: Arterial stiffness, wave reflections, and the risk of coronary artery disease. Circulation 2004;109:184–189.

15 Syeda B, Gottsauner-Wolf M, Denk S, Pichler P, Khorsand A, Glogar D: Arterial compliance: a diagnostic marker for atherosclerotic plaque burden? Am J Hypertens 2003;16:356–362.

16 Nair GV, Waters D, Rogers W, Kowalchuk GJ, Stuckey TD, Herrington DM: Pulse pressure and coronary atherosclerosis progression in postmenopausal women. Hypertension 2005;45:53–57.

17 Vihert AM: Atherosclerosis of the aorta and coronary arteries in coronary heart disease. Bull World Health Organ 1976;53:585–596.

18 Farrar DJ, Bond MG, Sawyer JK, Green HD: Pulse wave velocity and morphological changes associated with early atherosclerosis progression in the aortas of cynomolgus monkeys. Cardiovasc Res 1984;18:107–118.

19 Farrar DJ, Green HD, Wagner WD, Bond MG: Reduction in pulse wave velocity and improvement of aortic distensibility accompanying regression of atherosclerosis in the rhesus monkey. Circ Res 1980;47:425–432.

20 Farrar DJ, Green HD, Bond MG, Wagner WD, Gobbee RA: Aortic pulse wave velocity, elasticity, and composition in a nonhuman primate model of atherosclerosis. Circ Res 1978;43:52–62.

21 Mitchell GF, DeStefano AL, Larson MG, Benjamin EJ, Chen MH, Vasan RS, et al: Heritability and a genome-wide linkage scan for arterial stiffness, wave reflection, and mean arterial pressure: the Framingham Heart Study. Circulation 2005;112:194–199.

22 Medley TL, Cole TJ, Gatzka CD, Wang WY, Dart A, Kingwell BA: Fibrillin-1 genotype is associated with aortic stiffness and disease severity in patients with coronary artery disease. Circulation 2002;19:810–815.

23 Medley TL, Kingwell BA, Gatzka CD, Pillay P, Cole TJ: Matrix metalloproteinase-3 genotype contributes to age-related aortic stiffening through modulation of gene and protein expression. Circ Res 2003;92:1254–1261.

24 Medley TL, Cole TJ, Dart AM, Gatzka CD, Kingwell BA: Matrix metalloproteinase-9 genotype influences large artery stiffness through effects on aortic gene and protein expression. Arterioscler Thromb Vasc Biol 2004;24:1479–1484.

25 Durier S, Fassot C, Laurent S, Boutouyrie P, Couetil JP, Fine E, et al: Physiological genomics of human arteries: quantitative relationship between gene expression and arterial stiffness. Circulation 2003;108:1845–1851.

26   Benetos A, Gautier S, Ricard S, Topouchian J, Asmar R, Poirier O, et al: Influence of angiotensin-converting enzyme and angiotensin II type 1 receptor gene polymorphisms on aortic stiffness in normotensive and hypertensive patients. Circulation 1996;94:698–703.

27   Ryan SM, Waack BJ, Weno BL, Heistad DD: Increases in pulse pressure impair acetylcholine-induced vascular relaxation. Am J Physiol 1995;268:H359–H363.

28   Antikainen R, Jousilahti P, Tuomilehto J: Systolic blood pressure, isolated systolic hypertension and risk of coronary heart disease, strokes, cardiovascular disease and all-cause mortality in the middle-aged population. J Hypertens 1998;16:577–583.

29   Rajkumar C, Cameron JD, Christophidis N, Jennings GL, Dart AM: Reduced systemic arterial compliance is associated with left ventricular hypertrophy and diastolic dysfunction in older people. J Am Geriatr Soc 1997;45:803–808.

30   Nitta K, Akiba T, Uchida K, Otsubo S, Otsubo Y, Takei T, et al: Left ventricular hypertrophy is associated with arterial stiffness and vascular calcification in hemodialysis patients. Hypertens Res 2004;27:47–52.

31   Lekakis JP, Zakopoulos NA, Protogerou AD, Papaioannou TG, Kotsis VT, Pitiriga V, et al: Arterial stiffness assessed by pulse wave analysis in essential hypertension: relation to 24-hour blood pressure profile. Int J Cardiol 2005;102:391–395.

32   Marcus ML, Koyanagi S, Harrison DG, Doty DB, Hiratzka LF, Eastham CL: Abnormalities in the coronary circulation that occur as a consequence of cardiac hypertrophy. Am J Med 1983;75: 62–66.

33   Kelly RP, Tunin R, Kass DA: Effect of reduced aortic compliance on cardiac efficiency and contractile function of in situ canine left ventricle. Circ Res 1992;71:490–502.

34   Watanabe H, Ohtsuka S, Kakihana M, Sugishita Y: Coronary circulation in dogs with an experimental decrease in aortic compliance. J Am Coll Cardiol 1993;21:1497–1506.

35   Kass DA, Saeki A, Tunin RS, Recchia FA: Adverse influence of systemic vascular stiffening on cardiac dysfunction and adaptation to acute coronary occlusion. Circulation 1996;93:1533–1541.

36   Langille DB, Joffres MR, MacPherson KM, Andreou P, Kirkland SA, MacLean DR: Prevalence of risk factors for cardiovascular disease in Canadians 55–74 years of age: results from the Canadian Heart Health Surveys, 1986–1992. CMAJ 1999;161(8 suppl):S3–S9.

37   Nielsen WB, Vestbo J, Jensen GB: Isolated systolic hypertension as a major risk factor for stroke and myocardial infarction and an unexploited source of cardiovascular prevention: a prospective population-based study. J Hum Hypertens 1995;9:175–180.

38   Himmelmann A, Hedner T, Hansson L, O'Donnell CJ, Levy D: Isolated systolic hypertension: an important cardiovascular risk factor. Blood Press 1998;7:197–207.

39   Dart AM, Kingwell BA: Pulse pressure – a review of mechanisms and clinical relevance. J Am Coll Cardiol 2001;37:975–984.

40   Belz GG: Elastic properties and windkessel function of the human aorta. Cardiovasc Drugs Ther 1995;9:73–83.

41   Kleschyov AL, Oelze M, Daiber A, Huang Y, Mollnau H, Schulz E, et al: Does nitric oxide mediate the vasodilator activity of nitroglycerin? Circ Res 2003;93:e104–e112.

42   Thatcher GR, Nicolescu AC, Bennett BM, Toader V: Nitrates and NO release: contemporary aspects in biological and medicinal chemistry. Free Radic Biol Med 2004;37:1122–1143.

43   Wilkinson IB, MacCallum H, Cockcroft JR, Webb DJ: Inhibition of basal nitric oxide synthesis increases aortic augmentation index and pulse wave velocity in vivo. Br J Clin Pharmacol 2002; 53:189–192.

44   Laurent S, Arcaro G, Benetos A, Lafleche A, Hoeks AP, Safar M: Mechanism of nitrate-induced improvement on arterial compliance depends on vascular territory. J Cardiovasc Pharmacol 1992;19:641–649.

45   Simon AC, Levenson JA, Levy BY, Bouthier JE, Peronneau PP, Safar ME: Effect of nitroglycerin on peripheral large arteries in hypertension. Br J Clin Pharmacol 1982;14:241–246.

46   Starmans-Kool MJ, Kleinjans HA, Lustermans FA, Kragten JA, Breed JG, Van Bortel LM: Treatment of elderly patients with isolated systolic hypertension with isosorbide dinitrate in an asymmetric dosing schedule. J Hum Hypertens 1998;12:557–561.

47   Bouthier JD, Safar ME, Benetos A, Simon AC, Levenson JA, Hugues CM: Haemodynamic effects of vasodilating drugs on the common carotid and brachial circulations of patients with essential hypertension. Br J Clin Pharmacol 1986;21:137–142.

48   Duchier J, Iannascoli F, Safar M: Antihypertensive effect of sustained-release isosorbide dinitrate for isolated systolic systemic hypertension in the elderly. Am J Cardiol 1987;60:99–102.

49   Augier T, Bertolotti C, Friggi A, Charpiot P, Barlatier A, Bodard H, et al: Therapeutic effects of nitric oxide-donor isosorbide dinitrate on atherosclerosis-induced alterations in hemodynamics and arterial viscoelasticity are independent of the wall elastic component. J Cardiovasc Pharmacol 1996;27:752–759.

50   Levenson JA, Bouthier JE, Chau NP, Roland E, Simon AC: Effects of nicorandil on arterial and venous vessels of the forearm in systemic hypertension. Am J Cardiol 1989;63:40J–43J.

51   Simon AC, Levenson J, Bouthier JD, Safar ME: Effects of chronic administration of enalapril and propranolol on the large arteries in essential hypertension. J Cardiovasc Pharmacol 1985;7:856–861.

52   Ting CT, Chen CH, Chang MS, Yin FC: Short- and long-term effects of antihypertensive drugs on arterial reflections, compliance, and impedance. Hypertension 1995;26:524–530.

53   Kelly R, Daley J, Avolio AP, O'Rourke MF: Arterial dilation and reduced wave reflection: benefit of dilevalol in hypertension. Hypertension 1989;14:14–21.

54   Van Merode T, van Bortel LM, Smeets FA, Mooij JM, Bohm RO, Rahn KH, et al: Verapamil and nebivolol improve carotid artery distensibility in hypertensive patients. J Hypertens Suppl 1989; 7:S262–S263.

55   Boutouyrie P, Bussy C, Hayoz D, Hengstler J, Dartois N, Laloux B, et al: Local pulse pressure and regression of arterial wall hypertrophy during long-term antihypertensive treatment. Circulation 2000;101:2601–2606.

56   Asmar R, Kerihuel JC, Girerd XJ, Safar M: Effect of bisoprolol on blood pressure and arterial hemodynamics in systemic hypertension. Am J Cardiol 1991;68:61–64.

57   McEniery CM, Schmitt M, Qasem A, Webb DJ, Avolio AP, Wilkinson IB, et al: Nebivolol increases arterial distensibility in vivo. Hypertension 2004;44:305–310.

58   Haouzi A, Berglund H, Pelikan PC, Maurer G, Siegel RJ: Heterogeneous aortic response to acute β-adrenergic blockade in Marfan syndrome. Am Heart J 1997;133:60–63.

59   Rios AS, Silber EN, Bavishi N, Varga P, Burton BK, Clark WA, et al: Effect of long-term β-blockade on aortic root compliance in patients with Marfan syndrome. Am Heart J 1999;137:1057–1061.

60   Delerme S, Boutouyrie P, Laloux B, Gautier I, Benetos A, Asmar R, et al: Aortic stiffness is reduced beyond blood pressure lowering by short- and long-term antihypertensive treatment: a meta-analysis of individual data in 294 patients (abstract). Hypertension 1998;32:789.

61   Laurent S, Kingwell B, Bank A, Weber M, Struijker-Boudier H: Clinical applications of arterial stiffness: therapeutics and pharmacology. Am J Hypertens 2002;15:453–458.

62   Asmar RG, Benetos A, Chaouche-Teyara K, Raveau-Landon CM, Safar ME: Comparison of effects of felodipine versus hydrochlorothiazide on arterial diameter and pulse-wave velocity in essential hypertension. Am J Cardiol 1993;72:794–798.

63   De Cesaris R, Ranieri G, Filitti V, Andriani A: Large artery compliance in essential hypertension. Effects of calcium antagonism and β-blocking. Am J Hypertens 1992;5:624–628.

64   Meune C, Mahe I, Mourad JJ, Cohen-Solal A, Levy B, Kevorkian JP, et al: Aspirin alters arterial function in patients with chronic heart failure treated with ACE inhibitors: a dose-mediated deleterious effect. Eur J Heart Fail 2003;5:271–279.

65   Weber T, Eber B, Auer J: Aspirin, ACE inhibitors and arterial stiffness. Eur J Heart Fail 2004;6: 117–118.

66   Hermida RC, Ayala DE, Calvo C, Lopez JE: Aspirin administered at bedtime, but not on awakening, has an effect on ambulatory blood pressure in hypertensive patients. J Am Coll Cardiol 2005;46:975–983.

67   Von der Weid PY, Hollenberg MD, Fiorucci S, Wallace JL: Aspirin-triggered, cyclooxygenase-2-dependent lipoxin synthesis modulates vascular tone. Circulation 2004;110:1320–1325.

68   Vlachopoulos C, Dima I, Aznaouridis K, Vasiliadou C, Ioakeimidis N, Aggeli C, et al: Acute systemic inflammation increases arterial stiffness and decreases wave reflections in healthy individuals. Circulation 2005;112:2193–2200.

69   Zieman SJ, Melenovsky V, Kass DA: Mechanisms, pathophysiology, and therapy of arterial stiff-ness. Arterioscler Thromb Vasc Biol 2005;25:932–943.
70   Bolton WK, Cattran DC, Williams ME, Adler SG, Appel GB, Cartwright K, et al: Randomized trial of an inhibitor of formation of advanced glycation end products in diabetic nephropathy. Am J Nephrol 2004;24:32–40.
71   Wolffenbuttel BH, Boulanger CM, Crijns FR, Huijberts MS, Poitevin P, Swennen GN, et al: Breakers of advanced glycation end products restore large artery properties in experimental diabetes. Proc Natl Acad Sci USA 1998;95:4630–4634.
72   Kass DA, Shapiro EP, Kawaguchi M, Capriotti AR, Scuteri A, deGroof RC, et al: Improved arte-rial compliance by a novel advanced glycation end-product crosslink breaker. Circulation 2001; 104:1464–1470.
73   Kanauchi M, Tsujimoto N, Hashimoto T: Advanced glycation end products in nondiabetic pa-tients with coronary artery disease. Diabetes Care 2001;24:1620–1623.
74   Bakris GL, Bank AJ, Kass DA, Neutel JM, Preston RA, Oparil S: Advanced glycation end-product cross-link breakers: a novel approach to cardiovascular pathologies related to the aging process. Am J Hypertens 2004;17:23S–30S.
75   Kingwell BA, Medley TL, Waddell TK, Cole TJ, Dart AM, Jennings GL: Large artery stiffness: structural and genetic aspects. Clin Exp Pharmacol Physiol 2001;28:1040–1043.

Bronwyn Kingwell, A/Prof.
Baker Heart Research Institute
PO Box 6492, St Kilda Road Central
Melbourne, Vic 8008 (Australia)
Tel. +61 3 9276 3261, Fax +61 3 9276 2461, E-Mail b.kingwell@alfred.org.au

Safar ME, Frohlich ED (eds): Atherosclerosis, Large Arteries and Cardiovascular Risk.
Adv Cardiol. Basel, Karger, 2007, vol 44, pp 139–149

....

Central Pulse Pressure and Atherosclerotic Alterations of Coronary Arteries

Nicolas Danchin[a]   *Jean-Jacques Mourad*[b]

[a]Department of Cardiology, Hôpital Européen Georges Pompidou, Paris, and
[b]Department of Internal Medicine, Hôpital Avicenne, Bobigny, France

Abstract

Central pulse pressure is more likely to reflect the haemodynamic conditions to which the heart and coronary arteries are subjected than is peripheral pulse. We reviewed the data currently available on the correlations between central pulse pressure and both the presence and extent of coronary artery disease, as well as clinical outcomes. Five clinical studies have reported an association between central pulse pressure and the presence of coronary artery disease documented by coronary angiography. Four studies, including three of the previous ones, also found a correlation between central pulse pressure and the extent of coronary artery disease. In one of these studies, however, the correlation was present only in men, whereas no link was found between pulse pressure and coronary artery disease in women. After coronary angioplasty, increased central pulse pressure has been found correlated with the occurrence of restenosis after balloon angioplasty, but not after stent implantation. Finally, the ASCOT-CAFE trial found a positive correlation between pulse pressure and the occurrence of cardiovascular events, confirming the prognostic significance of this parameter.

Although there is epidemiologic evidence of a relationship between brachial pulse pressure and cardiovascular events, including coronary events, conflicting data have also been reported [1–4]. This may be because brachial pulse pressure is likely to be a less reliable index of the condition of the coronary arteries than central pulse pressure. In the present article, we will review the data currently available on the links between central and peripheral pulse pressure, as well as the data on the correlations between central pulse pressure and the presence and extent of coronary artery disease.

Central versus Peripheral Pulse Pressure

Differences between central and peripheral arterial pressures have been described in detail elsewhere [5–8] (Chapter 1). Schematically, the arterial tree can be divided into two compartments (central and peripheral). Brachial pressure represents blood pressure in the peripheral compartment, while aortic (or carotid) pressure represents blood pressure in the central compartment. While diastolic and mean arterial pressures remain more or less constant throughout the arterial tree, the level of systolic blood pressure varies according to the nature of the arteries where it is measured. Thus, systolic blood pressure (and consequently pulse pressure) is notably higher in peripheral than in central arteries (by approximately 14 mm Hg in humans). This difference results from a difference in the summation of the forward and backward pressure waves along the arterial tree, as detailed in Chapter 1. Under physiologic conditions in younger subjects, the backward pressure wave returns to the central arteries during diastole, which explains why pulse pressure is higher in the peripheral than in the central arteries (pulse pressure amplification). However, when reflection occurs earlier, the backward (reflected) wave will reach the central compartment at an earlier stage, during systole. The consequence of this altered timing is an increase in systolic blood pressure and a decrease in diastolic blood pressure, resulting in an increased pulse pressure. Earlier reflection of the pressure wave may be the consequence of increased pulse wave velocity, such as is observed with stiffer and/or calcified arteries, but also of changes in the more peripheral arteries, that will affect their capacity to reflect the pressure wave. Arteriolar constriction, remodeling, and rarefaction can thus increase systolic blood pressure and pulse pressure. In addition, more proximal reflection sites, which have limited impact under normal conditions, may influence wave reflection in certain pathological conditions, such as extensive atherosclerotic disease of the arteries; in particular, the presence of calcifications at the bifurcation of the main branches of the aorta may constitute reflection sites which are more proximal to the ascending aorta and therefore increase pulse pressure. These will influence central pulse pressure whereas peripheral pulse pressure will not be directly affected.

Interpreting the significance of elevated pulse pressure is difficult. Indeed, increased pulse pressure per se is likely to have untoward effects on the coronary circulation because an elevated systolic blood pressure increases vascular load, while a lower diastolic blood pressure will reduce coronary perfusion; but in addition, an increased pulse pressure may correspond to the presence of vascular disease (and in particular, atherosclerosis of the aorta). Therefore, whereas hypertension is a well-known cardiovascular risk factor, pulse pressure might represent more of a marker of preclinical disease [9], as the correla-

Table 1. Central pulse pressure in patients with or without coronary artery disease (CAD) demonstrated by coronary angiography

Study (first author)	Pulse pressure in patients without CAD, mm Hg	Pulse pressure in patients with CAD, mm Hg	p value
Lee [12]	51±16	81±15	<0.0001
Nishijima [14]	69±21	77±22	0.003
Hayashi [15]	66.5±23	74±20	<0.03
Waddell [16][1]	38±1	45±2/53±3[2]	<0.01
Danchin [17]	56±17	61±20	<0.03

[1] Central blood pressure measured non-invasively using carotid blood pressure.

[2] Two groups with CAD of increasing severity.

tions between the presence of atheroma of the thoracic aorta and the presence of coronary artery disease have been well documented. Whatever the case, however, it is obvious that central pulse pressure is more likely to reflect the hemodynamic conditions to which the heart and coronary arteries are subjected than is peripheral pulse.

Central Pulse Pressure and Presence and Extent of Coronary Artery Disease (tables 1, 2)

Over the past 10 years, several studies in different types of populations have shown that central pulse pressure could be related to the presence and extent of coronary artery disease.

Experimental studies have shown that increases in pulse pressure resulted in impaired acetylcholine-induced vascular relaxation [10], suggesting that increased pulse pressure might be involved in the first steps of the process of atherosclerosis. More recently, it has been shown that high pulse pressure on ambulatory recordings was associated with increases in biological markers of thrombogenesis and altered flow-mediated vasodilation in patients with coronary artery disease [11].

To the best of our knowledge, Lee et al. [12], who studied a population of patients undergoing left heart catheterization before intervention for mitral valve stenosis, were the first, in 1998, to show an association between the presence of coronary artery disease and high pulse pressure, measured either at the

Table 2. Central pulse pressure in relation to severity of coronary artery disease (CAD)

Study (first author)	Definition of the groups studied	Central pulse pressure mm Hg	p value
Waddell [16][1]	No CAD, 50–89% stenosis, ≥90% stenosis	38±1/45±2/53±3	<0.01
Danchin [17][2]	No CAD, 1–2 stenoses, ≥3 stenoses	51±16/54±18/64±20	<0.001
Philippe [18]	1-, 2-, and 3-vessel disease	55±18/64±19/66±19	<0.03
Jankowski [19]	1-, 2-, and 3-vessel disease	63±16/65±18/72±19	<0.001

[1] Central blood pressure measured non-invasively using carotid blood pressure.
[2] Male population.

aortic or brachial levels. Central pulse pressure was 81 ± 15 mm Hg in the 48 patients with coronary disease versus 51 ± 16 mm Hg in those with no coronary stenosis. Brachial pulse pressure was also significantly higher in patients with coronary artery disease.

Nearly simultaneously, Gatzka et al. [13] showed that aortic stiffness was higher in patients with chest pain and positive exercise tests, compared with controls.

Nishijima et al. [14] included 293 patients who had undergone coronary angiography for suspected coronary artery disease, and without history of myocardial infarction or presence of local asynergy on left ventriculography. Aortic pressures were recorded in the ascending aorta by means of fluid-filled catheters. There was no significant difference between the group of 102 patients with and the one without coronary artery disease as regards systolic, diastolic and mean blood pressure in the ascending aorta. However, central pulse pressure and fractional pulse pressure, defined as the ratio of pulse pressure to mean blood pressure, were significantly higher, while just a trend was noted for peripheral pulse pressure. When pulsatility was analyzed by tertiles, the odds ratio (OR) for the presence of coronary artery disease, after adjustment for potential confounders, was 2.90 (95% confidence interval (CI): 1.43–5.89) for the second tertile, and 3.47 (95% CI: 1.52–7.95) for the third tertile. Conversely, no significant relationship was found between peripheral pulsatility and the presence of coronary artery disease.

In another Japanese population of 190 patients undergoing coronary angiography, Hayashi et al. [15] analyzed aortic pressures and waveform in relation to coronary heart disease. Central pulse pressure was higher in patients with coronary artery disease (74 ± 20 vs. 66.5 ± 23 mm Hg, p < 0.03). In addition, the inflection time of the aortic pressure waveform, an indicator of large artery function and reflection in the arterial system, was a strong correlate of the presence of coronary atherosclerosis, even after multivariable adjustment.

Concordant findings were reported by Waddell et al. [16] in a cohort of 114 men with coronary artery disease (defined as the presence of at least one ≥50% stenosis on one of the main coronary arteries), compared with 57 age-matched men controls. In addition, coronary artery disease patients were further subdivided into those with moderate disease (n = 57; stenosis severity 50–89%) and those with severe (≥90%) stenoses (n = 57). Central pressure was recorded non-invasively by measuring carotid pressure. Brachial pulse pressure was higher in patients than in controls, but there was no significant difference between the two groups of coronary patients according to the severity of the disease. In contrast, carotid pulse pressure was significantly different in all three groups, and highest in the group with the most severe stenoses. In this study, however, coronary artery disease severity was defined in a rather unusual way, by taking into account the degree of stenosis, but not the extent of coronary disease.

In a larger, multicenter study involving 1,337 patients with suspected coronary artery disease and referred for a first diagnostic angiogram, we analyzed the correlations between the presence and extent of coronary artery disease and aortic pulse pressure in the subset of 280 patients receiving no medications with antihypertensive properties [17]. Blood pressure was measured by fluid-filled catheters in the ascending aorta. Coronary artery disease was defined by the presence of at least one ≥50% stenosis on any of the coronary arteries or their main branches. The extent of coronary artery disease was further characterized by the number of ≥50% stenoses for each patient. In the whole population, brachial pulse pressure was only slightly and not significantly higher in patients with coronary artery disease. In contrast, aortic pulse pressure was 5 mm Hg higher in the population with coronary artery disease (p < 0.03). The size of the population allowed analyzing separately the data according to gender. Interestingly, the correlation between increased central pulse pressure and presence of coronary artery disease was present only in men. Moreover, the extent of coronary disease was also correlated with pulse pressure in men, but not in women: men with no disease, 51 ± 16 mm Hg; 1 or 2 coronary stenoses, 54 ± 18 mm Hg; >2 stenoses, 64 ± 20 mm Hg (p < 0.001). Because several baseline variables were different between patients with or without coronary artery disease, a multiple regression analysis was performed to determine whether aortic pulse pressure was an independent correlate of coronary artery disease. In women, there was no significant association between pulse pressure and coronary artery disease. In contrast, in men, a 1-mm Hg increase in central pulse pressure was associated with an OR of 1.02 for the presence of coronary artery disease (p < 0.05). The association between pulse pressure and coronary artery disease in men persisted even after the other components of blood pressure (systolic, diastolic or mean blood pressure) were forced into the multivariable model.

Philippe et al. [18] also analyzed the correlations between pulse pressure and extent of coronary disease, in 99 patients with documented coronary stenoses that were scheduled for percutaneous transluminal coronary interventions. Most of the patients were men. The extent of coronary artery disease was categorized by the number of major vessels involved (one, two or three diseased vessels). Aortic, but not brachial pulse pressure was significantly related to the extent of coronary disease: one-vessel disease, 55 ± 18 mm Hg; two-vessel disease, 64 ± 19 mm Hg; three-vessel disease, 66 ± 19 mm Hg (p < 0.03). Using multiple regression analysis, only male gender and the level of aortic pulse pressure were significant correlates of the extent of coronary artery disease. Conversely, using aortic pulse pressure as a dependent variable, higher mean aortic pressure, lower heart rate, female gender, and number of diseased vessels were independent correlates of pulse pressure in a multiple linear regression model. Of note, 11 patients had subsequent restenosis; no association was found between restenosis and either brachial or central pulse pressure.

Jankowski et al. [19] studied a group of 445 patients (including 95 women) with angiographically documented coronary artery disease and a left ventricular ejection fraction ≥55%. The extent of coronary artery disease was also defined as the number of diseased major coronary vessels. A strong association was found between aortic pulse pressure and extent of coronary artery disease: one-vessel disease, 63 ± 16 mm Hg; two-vessel disease, 65 ± 18 mm Hg; three-vessel disease, 72 ± 19 mm Hg (p < 0.001). Fractional systolic and diastolic pressures were also associated with the number of diseased vessels. By multivariable analyses, a 10-mm Hg increase in aortic pulse pressure was associated with an OR of 1.15 (95% CI: 1.01–1.30) for the presence of triple vessel disease. Brachial pulse pressure was significantly associated with the number of diseased vessels by univariate analysis (p < 0.05), but not by multivariate analysis. The male and female populations were not analyzed separately.

Finally, the findings linking the presence and extent of coronary artery disease with central pulse pressure are corroborated by a study showing increased central pulse pressure in hypercholesterolemic patients compared with controls, suggesting that a relationship between central pulse pressure and coronary artery disease might already exist at a very early stage of the atherosclerotic disease [20].

Central Pulse Pressure and Clinical Outcomes

In coronary patients, only a few studies have assessed the prognostic value of brachial or central pulse pressure in terms of clinical outcomes [21–26]. In the Balloon Angioplasty Revascularization Investigation (BARI) trial [21], brachial pulse pressure was shown to be an important prognostic indicator in patients with known coronary artery disease undergoing myocardial revascularization. Likewise, investigators of the Survival and Ventricular Enlargement (SAVE) trial also found a strong prognostic significance for brachial pulse pressure measured before hospital discharge in patients having sustained large myocardial infarctions [22].

As regards central pulse pressure, several studies [23–25] found an association between high pulse pressure and restenosis after coronary angioplasty. Nakayama et al. [23] studied 53 patients with preserved left ventricular function undergoing balloon angioplasty; 23 of them subsequently had restenosis at the angioplasty site. Fractional pulse pressure in the ascending aorta was significantly associated with the risk of restenosis; restenosis rates were 18, 33 and 78%, respectively, for tertiles 1–3 of aortic pulsatility. Lu et al. [24] also analyzed a population of 87 patients >60 years of age and with preserved left ventricular function, undergoing balloon angioplasty. Restenosis was found in 39 patients and was associated with higher levels of central pulse pressure (78 ± 12 mm Hg vs. 66 ± 15 mm Hg, p < 0.001). The ORs for restenosis were 5.88 (95% CI: 2.17–15.93) for a pulse pressure >66 mm Hg and 13.72 (95% CI: 4.81–39.05) for a fractional pulse pressure >0.72. In addition to the two previously described studies, another one [25] analyzed the correlation between the inflection time on the aortic waveform, a marker of arterial stiffness, and the risk of restenosis in 74 patients having undergone balloon coronary angioplasty. Restenosis was observed in 26, 33 and 74% according to the tertiles of inflection time and a shorter inflection time was an independent correlate of restenosis after multivariable analysis. Overall, there is concordant evidence of a link between central pulse pressure and the risk of restenosis after balloon angioplasty. After stent implantation, which is the currently used angioplasty technique, however, no such relationship was evidenced in the small cohort of patients with restenosis in the study by Philippe et al. [18].

More relevant to current clinical practice are the results from Chirinos et al. [26], who followed a cohort of 324 men having undergone coronary angiography for an average of 3 years. All patients had coronary artery disease defined by the presence of at least one >10% stenosis. Patients with concomitant valvular disease were excluded. During the follow-up period, 20% of the patients died and 43% had at least one major adverse cardiac event (death, myocardial infarction, unstable angina, unscheduled myocardial revasculariza-

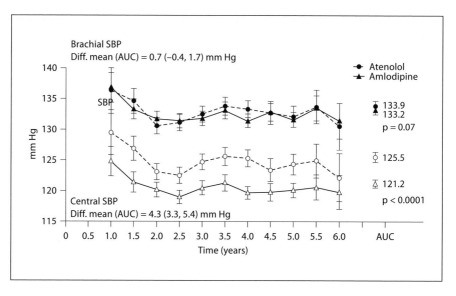

Fig. 1. Peripheral and central SBP on amlodipine and atenolol-based therapy in the ASCOT-CAFE substudy [27].

tion or stroke). Central pulse pressure correlated with the risk of both death and major cardiac events. After adjustment on left ventricular function and mean aortic pressure, the OR for all-cause mortality was 1.18 (95% CI: 1.05–1.33, p < 0.005), and the OR for any major cardiac event was 1.09 (95% CI: 1.00–1.17, p < 0.05) for each 10 mm Hg increment in pulse pressure. In addition, an inverse correlation was found between adverse events and diastolic blood pressure, and this particularly for patients with three-vessel disease. When adjusted for each other, both aortic mean blood pressure and aortic pulse pressure were independent correlates of mortality. Brachial pulse pressure was not a predictor of major adverse cardiac events.

The importance of integrating central pressure in a comprehensive approach of recent trials findings has been highlighted by the ASCOT-CAFE trial [27]: A total of 2,199 patients were recruited for this substudy from the main ASCOT patient population, and were well-matched. The difference in peripheral SBP between the amlodipine-based regimen and atenolol-based regimen in ASCOT CAFE was only 0.7 mm Hg (NS) compared with 2.7 mm Hg in the full study. The central arterial SBP was shown to be 4.3 mm Hg lower (fig. 1) for the amlodipine-based regimen (solid line in fig. 1) than for the atenolol-based regimen (dotted line in fig. 1). While peripheral PP was 0.9 mm Hg greater in the amlodipine-based regimen, it was found to be 3.0 mm Hg lower centrally. Unadjusted for patient characteristics, both peripheral PP and central PP predicted ASCOT CAFE study outcomes with a p value of <0.0001. Since the pressures are dependent on risk factors, the results were adjusted for baseline differences in these parameters. When corrected this way, central PP remained significantly related to outcome (p = 0.048).

The most solid result of the ASCOT CAFE trial was the demonstration of the amlodipine-based regimen's greater central arterial pressure-lowering effect versus the atenolol-based regimen. Since central PP was correlated with long-term outcomes, this may help explain the benefit of the amlodipine-based regimen. Other demonstrations of superiority, based on the results of similar trials, such as the LIFE study [28], should be reconsidered in terms of underlying explicative mechanisms.

Conclusion

Overall, there are concordant data showing an association between aortic or central pulse pressure and both the presence and extent of coronary artery disease. Whether this association is found only, or mainly, in men, as suggested by one study, will need further research, as most of the studies so far have involved only small populations of women. Several studies also indicate that, in patients with documented coronary artery disease, an increased pulse pressure is a correlate of worse clinical outcomes. In patients undergoing balloon coronary angioplasty, the risk of restenosis may be increased when pulse pressure is higher. More importantly, in men with coronary artery disease the risk of death increases at higher levels of central pulse pressure. These data suggest that high pulse pressure is not only a marker of preclinical cardiovascular disease, but possibly also a true risk factor for adverse clinical events in patients with coronary artery disease.

References

1   Franklin SS, Khan SA, Wong ND, Larson MG, Levy D: Is pulse pressure useful in predicting risk for coronary heart disease? The Framingham Heart Study. Circulation 1999;100:354–360.
2   Gasowski J, Fagard RH, Staessen JA, et al for the INDANA Project Collaborators: Pulsatile blood pressure component of mortality in hypertension: a meta-analysis of clinical trial control groups. J Hypertens 2002;20:145–151.
3   Benetos A, Zureik M, Morcer J, et al: A decrease in diastolic blood pressure combined with an increase in systolic blood pressure is associated with a higher cardiovascular mortality in men. J Am Coll Cardiol 2000;35:673–680.
4   Lewington S, Clarke R, Oizilbash N, Peto R, Collins R for the Prospective Study Collaboration: Age-specific relevance of usual blood pressure to vascular mortality: a meta-analysis of individual data for one million adults in 61 prospective studies. Lancet 2002;360:1903–1913.

5   Safar ME, Levy BI, Struijker-Boudier H: Current perspectives on arterial stiffness and pulse pressure in hypertension and cardiovascular disease. Circulation 2003;107:2864–2869.

6   Safar M: Central versus peripheral blood pressure measurements. Hypertension 2005;45:e14.

7   Dart AM, Kingwell BA: Pulse pressure. A review of mechanisms and clinical relevance. J Am Coll Cardiol 2001;37:975–984.

8   O'Rourke MF: Ascending aortic pressure wave indices and cardiovascular disease. Am J Hypertens 2004;17:721–723.

9   De Simone G, Roman MJ, Alderman MH, Galderisi M, de Divitiis O, Devereux RB: Is high pulse pressure a marker of preclinical cardiovascular disease? Hypertension 2005;45:575–579.

10   Ryan SM, Waack BJ, Weno BL, Heistad DD: Increases in pulse pressure impair acetylcholine-induced vascular relaxation. Am J Physiol 1995;268:H359–H363.

11   Lee KW, Blann AD, Lip GYH: High pulse pressure and nondipping circadian blood pressure in patients with coronary artery disease: relationship to thrombogenesis and endothelial damage/dysfunction. Am J Hypertens 2005;18:104–115.

12   Lee TM, Lin YJ, Su SF, Chien KL, Chen MF, Liau CS, Lee YT: Relation of systemic arterial pulse pressure to coronary atherosclerosis in patients with mitral stenosis. Am J Cardiol 1997;80:1035–1039.

13   Gatzka CD, Cameron JD, Kingwell BA, Dart AM: Relation between coronary artery disease, aortic stiffness, and left ventricular structure in a population sample. Hypertension 1998;32:575–578.

14   Nishijima T, Nakayama Y, Tsumura K, et al: Pulsatility of ascending aortic blood pressure waveform is associated with an increased risk of coronary heart disease. Am J Hypertens 2001;14:469–473.

15   Hayashi T, Nakayama Y, Tsumura K, Yoshimaru K, Ueda H: Reflection in the arterial system and the risk of coronary heart disease. Am J Hypertens 2002;15:405–409.

16   Waddell TK, Dart AM, Medley TL, Cameron JD, Kingwell BA: Carotid pressure is a better predictor of coronary artery disease severity than brachial pressure. Hypertension 2001;38:927–931.

17   Danchin N, Benetos A, Lopez-Sublet M, Demicheli T, Safar M, Mourad JJ for the ESCAPP Investigators: Aortic pulse pressure is related to the presence and extent of coronary artery disease in men undergoing diagnostic coronary angiography: a multicenter study. Am J Hypertens 2004;17:129–133.

18   Philippe F, Chemaly E, Blacher J, Mourad JJ, Dibie A, Larrazet F, Laborde F, Safar ME: Aortic pulse pressure and extent of coronary artery disease in percutaneous transluminal coronary angioplasty candidates. Am J Hypertens 2002;15:672–677.

19   Jankowski P, Kawecka-JAszcz K, Bryniarski L, et al: Fractional diastolic and systolic pressure in the ascending aorta are related to the extent of coronary artery disease. Am J Hypertens 2004;17:641–646.

20   Wilkinson IB, Prasad K, Hall IR, et al: Increased central pulse pressure and augmentation index in subjects with hypercholesterolemia. J Am Coll Cardiol 2002;39:1005–1011.

21   Domanski MJ, Sutton-Tyrrell K, Mitchell GF, Faxon DP, Pitt B, Sopko G: Determinants and prognostic information provided by pulse pressure in patients with coronary artery disease undergoing revascularization. The Balloon Angioplasty Revascularization Investigation (BARI). Am J Cardiol 2001;87:675–679.

22   Mitchell GF, Moyé LA, Braunwald E, et al for the SAVE Investigators: Sphygmomanometrically determined pulse pressure is a powerful independent predictor of recurrent events after myocardial infarction in patients with impaired left ventricular function. Circulation 1997;96:2254–2260.

23   Nakayama Y, Tsumura K, Yamashita N, Yoshimaru K, Hayashi T: Pulsatility of ascending aortic pressure waveform is a powerful predictor of restenosis after percutaneous transluminal coronary angioplasty. Circulation 2000;101:470–472.

24   Lu TM, Hsu NW, Chen YH, Lee WS, Wu CC, Ding YA, Chang MS, Lin SJ: Pulsatility of ascending aorta and restenosis after coronary angioplasty in patients >60 years of age with stable angina pectoris. Am J Cardiol 2001;88:964–968.

25 Ueda H, Nakayama H, Tsumura K, Yoshimaru K, Hayashi T, Yoshikawa J: Inflection point of ascending aortic waveform is a powerful predictor of restenosis after percutaneous transluminal coronary angioplasty. Am J Hypertens 2002;15:823–826.

26 Chirinos JA, Zambrano JP, Chakko S, et al: Relation between ascending aortic pressures and outcomes in patients with angiographically demonstrated coronary artery disease. Am J Cardiol 2005;96:645–648.

27 Williams B: Differential impact of blood pressure-lowering drugs on central arterial pressure influences clinical outcomes. Principal results of the conduit artery function evaluation (CAFE) study in ASCOT. Circulation 2005;112:3362.

28 Dahlof B, Devereux RB, Kjeldsen SE, et al: Cardiovascular morbidity and mortality in the Losartan Intervention For Endpoint reduction in hypertension study (LIFE): a randomised trial against atenolol. Lancet 2002;359:995–1003.

Nicolas Danchin
Service de Cardiologie, Hôpital Européen Georges Pompidou
20, rue Leblanc, FR–75015 Paris (France)
Tel. +33 156 09 25 71, Fax +33 156 09 25 72
E-Mail nicolas.danchin@egp.aphp.fr

Safar ME, Frohlich ED (eds): Atherosclerosis, Large Arteries and Cardiovascular Risk.
Adv Cardiol. Basel, Karger, 2007, vol 44, pp 150–159

··························

Does Brachial Pulse Pressure Predict Coronary Events?

Paolo Verdecchia   *Fabio Angeli*

Unità di Ricerca Clinica, Cardiologia Preventiva, Struttura Complessa di
Cardiologia, Ospedale R. Silvestrini, Perugia, Italy

Abstract

Brachial pulse pressure (PP) is an established risk marker for cardiovascular disease.
PP is largely determined by the stroke volume in young subjects, although the progressive
amplification of pulse wave from central to peripheral arteries could make brachial PP
not representative of the central PP in the young. With advancing age, brachial PP better
reflects the progressive stiffening of aorta and the large elastic arteries. PP correlates with
vascular and cardiac hypertrophy, although the association with cardiac hypertrophy
seems more closely attributable to systolic blood pressure (BP). An association has been
noted in several longitudinal studies between PP and the incidence of major cardiovas
cular events. However, some longitudinal studies carried out in subjects with predominantly systolic and diastolic hypertension showed that PP is the dominant predictor of
coronary events, while mean BP is the major predictor of cerebrovascular events. Such an
assumption may not be held in subjects with isolated systolic hypertension, where a wide
PP seems to predict coronary and cerebrovascular events to a similar extent. From a pathophysiological standpoint, a wide PP might reflect diffuse atherosclerotic processes potentially involving also the large coronary arteries. Some data suggest that a wide PP could
also represent a direct and independent stimulus for progression of atherosclerosis.

Introduction

Brachial pulse pressure (PP), defined as the difference between systolic
and diastolic blood pressure (BP) at brachial level, is an established marker of
cardiovascular risk in different clinical settings [1]. PP increases with age [1–5]
and an important basic mechanism of this phenomenon is believed to be the

progressive stiffening of large elastic arteries with ageing [1–5]. PP showed a direct association with vascular [4–8] and cardiac hypertrophy [9, 10] in several studies, although the association with cardiac hypertrophy appeared to be more closely determined by systolic BP than by PP [11]. Of particular note, a significant association emerged in several longitudinal studies between brachial PP and the subsequent risk of major cardiovascular events and such association was often independent of systolic and diastolic BP [12–23]. For example, in the Framingham Study, 1,924 men and women aged between 50 and 79 years, without clinical evidence of coronary artery disease and not taking antihypertensive drugs at entry, were followed for more than 20 years. Overall, these subjects contributed 433 new cases of coronary artery disease. When systolic BP and diastolic BP were jointly entered into the multivariate analysis, the association with coronary artery disease risk was positive for systolic BP (HR 1.22; 95% CI 1.15–1.30) and negative for diastolic BP (HR 0.86; 95% CI 0.75–0.98). Furthermore, four subgroups were defined according to systolic BP levels (<120, 120–139, 140–159, and ≥160 mm Hg). Within each of these subgroups, the association with coronary heart disease risk was negative for diastolic BP and positive for PP.

In a previous study from our group, the association between PP and cardiovascular disease risk was also independent of potent prognostic markers including left ventricular mass at echocardiography and white-coat hypertension [14].

The aim of this review is to summarize the current evidence about the prognostic impact of PP on the cardiac events with particular emphasis on the additional prognostic information provided by ambulatory monitoring of PP.

Epidemiological Aspects

Despite the established prognostic value of PP, the majority of longitudinal studies examined a composite pool of cardiovascular events, with coronary and cerebrovascular end-points rarely tested separately. However, in a study carried out by Benetos et al. [15] in the general population, PP predicted cardiac but not cerebrovascular mortality. These data have been confirmed in the setting of the Medical Research Council (MRC) Mild Hypertension Trial, where coronary events were best predicted by high levels of systolic BP associated with low values of diastolic pressure (fig. 1) [19]. In that study, PP was a stronger predictor of coronary events than systolic, diastolic or mean BP in men [19]. PP was similar to systolic pressure as a predictor of coronary events while stroke was better predicted by mean BP [19]. Also a study by Khattar et al. [24] with intra-arterial BP monitoring provided some indirect evidence of

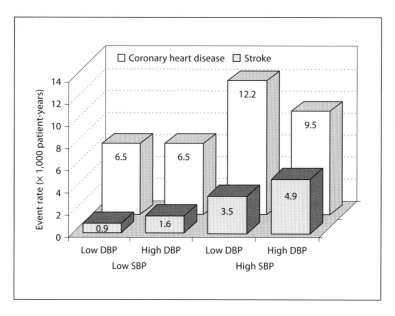

Fig. 1. In the MRC study, the highest incidence of coronary artery disease was noted in association with high values of systolic and low, rather than high, values of diastolic BP [modified from 19].

a greater predictive effect of PP on cardiac events than on cerebrovascular events.

Some years ago, we tested the hypothesis that the steady (i.e., mean BP) and pulsatile (i.e., PP) components of BP may exert a different prognostic impact on coronary artery disease and stroke in subjects with essential hypertension [25]. We analyzed data from the *Progetto Ipertensione Umbria Monitoraggio Ambulatoriale* (PIUMA) study, a prospective registry of morbidity and mortality in initially untreated subjects with essential hypertension who underwent 24-hour ambulatory BP monitoring as a part of their initial check-up. The analysis was carried out in 2,311 subjects who contributed 132 major cardiac events (1.20 per 100 person-years) and 105 cerebrovascular events (0.90 per 100 person-years) over a mean follow-up period of about 5 years. The incidence of coronary events increased with 24-hour ambulatory PP, but no appreciable rise was noted with ambulatory mean BP (fig. 2). In a multivariate analysis, after adjustment for the significant effect of several confounders (all $p < 0.01$), for each 10 mm Hg increase in 24-hour PP, there was an independent 35% increase in the risk of cardiac events. Furthermore, after adjustment for age, sex and diabetes (all $p < 0.05$), for every 10 mm Hg increase in 24-hour

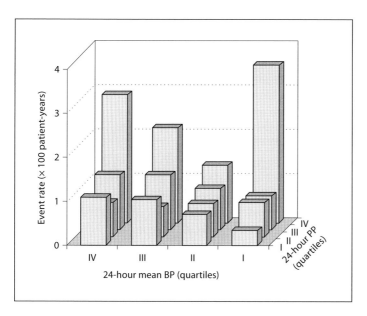

Fig. 2. The incidence of coronary events increased with 24-hour ambulatory PP, not with ambulatory mean BP. Cut-off points for quartiles: 96.0, 102.6 and 110.0 mmHg for mean BP; 44.0, 49.0 and 56.0 for PP [modified from 25].

mean BP there was an independent 42% increase in the risk of cerebrovascular events, with 24-hour PP not yielding independent significance. Twenty-four-hour PP was also an independent predictor of fatal cardiac events, and 24-hour mean BP of fatal cerebrovascular events.

These data led us to suggest that in subjects with predominantly systolic and diastolic hypertension, PP is the dominant predictor of coronary events, while mean BP is the major independent predictor of cerebrovascular events [25].

A meta-analysis of the prognostic value of PP in the European Working Party on Hypertension in the Elderly (EWPHE), Syst-Eur and Syst-China studies [20] showed a comparable predictive effect of PP on coronary events and stroke after adjustment for mean BP. However, the predictive effect of mean BP on both types of events was not statistically significant after adjustment for PP. A dominant predictive value of PP over mean BP on both coronary events and stroke was present only in the Syst-Eur and Syst-China studies, which included patients with isolated systolic hypertension, but not in the EWPHE study, which included subjects with predominantly systodiastolic hypertension.

In another meta-analysis of eight studies in elderly subjects with isolated systolic hypertension, the risk of death was directly associated with systolic BP and inversely associated with diastolic BP, thus emphasizing the prognostic value of PP [26]. In the large population of the Systolic Hypertension in the Elderly (SHEP) study, mean BP and PP were both independent determinants of stroke risk. However, even in this analysis the stroke risk increased to a greater extent with mean BP (by 20% for every 10 mm Hg) than with PP (by 11% for every 10 mm Hg) [18].

Overall, *these findings suggest that in subjects with predominantly systolic and diastolic hypertension, PP is the dominant predictor of coronary events while mean BP is the major predictor of stroke.* Such an assumption may not be held in subjects with isolated systolic hypertension, where PP may be a valid predictor of both coronary and cerebrovascular events.

Pathophysiology
A wide PP might be considered a prognostic marker for coronary artery disease by reflecting diffuse atherosclerotic processes potentially involving also the major coronary arteries. In addition, it could also represent a direct and independent stimulus for a further progression of atherosclerosis. In a recent study, PP showed a direct association with C-reactive protein and other markers of inflammation in hypertensive patients [27]. A potential basis for the strong impact of elevated PP on the risk of myocardial ischemia might also be the unfavorable balance between early reflection of the pressure wave in the aorta during systole, further increasing LV wall stress and oxygen requirement, and the potentially impaired coronary flow at low levels of diastolic BP [28].

It is worth noting, however, that brachial PP may not be a reliable marker of central PP, particularly in the young subjects, because of the progressive peripheral amplification of pressure wave, which tends to decrease with age and to increase with height [29, 30].

A study by Alfie et al. [31] provided details on the relation between PP and stroke volume at different ages in untreated hypertensive subjects. Before age 50, 24-hour PP showed a direct significant association with stroke volume and a negative association with arterial compliance, estimated by the ratio between stroke volume and PP. In contrast, after age 50, 24-hour PP correlated negatively with arterial compliance, without any significant relation with the stroke volume. Thus, the stroke volume is an important determinant of PP in young hypertensive subjects [31].

Additional Information Provided by Ambulatory Blood Pressure

Diagnosis and management of hypertension are traditionally based on BP measurements carried out in the hospital or physician's office. Over the last years, the great interest generated by ambulatory BP monitoring in clinical practice has increased medical interest about whether the clinic BP measures are the best ones to assess the cardiovascular risk in individual hypertensive patient.

For example, PP may be importantly affected by the alerting reaction evoked by the clinical visit. Several years ago, studies by Mancia et al. [32, 33] allowed to quantify for the first time the rise in intra-arterial BP evoked by the physician's visit, which approximated 4–75 mm Hg (mean 27) for systolic BP and 1–36 mm Hg (mean 15) for diastolic BP. Thus, the bigger rise in systolic than diastolic BP implied an increase in PP of about 12 mm Hg from before to during the visit.

The important conclusion of these studies is that clinic (office) PP may overestimate the usual levels of PP.

Indeed, some cross-sectional studies suggest that ambulatory PP correlates with organ damage more closely than clinic PP does. In the setting of the European Lacidipine Study on Atherosclerosis (ELSA) study, 24-hour PP was a strong and independent predictor of intima-media thickness in hypertensive patients and its predictive effect was superior to that of clinic PP [34].

In order to provide further insight into the prognostic value of ambulatory PP, we followed for about 4 years 2,010 initially untreated and uncomplicated subjects with essential hypertension included in the PIUMA study [35]. The crude rate of a composite pool of cardiovascular events (per 100 persons per year) in the 3 tertiles of the distribution of clinic PP was 1.38, 2.12 and 4.34, respectively, and that of fatal events was 0.12, 0.30 and 1.07 (log-rank test: both $p < 0.01$). In the 3 tertiles of the distribution of average 24-hour PP, the rate of total cardiovascular events was 1.19, 1.81 and 4.92, and that of fatal events was 0.11, 0.17 and 1.23 (log-rank test: both $p < 0.01$). For any level of clinic PP, the incidence of a composite pool of cardiovascular events increased with ambulatory PP. In contrast, for any level of 24-hour ambulatory PP there was no appreciable rise in the event rate with increasing clinic PP (fig. 3). In a multivariate analysis, after adjustment for the influence of concomitant risk factors, survival data were better fitted by the model containing ambulatory PP than by that containing clinic PP. In each of the 3 tertiles of clinic PP, cardiovascular morbidity and mortality increased from the first to the third tertile of average 24-hour ambulatory PP (log-rank test: all $p < 0.01$).

In summary, these data suggest that *the alerting reaction to office BP measurement weakens the relation between PP and total cardiovascular risk, and*

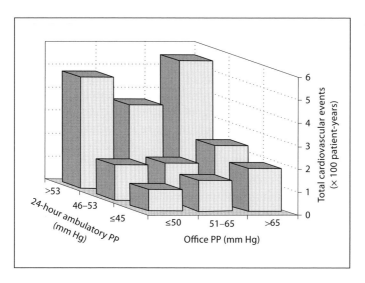

Fig. 3. For any level of clinic PP, the incidence of a composite pool of cardiovascular events increased with ambulatory PP. In contrast, for any level of 24-hour ambulatory PP there was no appreciable rise in the event rate with increasing clinic PP [adapted from 35].

that ambulatory PP provides a more precise estimate of risk [35]. These data have been confirmed in the setting of the Systolic Hypertension in Europe (Syst-Eur) study [36], carried out in elderly subjects with isolated systolic hypertension. In this study, 24-hour and nighttime PP showed an association with total and cardiovascular mortality, all cardiovascular events, stroke, and cardiac events, while daytime PP predicted cardiovascular mortality, all cardiovascular end-points, and stroke. In addition, 24-hour and nighttime ambulatory PP predicted cardiovascular outcome over and beyond clinic PP.

Therapeutic Implications

Despite the evidence on the prognostic impact of brachial PP on coronary and cerebrovascular events, no recommendations are available as to guide antihypertensive treatment on the basis of brachial PP. Furthermore, it is not clear whether some classes of antihypertensive drugs are more effective than others on arterial distensibility and compliance. Some data suggest that ACE inhibitors are particularly effective on arterial wall properties and aortic pulse wave velocity in hypertensive patients [36–38], but further research is needed in this area. A recent meta-regression analysis showed that ACE inhibitors confer specific protection against coronary heart disease independent of their antihypertensive effect [39]. Since that analysis addressed mega-trials in which systolic and diastolic BP were measured at brachial level [39], one potential mechanism of the superiority of ACE inhibitors on coronary events might be a greater BP response at central (aortic) level.

Acknowledgments

The authors gratefully thank Miss Francesca Saveri for secretarial assistance. The study has been supported by a grant from the *Associazione Umbra Cuore e Ipertensione*, Perugia, Italy.

References

1   Safar ME: Pulse pressure in essential hypertension: clinical and therapeutic implications. J Hypertens 1989;7:769–776.
2   Sleight P: Blood pressures, hearts, and U-shaped curves. Lancet 1988;i:235.
3   Franklin SS, Gustin WG, Wong ND, Larson MG, Weber MA, Kannel WB, Levy D: Hemodynamic patterns of age-related changes in blood pressure: the Framingham Study. Circulation 1997;96:308–315.
4   Boutouyrie P, Bussy C, Lacolley P, Girerd X, Laloux B, Laurent S: Association between local pulse pressure, mean blood pressure and large-artery remodeling. Circulation 1999;100:1387–1393.
5   James MA, Watt PA, Potter JF, Thurston H, Swales JD: Pulse pressure and resistance artery structure in the elderly. Hypertension 1995;26:301–306.
6   Franklin SS, Sutton-Tyrrel K, Belle S, Weber M, Kuller LH: The importance of pulsatile components of hypertension in predicting carotid stenosis in older adults. J Hypertens 1997;15:1143–1150.
7   Boutouyrie P, Bussy C, Hayoz D, et al: Local pulse pressure and regression of arterial wall hypertrophy during long-term antihypertensive treatment. Circulation 2000;101:2601–2606.
8   Matthews KA, Owens JF, Kuller LH, Sutton-Tyrrell K, Lassila HC, Wolfson SK: Stress-induced pulse pressure change predicts women's carotid atherosclerosis. Stroke 1998;29:1525–1530.
9   Khattar RS, Acharya DU, Kinsey C, Senior R, Lahiri A: Longitudinal association of ambulatory pulse pressure with left ventricular mass and vascular hypertrophy in essential hypertension. J Hypertens 1997;15:737–743.
10 Darné B, Girerd X, Safar ME, Cambien F, Guize L: Pulsatile versus steady component of blood pressure: a cross-sectional and prospective analysis of cardiovascular mortality. Hypertension 1989;13:392–400.
11 Verdecchia P, Schillaci G, Borgioni C, Gattobigio R, Ambrosio G, Porcellati C: Prevalent influence of systolic over pulse pressure on left ventricular mass in essential hypertension. Eur Heart J 2002 23:658–665.
12 Pannier B, Brunel P, el Aroussy W, Lacolley P, Safar ME: Pulse pressure and echocardiographic findings in essential hypertension. J Hypertens 1989;7:127–132.
13 Madhavan S, Ooi WL, Cohen H, Alderman MH: Relation of pulse pressure and blood pressure reduction to the incidence of myocardial infarction. Hypertension 1994;23:395–401.
14 Verdecchia P, Porcellati C, Schillaci G, Borgioni C, Ciucci A, Battistelli M, Guerrieri M, Gatteschi C, Zampi I, Santucci A, Santucci C, Reboldi G: Ambulatory blood pressure: an independent predictor of prognosis in essential hypertension. Hypertension 1994;24:793–801.

15 Benetos A, Safar M, Rudnichi A, Smulyan H, Richard JL, Ducimetière P, Guize: Pulse pressure. A predictor of long-term cardiovascular mortality in a French male population. Hyertension 1997;30:1410–1415.

16 Mitchell GF, Moyé LA, Braunwald E, Rouleau JL, Bernstein V, Geltman EM, Flaker GC, Pfeffer MA for the SAVE Investigators: Sphygmomanometrically determined pulse pressure is a powerful independent predictor of recurrent events after myocardial infarction in patients with impaired left ventricular function. Circulation 1997;96:4254–4260.

17 Franklin SS, Khan SA, Wong ND, Larson MG, Levy D: Is pulse pressure useful for predicting risk for coronary heart disease? The Framingham Heart Study. Circulation 1999;100:354–360.

18 Domanski MJ, Davis BR, Pfeffer MA, Kastantin M, Mitchell GF: Isolated systolic hypertension. Prognostic information provided by pulse pressure. Hypertension 1999;34:375–380.

19 Millar JA, Lever AF, Burke V: Pulse pressure as a risk factor for cardiovascular events in the MRC Mild Hypertension Trial. J Hypertens 1999;17:1065–1072.

20 Blacher J, Staessen JA, Girerd X, Gasowski J, Thijs L, Liu L, Wang Ji G, Fagard RH, Safar ME: Pulse pressure not mean pressure determines cardiovascular risk in older hypertensive patients. Arch Intern Med 2000;160:1085–1089.

21 Vaccarino V, Holford TR, Krumholz HM: Pulse pressure and risk for myocardial infarction and heart failure in the elderly. J Am Coll Cardiol 2000;36:130–138.

22 Domanski M, Norman J, Wolz M, Mitchell G, Pfeffer M: Cardiovascular risk assessment using pulse pressure in the First National Health and Nutrition Examination Survey (NHANES I). Hypertension 2001;38:793–797.

23 Blacher J, Staessen JA, Girerd X, Gasowski J, Thijs L, Liu L, Wang JG, Fagard RH, Safar ME: Pulse pressure not mean pressure determines cardiovascular risk in older hypertensive patients. Arch Intern Med 2000;160:1085–1089.

24 Khattar R, Swales JD, Banfield A, Dore C, Senior R, Lahiri A: Prediction of coronary and cerebrovascular morbidity and mortality by direct continuous ambulatory blood pressure monitoring in essential hypertension. Circulation 1999;100:1071–1076.

25 Verdecchia P, Schillaci G, Reboldi G, Franklin SS, Porcellati C: Different prognostic impact of 24-hour mean blood pressure and pulse pressure on stroke and coronary artery disease in essential hypertension. Circulation 2001;103:2579–2584.

26 Staessen JA, Gasowski J, Wang JG, Thijs L, Den Hond E, Boissel JP, Coope J, Ekbom T, Gueyffier F, Liu L, Kerlikowske K, Pocock S, Fagard RH: Risks of untreated and treated isolated systolic hypertension in the elderly: meta-analysis of outcome trials. Lancet 2000;355:865–872.

27 Manabe S, Okura T, Watanabe S, Higaki J: Association between carotid haemodynamics and inflammation in patients with essential hypertension. J Hum Hypertens 2005;19:787–791.

28 Kelly R, Hayward C, Avolio A, et al: Noninvasive determination of age-related changes in the human arterial pulse. Circulation 1989;80:1652–1659.

29 Nichols AA, Avolio AP, Kelly RP, O'Rourke MF: Effects of age and hypertension on wave travel and reflections; in O'Rourke MF, Safar ME, Dzau JV (eds): Arterial Vasodilatation: Mechanisms and Therapy. London, Arnold, 1993, p 32.

30 Asmar R, Brisac AM, Courivaus JM, Lecor B, London GM, Safar ME: Influence of gender on the level of pulse pressure: the role of large conduit arteries. Clin Exp Hypertens 1997;5–6:793–811.

31 Alfie J, Waisman GD, Galarza CR, Camera MI: Contribution of stroke volume to the change in pulse pressure pattern with age. Hypertension 1999;34:808–812.

32 Mancia G, Bertineri G, Grassi G, Parati G, Pomidossi G, Ferrari A, Gregorini L, Zanchetti A: Effects of blood pressure measured by the doctor on patient's blood pressure and heart rate. Lancet 1983;ii:695–698.

33 Mancia G: Parati G, Pomidossi G, Grassi G, Casadei R, Zanchetti A: Alerting reaction and rise in blood pressure during measurement by physician and nurse. Hypertension 1987;9:209–215.

34 Zanchetti A, Bond MG, Hennig M, Neiss A, Mancia G, Dal Palu C, Hansson L, Magnani B, Rahn KH, Reid J, Rodicio J, Safar M, Eckes L, Ravinetto R: Risk factors associated with alterations in carotid intima-media thickness in hypertension: baseline data from the European Lacidipine Study on Atherosclerosis. J Hypertens 1998;16:949–961.

35 Verdecchia P, Schillaci G, Borgioni C, Ciucci A, Pede S, Porcellani C: Ambulatory pulse pressure: a potent predictor of total cardiovascular risk in hypertension. Hypertension 1998;32:983–938.

36 Benetos A, Vasmant D, Thiery P, Safar M: Effects of ramipril on arterial hemodynamics. J Cardiovasc Pharmacol 1991;18:S153–S156.
37 Asmar RG, Pannier B, Santoni JP, et al: Reversion of cardiac hypertrophy and reduced arterial compliance after converting enzyme inhibition in essential hypertension. Circulation 1988;78: 941–950.
38 Shimamoto H, Shimamoto Y: Lisinopril improves aortic compliance and renal flow: comparison with nifedipine. Hypertension 1995;25:327–334.
39 Verdecchia P, Reboldi G, Angeli F, Gattobigio R, Bentivoglio M, Thijs L, Staessen JA, Porcellati C: Angiotensin-converting enzyme inhibitors and calcium channel blockers for coronary heart disease and stroke prevention. Hypertension 2005;46:386–392.

Paolo Verdecchia, MD, FACC, FAHA
Unità di Ricerca Clinica, Cardiologia Preventiva
Struttura Complessa di Cardiologia, Ospedale R. Silvestrini
IT–06100 Perugia (Italy)
Tel. +39 075 578 2213/5782207, Mobile +39 348 331 8077
Fax +39 075 578 2214, E-Mail verdec@tin.it

Safar ME, Frohlich ED (eds): Atherosclerosis, Large Arteries and Cardiovascular Risk.
Adv Cardiol. Basel, Karger, 2007, vol 44, pp 160–172

······················

Does Arterial Stiffness Predict Atherosclerotic Coronary Events?

Carmel M. McEniery[a] *John R. Cockcroft*[b]

[a]Clinical Pharmacology Unit, University of Cambridge, Addenbrooke's Hospital, Cambridge, and [b]Wales Heart Research Institute, Cardiff University, University Hospital, Cardiff, UK

Abstract

Coronary heart disease is a major cause of death and morbidity. Due to the increased longevity of most developed societies, there is an increasing overlap between arteriosclerosis associated with normal vascular ageing and atherosclerosis associated with cardiovascular risk factors. There is therefore a need for improvements, both in the early identification of individuals at risk, and in cardiovascular risk stratification. Arterial stiffness is an important determinant of cardiovascular risk and can now be measured simply and noninvasively in large populations. This review will therefore focus on the current evidence as to the predictive value of arterial stiffness in relation to coronary events and also on the possible pathophysiological mechanisms linking arterial stiffness and atherosclerosis.

Copyright © 2007 S. Karger AG, Basel

Introduction

Atherosclerotic coronary heart disease (CHD) is one of the leading causes of death worldwide. Therefore, the early detection of occult atheroma, or those individuals who are at significantly increased risk, is necessary for successful primary prevention of myocardial infarction and angina. Moreover, significant CHD can exist without overt clinical signs or symptoms. Indeed, a significant number of first myocardial infarctions occur in individuals in whom traditional cardiovascular risk factors are only slightly elevated [1, 2]. Therefore, early identification of novel cardiovascular risk markers and more accurate risk stratification is required. As described in previous chapters, arterial stiffness is considered a key risk factor for cardiovascular disease, and can be assessed in large populations, using relatively simple, non-invasive methods. This chapter will review the evidence surrounding the predictive value of arterial stiffness in relation to atherosclerotic coronary events.

Cross-Sectional Studies

A logical first step in defining the value of arterial stiffness as a predictor of atherosclerotic coronary events is to determine whether large artery stiffness is increased in subjects who have already experienced a coronary event compared to healthy individuals. Hirai et al. [3] were amongst the first to examine this question. They assessed β stiffness index (a measure of aortic stiffness) in 49 patients who had suffered a myocardial infarction and 19 controls, and demonstrated that aortic stiffness was significantly higher in patients relative to controls.

Two further studies have examined the relationship between arterial stiffness and restenosis post-angioplasty [4, 5]. Both were invasive and demonstrated a significant relationship between restenosis and aortic pulsatility [4], and with aortic augmentation index [5]. Nishijima et al. [4] studied 53 consecutive patients admitted for revascularization who had had successful coronary balloon angioplasty and coronary angiography 3 months after angioplasty. They evaluated the morphology of the invasively measured ascending aortic pressure wave. In order to quantify the relative magnitude of the pulsatile aortic pressure they normalized it to mean pressure and defined this value as the fractional pulse pressure. This surrogate measure of aortic stiffness was a powerful predictor of restenosis, even after adjustments for age, sex, cardiovascular risk factors, vessel size and previous myocardial infarction. The odds ratio for restenosis was 33.5% in the highest tertile of fractional pulse pressure compared to the lowest tertile and the authors calculated that for each 0.1 increase in fractional pulse pressure, the odds ratio of restenosis rose by 88%.

In a similar study, Ueda et al. [5] investigated the predictive value of the invasively measured aortic augmentation index in 74 consecutive patients undergoing revascularization using similar inclusion criteria as the study of Nishijima et al. [4]. They assessed aortic stiffness by measuring time to the inflection point on the aortic pressure wave form – so-called 'T_R', which provides a surrogate measure of aortic pulse wave velocity (T_R falls as pulse wave velocity increases). The odds ratio of restenosis was ~7 in the lowest tertile relative to the highest, and a 20-ms increase in inflection time increased the odds ratio of restenosis by 70%. One potential limitation of these studies is that they used fluid-filled pressure catheters which are less accurate than high-fidelity pressure transducers due to a poorer frequency response. Nevertheless, they do emphasize the value of surrogate measures of aortic stiffness in predicting the risk of restenosis post-angioplasty.

Arterial stiffness also appears to be increased in subjects with microvascular CHD. In a more recent study, Arroyo-Espliguero et al. [6] assessed carotid artery stiffness using Doppler ultrasound in a cohort of 30 patients with syndrome X. Carotid stiffness was significantly increased in those with syndrome X compared with control subjects. Although distensibility also tended to be lower in the syndrome X group, this did not reach statistical significance.

The risk of myocardial infarction is greatest in individuals with pre-existing coronary artery disease and a number of small studies have demonstrated significant relationships between invasive [4, 7, 8] and non-invasive [9, 10] measurements of arterial stiffness and the extent and severity of coronary atheromatous disease. Jankowski et al. [8] studied 445 patients with angiographically confirmed coronary artery disease and measured ascending aortic pressure during catheterization. They used fractional aortic diastolic and systolic pressure derived from the invasively acquired aortic waveforms. Fractional systolic and fractional diastolic pressure differentiated patients with one-, two-, and three-vessel coronary artery disease. Interestingly, none of the brachial pressure indices was independently related to the extent of coronary atherosclerosis.

A recent large multi-centre study involving 1,337 patients at high risk of coronary artery disease from 75 centres demonstrated a significant relationship between invasively measured central aortic pulse pressure and both the presence and severity of angiographically determined coronary artery disease [11]. McLeod et al. [9] assessed pulse wave velocity and augmentation index in a group of patients undergoing intravascular ultrasound of their coronary arteries. They demonstrated a significant relationship between carotid-radial pulse wave velocity and plaque load. Interestingly, aortic augmentation index measured non-invasively did not correlate with plaque load, which is in contrast to an earlier study using invasive measurements of augmentation index [12]. Moreover, in a large non-invasive study performed in 465 consecutive male patients undergoing coronary angiography for symptoms of suspected coronary artery disease, Weber et al. [10] found a significant association between the presence and severity of coronary artery disease and central aortic augmentation index. Taken together, the results from the studies to date are consistent with the hypothesis that central aortic stiffness may promote the development of coronary artery disease and that therapeutic intervention targeted at reducing arterial stiffness may be of benefit in patients with coronary artery disease.

Table 1. Prospective longitudinal studies examining the relationship between aortic pulse wave velocity and outcome

Reference	Patient group	Presence of CHD	Subjects (male/female)	Age years	Duration of follow-up, years	End-points	Major findings
Blacher [13]	ESRD	Yes	241 (147/94)	52	6	All-cause and CV mortality	Aortic PWV significantly associated with all-cause and CV mortality
Laurent [14]	Hypertensives	Yes	1,980 (1,297/983)	50	9	All-cause and CV mortality	Aortic PWV significantly associated with all-cause and CV mortality Aortic PWV significantly associated with CV mortality in patients without history of CV disease
Cruickshank [15]	Type 2 diabetes	Yes	397 (239/158)	60	10	All-cause and CV mortality	PWV-independent predictor of all-cause and CV mortality
Boutouyrie [19]	Hypertensives	No	1,045 681/364	51	5.7	Fatal or non-fatal CHD event	Aortic PWV-independent predictor of primary coronary events Aortic PWV-independent predictor of CV events
Meaume [17]	Elderly hospitalized	Yes	141 38/103	87	2.5	All-cause and CV mortality	Aortic PWV significantly associated with CV mortality (SBP/PP not associated) Past history of MI also significantly associated with all-cause and CV mortality
Sutton-Tyrrell [18]	Well-functioning older adults	Yes	2,488 (1,186/1,302)	74	4.6	All-cause and CV mortality and CHD events	Aortic PWV significantly associated with all-cause and CV mortality Aortic PWV significantly associated with CHD events and stroke, but not CHF Association remained when individuals with prevalent CVD at baseline excluded from the analysis

Longitudinal Studies

Although cross-sectional studies provide useful information concerning the relationship between arterial stiffness and coronary events, prospective longitudinal studies with hard end-points are required to attribute a causal role of arterial stiffening in disease pathophysiology.

Evidence that Aortic Pulse Wave Velocity Predicts Outcome in Patient Groups

The results of a number of longitudinal follow-up studies clearly demonstrate that arterial stiffness, assessed by measuring the aortic pulse wave velocity, is a key, independent determinant of both total and cardiovascular mortality. The first such study, published by Blacher et al. [13] in 1999, consisted of 241 patients with end-stage renal disease, with an average age of 52 years at baseline. Over a mean follow-up of 6 years, 73 deaths were recorded, including 48 fatal cardiovascular events of which 15 were due to CHD. Aortic pulse wave velocity, determined from transcutaneous Doppler flow recordings at the aortic arch and the femoral artery, emerged as a significant and independent predictor of total and cardiovascular mortality, along with age, and diastolic blood pressure which was inversely associated with outcome. These findings were extended to two other patient groups – essential hypertension [14] and type 2 diabetes [15]. In 1,980 patients with essential hypertension, followed-up for an average of 9 years, 107 fatal events were recorded, 46 of which were due to cardiovascular events and 19 deaths related to CHD. The significant determinants of mortality were pulse wave velocity, age, heart rate and a previous history of cardiovascular disease. Aortic pulse wave velocity was also assessed in 397 patients with type 2 diabetes (mean age 60 years). The patients were followed up for 10 years and aortic pulse wave velocity found to be significantly and independently related to total and cardiovascular mortality, together with age and female gender.

Although these studies provide good evidence that aortic pulse wave velocity is an important and novel marker of cardiovascular risk, many of the patients had pre-existing cardiovascular conditions, which may have confounded the results. Indeed, in the renal failure cohort, the incidence of previous cardiovascular events was significantly increased in those individuals who fell within the highest tertile of pulse wave velocity (48%), compared with those in the lowest tertile (6%). Moreover, in the diabetic cohort, the incidence of ischaemic heart disease was significantly higher in non-survivors (21%) compared with survivors (4%). However, in a sub-analysis of the hypertensive cohort, including only those patients with no previous history of cardiovascular disease (n = 1,798), the independent association between aortic pulse wave velocity and cardiovascular mortality remained.

Table 2. Prospective longitudinal studies examining the relationship between other indices of large artery properties and outcome

Reference	Measure	Patient group	Presence of CHD	Subjects (male/female)	Age years	Duration of follow-up, years	End-points	Major findings
Franklin [16]	PPP	Framingham Cohort	No	1,924 (830/1,094)	61	14.3	Incident CHD	Greater increase in CDH risk with increase in PP
Schram [43]	PPP	Type 2 diabetes	Yes	208	66	8.6	CV mortality	PPP significantly associated with CV mortality
Safar [22]	CPP	ESRD	Yes	180 (108/72)	54	4.3	All-cause mortality	Carotid (central) PP more powerful predictor of all-cause mortality than brachial PP
London [23]	AIx	ESRD	Yes	180 (108/72)	54	4.3	All-cause and CV mortality	AIx significantly associated with all-cause and CV mortality
Chirinos [24]	AP/AIx	Established CAD	Yes	297 (297/0)	64	3.2	MACEs	AP and AIx significantly associated with occurrence of MACEs AP significantly associated with all-cause mortality
Matsuoka [25]	Brachial-ankle PWV	Elderly adults	Not reported	298 (120/178)	79	3.4	CV mortality	Brachial-ankle PWV significantly associated with CV mortality

Does Arterial Stiffness Predict Atherosclerotic Coronary Events?

Evidence that Aortic Pulse Wave Velocity Predicts Outcome in Older Individuals

Systolic blood pressure rises continuously throughout life, whereas diastolic blood pressure tends to level off and may even decline in persons over 50 years of age [16]. Consequently, pulse pressure increases as a function of chronological age, a process attributed to large artery stiffening. Systolic blood pressure and pulse pressure are considered major markers of cardiovascular risk in older individuals [16]. More recently, two prospective longitudinal studies have extended these findings by demonstrating that aortic pulse wave velocity is also an important determinant of outcome in older individuals. In 141 elderly, hospitalized individuals (mean age 87), followed up over 2.5 years [17], 56 deaths were recorded, including 27 fatal cardiovascular events. Aortic pulse wave velocity independently predicted cardiovascular but not total mortality. However, a previous history of myocardial infarction was also a significant predictor of both cardiovascular and total mortality in this population. Interestingly, systolic and pulse pressure had no predictive value when included with pulse wave velocity in regression models. These findings were recently confirmed and extended in a much larger cohort of 2,488 well-functioning, older adults, recruited from the general population [18]. The mean age of the cohort was 74 years and the average length of follow-up was 4.6 years. In all, 265 deaths were recorded, including 111 from cardiovascular causes. Again, aortic pulse wave velocity emerged as a significant predictor of both cardiovascular and total mortality.

Evidence that Aortic Pulse Wave Velocity Predicts Coronary Events

Although there is a clear link between aortic pulse wave velocity and outcome in patient groups and older individuals, the evidence supporting a direct relationship between arterial stiffness and coronary events is somewhat limited. This is most probably due to relatively small samples sizes in most studies to date, which preclude meaningful sub-analyses concerning CHD events. However, in a separate analysis of the cohort of patients with essential hypertension described above, 1,045 patients with no previous history of cardiovascular disease (mean age 51 years) were followed up over an average of 5.7 years [19]. Ninety-seven fatal and non-fatal cardiovascular events were recorded, including 53 coronary events. Aortic pulse wave velocity emerged as a significant predictor of primary coronary events in this population. In another sub-analysis of the cohort of well-functioning older adults [18], a higher aortic pulse wave velocity independently predicted coronary events. Although ~25% of patients had pre-existing cardiovascular disease, when these individuals were excluded from the analyses, the association between pulse wave velocity and coronary events remained.

Other Indices

A number of longitudinal studies have examined the importance of other arterial haemodynamic indices in determining outcome. Brachial pulse pressure is often used as a surrogate measure of large artery stiffness and there is overwhelming evidence described elsewhere, demonstrating an independent relationship between brachial pulse pressure and cardiovascular risk. However, pulse pressure measured at the brachial artery does not always provide an accurate indication of central pulse pressure, due to the phenomenon of pressure amplification within the arterial system. This is important clinically, because the left ventricle, kidney, and brain are exposed to *central*, not peripheral pressure [20, 21].

Only one study has examined the importance of central pulse pressure in predicting events and only total mortality was considered. In a cohort of 180 patients with end-stage renal failure (mean age 54 years) [22], carotid pulse pressure was a more powerful predictor of outcome than peripheral pulse pressure. Using the same cohort of patients, carotid augmentation index also independently predicted both cardiovascular and total mortality [23].

Central pressure augmentation and augmentation index were also examined in a cohort of 297 male subjects (mean age 64 years), all of whom were undergoing clinically indicated coronary angiography [24]. Both augmentation pressure and augmentation index were significantly associated with the occurrence of a major adverse cardiovascular event, and augmentation pressure was also significantly associated with all-cause mortality. Finally, in a Japanese population of 297 elderly adults (mean age 79 years), brachial-ankle pulse wave velocity was significantly associated with cardiovascular mortality [25].

Despite relatively few studies, there is a growing body of evidence which clearly demonstrates that arterial stiffness, assessed by measuring the aortic pulse wave velocity, is a key predictor of cardiovascular and all-cause mortality in a number of patient groups and older individuals, including those with no prior history of cardiovascular disease. Moreover, other haemodynamic indices which relate to large artery properties, such as central pulse pressure, augmentation index and brachial-ankle pulse wave velocity, are also important determinants of risk. Although longitudinal studies provide much greater evidence of causality concerning the importance of arterial stiffness in the pathophysiology of cardiovascular disease, intervention studies are now required to establish causation fully and to reduce the excess cardiovascular risk associated with arterial stiffening.

Pathophysiological Mechanisms

There is clearly a close, yet complex, relationship between the stiffness of the large arteries and the process of atherosclerosis. Arterial stiffening and atherosclerosis often co-exist, and several studies have identified a correlation between atherosclerotic burden and aortic stiffness. Moreover, as already discussed, arterial stiffness is a predictor of future cardiovascular, and indeed coronary, events. These observations have led many to think of arterial stiffness as simply a marker of atherosclerotic disease. Although they may share common risk factors such as hypertension and cigarette smoking, pathologically, and clinically, atherosclerosis and arteriosclerosis must be considered as distinct clinical entities. Furthermore, stiffening of the large arteries may also promote cardiovascular disease by a number of mechanisms [26, 27].

As the aorta stiffens, pulse pressure rises, due to reduced buffering capacity, but also augmentation of systolic pressure by a faster return of reflected pressure waves from the periphery. This rise in central systolic pressure promotes left ventricular hypertrophy and ventricular stiffening ultimately leading to diastolic dysfunction and heart failure [27]. Indeed, left ventricular mass is more closely related to pulse pressure in the aorta than that measured more commonly in the brachial artery [28]. The concomitant fall in diastolic pressure reduces coronary blood flow, exacerbating the situation, and predisposing to ischaemia. The widened pulse pressure is transmitted to other arteries such as the carotid, which then undergo a process of remodelling to reduce wall stress, leading to intima-media thickening [29]. Arterial stiffening also increases cyclical stresses within the arterial wall, accelerating elastic fibre fatigue fracture, further stiffening the vessel and creating a vicious circle.

Endothelial Function

The endothelium is a monolayer of cells lining the vascular tree, which we now recognize to play a pivotal role in cardiovascular homeostasis. These cells release a number of vasoactive mediators including nitric oxide and endothelin-1. In addition to being a potent vasodilator, nitric oxide has a number of important anti-atherosclerotic actions including inhibition of platelet aggregation, expression of adhesion molecules, and smooth muscle cell proliferation. Although a number of pharmacological and chemical stimuli regulate endothelial nitric oxide production, shear stress is one of the more important physiological stimuli for nitric oxide production in vivo.

As arteries stiffen, the mean shear stress may increase but shear stress rate falls [30], thus reducing endothelial nitric oxide production – a key initiating event in atheroma formation. Indeed, it is well recognized that atheroma in the carotid arteries predominantly occurs at sites of low shear stress rate [31].

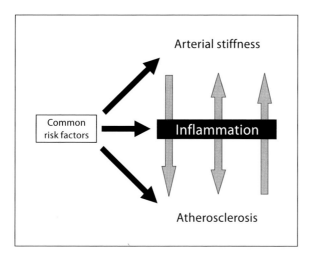

Fig. 1. Possible links between arterial stiffness and atherosclerosis.

Moreover, endothelial dysfunction, characterized by decreased bioavailability of nitric oxide, predicts the risk of future cardiovascular and coronary events in subjects with known coronary artery disease [32, 33], and those with hypertension [34].

Reduced nitric oxide production may also lead to further arterial stiffening. We have recently demonstrated that blockade of nitric oxide synthesis leads to an increase in local arterial stiffness [35, 36], supporting the hypothesis that endothelium-derived NO regulates arterial stiffness in vivo. Interestingly, recent data suggest a correlation between arterial stiffness and endothelial function both in the coronary [37] and peripheral [38] circulations.

Inflammation

Atherosclerosis is increasingly recognized as an inflammatory condition. Indeed, levels of the acute phase reactant C-reactive protein predict the risk of future cardiovascular events in subjects with coronary artery disease and in otherwise healthy individuals [39]. More recently, we and others have shown a relationship between C-reactive protein and large artery stiffness in healthy individuals free from overt atherosclerotic disease or traditional cardiovascular risk factors [40, 41]. Interestingly, acute systemic inflammation either experimental or disease-related [40, 42] leads to reversible aortic stiffening. This strongly suggests that inflammation plays a role in arterial stiffening, possibly due to endothelial dysfunction. However, whether inflammation drives both atherosclerosis and arterial stiffening, whether they all share common risk factors or whether atherosclerosis leads to inflammation which in turn increases arterial stiffness remains unclear (fig. 1).

To summarize: The incidence of atherosclerotic coronary disease is set to increase significantly over the next decade, due in large part to the increased longevity of many modern societies. Primary prevention of coronary disease is therefore a major priority for the future, and will require improved methods of risk stratification. Measurements of traditional risk factors may not provide adequate risk stratification within elderly populations where there is a substantial overlap between 'normal vascular ageing' and disease states leading to 'premature vascular ageing'.

Arterial stiffness is emerging as an important risk factor for CHD and can be non-invasively measured in large populations by a number of methods. Using such techniques, cross-sectional and longitudinal studies have demonstrated the value of arterial stiffness in terms of predicting atherosclerotic coronary events. In order to maximize the predictive power of measuring arterial stiffness in clinical practice, longitudinal studies need to be undertaken in order to ascertain which risk factors are the most important determinants of its progression. In addition, a better understanding of the pathophysiological mechanisms involved in mediating arterial stiffness and atherosclerotic coronary disease will allow improved targeting of therapeutic strategies in the future.

Finally, little doubt remains that the assessment of arterial stiffness will make a major contribution to the improved management of atherosclerotic coronary disease in the clinical arena and its assessment should be included in all future large intervention studies. The choice of technique will be influenced by a number of factors including, cost, ease of use, and most importantly, robust outcome data.

References

1   Downs JR, et al: Primary prevention of acute coronary events with lovastatin in men and women with average cholesterol levels: results of AFCAPS/TexCAPS. Air Force/Texas Coronary Atherosclerosis Prevention Study. JAMA 1998;279:1615–1622.
2   Sacks FM, et al: Coronary heart disease in patients with low LDL-cholesterol: benefit of pravastatin in diabetics and enhanced role for HDL-cholesterol and triglycerides as risk factors. Circulation 2002;105:1424–1428.
3   Hirai T, et al: Stiffness of systemic arteries in patients with myocardial infarction. Circulation 1989;80:78–86.
4   Nishijima T, et al: Pulsatility of ascending aortic blood pressure waveform is associated with an increased risk of coronary heart disease. Am J Hypertens 2001;14:469–473.
5   Ueda H, et al: Inflection point of ascending aortic waveform is a powerful predictor of restenosis after percutaneous transluminal coronary angioplasty. Am J Hypertens 2002;15:823–826.

6   Arroyo-Espliguero R, et al: Chronic inflammation and increased arterial stiffness in patients with cardiac syndrome X. Eur Heart J 2003;24:2006–2011.

7   Philippe F, et al: Aortic pulse pressure and extent of coronary artery disease in percutaneous transluminal coronary angioplasty candidates. Am J Hypertens 2002;15:672–677.

8   Jankowski P, et al: Fractional diastolic and systolic pressure in the ascending aorta are related to the extent of coronary artery disease. Am J Hypertens 2004;17:641–646.

9   McLeod AL, et al: Non-invasive measures of pulse wave velocity correlate with coronary arterial plaque load in humans. J Hypertens 2004;22:363–368.

10 Weber T, et al: Arterial stiffness, wave reflections, and the risk of coronary artery disease. Circulation 2004;109:184–189.

11 Danchin N, et al: Aortic pulse pressure is related to the presence and extent of coronary artery disease in men undergoing diagnostic coronary angiography: a multicenter study. Am J Hypertens 2004;17:129–133.

12 Hayashi T, et al: Reflection in the arterial system and the risk of coronary heart disease. Am J Hypertens 2002;15:405–409.

13 Blacher J, et al: Impact of aortic stiffness on survival in end-stage renal disease. Circulation 1999;99:2434–2439.

14 Laurent S, et al: Aortic stiffness is an independent predictor of all-cause and cardiovascular mortality in hypertensive patients. Hypertension 2001;37:1236–1241.

15 Cruickshank K, et al: Aortic pulse-wave velocity and its relationship to mortality in diabetes and glucose intolerance: an integrated index of vascular function? Circulation 2002;106:2085–2090.

16 Franklin SS, et al: Hemodynamic patterns of age-related changes in blood pressure: the Framingham Heart Study. Circulation 1997;96:308–315.

17 Meaume S, et al: Aortic pulse wave velocity predicts cardiovascular mortality in subjects >70 years of age. Arterioscler Thromb Vasc Biol 2001;21:2046–2050.

18 Sutton-Tyrrell K, et al: Elevated aortic pulse wave velocity, a marker of arterial stiffness, predicts cardiovascular events in well-functioning older adults. Circulation 2005;111:3384–3390.

19 Boutouyrie P, et al: Aortic stiffness is an independent predictor of primary coronary events in hypertensive patients: a longitudinal study. Hypertension 2002;39:10–15.

20 Nichols WW, O'Rourke MF: McDonald's Blood Flow in Arteries: Theoretic, Experimental and Clinical Principles, ed 5. London, Arnold, 2005.

21 O'Rourke MF, Safar ME: Relationship between aortic stiffening and microvascular disease in brain and kidney: cause and logic of therapy. Hypertension 2005;46:200–204.

22 Safar ME, et al: Central pulse pressure and mortality in end-stage renal disease. Hypertension 2002;39:735–738.

23 London GM, et al: Arterial wave reflections and survival in end-stage renal failure. Hypertension 2001;38:434–438.

24 Chirinos JA, et al: Aortic pressure augmentation predicts adverse cardiovascular events in patients with established coronary artery disease. Hypertension 2005;45:980–985.

25 Matsuoka O, et al: Arterial stiffness independently predicts cardiovascular events in an elderly community – Longitudinal Investigation for the Longevity and Aging in Hokkaido County (LILAC) study. Biomed Pharmacother 2005;59(suppl 1):S40–S44.

26 Najjar SS, Scuteri A, Lakatta EG: Arterial aging: is it an immutable cardiovascular risk factor? Hypertension 2005;46:454–462.

27 Lakatta EG, Levy D: Arterial and cardiac aging: major shareholders in cardiovascular disease enterprises. I. Aging arteries: a 'set up' for vascular disease. Circulation 2003;107:139–146.

28 Covic A, et al: Analysis of the effect of hemodialysis on peripheral and central arterial pressure waveforms. Kidney Int 2000;57:2634–2643.

29 Dao HH, et al: Evolution and modulation of age-related medial elastocalcinosis: impact on large artery stiffness and isolated systolic hypertension. Cardiovasc Res 2005;66:307–317.

30 Bergel DH, Cardiovascular Fluid Dynamics, vol 1. London, Academic Press, 1972.

31 Gow BS: The influence of vascular smooth muscle on the viscoelastic properties of blood vessels; in Bergel DH (ed): Cardiovascular Fluid Dynamics. London, Academic Press, 1972, pp 66–97.

32 Schachinger V, Britten MB, Zeiher AM: Prognostic impact of coronary vasodilator dysfunction on adverse long-term outcome of coronary heart disease. Circulation 2000;101:1899–1906.

33 Suwaidi JA, et al: Long-term follow-up of patients with mild coronary artery disease and endo-thelial dysfunction. Circulation 2000;101:948–954.

34 Perticone F, et al: Prognostic significance of endothelial dysfunction in hypertensive patients. Circulation 2001;104:191–196.

35 Wilkinson IB, et al: Nitric oxide regulates local arterial distensibility in vivo. Circulation 2002; 105:213–217.

36 Schmitt M, et al: Basal NO locally modulates human iliac artery function in vivo. Hypertension 2005;46:227–231.

37 Ichigi Y, et al: Increased ambulatory pulse pressure is a strong risk factor for coronary endothe-lial vasomotor dysfunction. J Am Coll Cardiol 2005;45:1461–1466.

38 Ceravolo R, et al: Pulse pressure and endothelial dysfunction in never-treated hypertensive pa-tients. J Am Coll Cardiol 2003;41:1753–1758.

39 Libby P: Inflammation in atherosclerosis. Nature 2002;420:868–874.

40 Yasmin MC, Wallace S, Mackenzie IS, Cockcroft JR, Wilkinson IB: C-reactive protein is associ-ated with arterial stiffness in apparently healthy individuals. Arterioscler Thromb Vasc Biol 2004;24:969–974.

41 Duprez DA, et al: Relationship between C-reactive protein and arterial stiffness in an asymp-tomatic population. J Hum Hypertens 2005;19:515–519.

42 Booth A, et al: Inflammation and arterial stiffness in systemic vasculitis. Arthritis Rheum 2004; 50:581–588.

43 Schram MT, et al: Diabetes, pulse pressure and cardiovascular mortality: the Hoorn Study. J Hy-pertens 2002;20:1743–1751.

John R. Cockcroft
Department of Cardiology, Wales Heart Research Institute
University Hospital, Cardiff CF14 4XN (UK)
Tel. +44 29 2074 3489, Fax +44 29 2074 3500
E-Mail cockcroftjr@Cardiff.ac.uk

Safar ME, Frohlich ED (eds): Atherosclerosis, Large Arteries and Cardiovascular Risk.
Adv Cardiol. Basel, Karger, 2007, vol 44, pp 173–186

·······················

Carotid Atherosclerosis, Arterial Stiffness and Stroke Events

Enrico Agabiti-Rosei   Maria Lorenza Muiesan

Internal Medicine, Department of Medical and Surgical Sciences,
University of Brescia, Brescia, Italy

Abstract

Assessment of intima-media thickness or of measures of large arteries compliance may identify patients at increased risk for stroke. In fact, carotid atherosclerosis and arterial stiffness are both related to risk factors associated with the occurrence of stroke. In addition, several cross-sectional studies have shown that risk factors associated with the occurrence of stroke have been correlated with carotid atherosclerosis development and progression and with increased arterial stiffness. Some studies have also shown that aortic stiffness is associated with the extent of atherosclerosis in the carotid and in other vascular beds. More importantly, longitudinal studies have demonstrated that carotid atherosclerosis and arterial stiffness are independent predictors of stroke (and other cardiovascular events). Interventional studies have demonstrated that treatment with statins, calcium antagonists, ACE inhibitors, and insulin sensitizers may be particularly effective on slowing the progression or favoring the regression of atherosclerotic changes, and may reduce large artery stiffness. It remains to be proven, in large prospective studies, whether the regression of increased arterial stiffness or of carotid intima-media thickness and plaque have a prognostic significance, i.e. are associated with a reduction of the risk of cerebrovascular events.

Introduction

Several cross-sectional studies have shown that risk factors associated with the occurrence of stroke have been correlated with carotid atherosclerosis development and progression and with increased arterial stiffness [1, 2]. Some studies have also shown that aortic stiffness is associated with the extent of atherosclerosis in the carotid and in other vascular beds.

More importantly, longitudinal studies have demonstrated that carotid atherosclerosis and arterial stiffness are independent predictors of stroke (and other cardiovascular events) [1–4]. Based on these important results, current research is focused on markers of subclinical arterial disease that may be measured by non-invasive investigation, i.e. arterial stiffness, carotid intima-media thickness (IMT) and plaque.

Carotid Atherosclerosis (IMT and Plaque)

Methodological Aspects
Carotid ultrasound is routinely used for the evaluation of patients with clinical signs (carotid bruits) or symptoms of cerebrovascular ischemia. Direct visualization of carotid and vertebral arteries is accurate and reproducible, and may allow the identification of plaques; in addition, duplex ultrasound is used to evaluate alterations in the Doppler peak systolic velocities and waveform, in order to measure degree of stenosis, and changes of flow direction in the vertebral arteries. Ultrasonic plaque morphology may add useful information on plaque stability and may correlate with symptoms. Definition of plaques is based on either arbitrary cutpoint of IMT, or on visual inspection and presence of acoustic shadows, or on changes in flow; these different methods can make difficult the evaluation of changes in plaque during interventional studies.

Values of carotid IMT measured at autopsy by ultrasound are similar to those calculated by direct measurement. In patients with preclinical disease, high-resolution ultrasound of the carotid arteries has been widely used for the measurement of intima-media complex (combined thickness of intima and media) in the arterial wall, in order to assess the prevalence, the main determinants and the progression of early vascular lesions [5, 6].

Quantitative analysis of IMT is reliable when sonographers are trained rigorously and reproducibility of scan measurements is evaluated over time; when these aspects are taken into account, measurement of IMT can be used in clinical trials and in routine clinical practice for cardiovascular risk assessment [7, 8].

There are different protocols and methods for measuring IMT [2, 7]. Measurements may be obtained by manual cursor placement or by automated computerized edge detection.

The most frequently used measurements in epidemiological and interventional clinical trials are: (1) mean maximum thickness (M_{max}) of up to 12 different sites (right and left, near and far walls, distal common, bifurcation and proximal internal carotid); (2) overall single maximum IMT (T_{max}), and (3) mean of the maximum IMT of the 4 far walls in the common, bifurcation or internal carotid segment, considered separately or pooled together for the carotid bifurcations and distal common carotid arteries (CBM_{max}).

Measurement of IMT at multiple sites frequently includes plaque thickness.

Some concern still exists regarding the clinical significance of these measures, since far wall common carotid thickness analysis by computerized edge detection may imply the risk of missing important information on other segments of the carotid tree. In addition, a diffuse thickening of the arterial wall may be observed in some patients and several focal plaques in others, so that multiple site IMT measurements could detect both alterations.

Intima-media thickening could represent an early phase in the development of atherosclerotic plaque: according to the results of the EVA (Etude du Vieillissement Artériel) study, in a sample of 1,010 subjects (age range 59–71 years), the higher IMT was a strong predictor of the occurrence of a new plaque during a mean follow-up of 4.4 years [9].

Clinical and epidemiological studies have given useful information on the reproducibility of IMT measured by ultrasound. Salonen et al. [10] have indicated that between-observers and intra-observers variation coefficients resulted in 10.5 and 8.3%, respectively. In the ACAPS study [11] mean replicate difference was 0.11 mm and in the MIDAS [12] 0.12 mm. More recently, in the ELSA (European Lacidipine Study of Atherosclerosis) that included more than 2,000 patients, the cross-sectional reproducibility of ultrasound measurements at baseline was calculated: the overall coefficient of reliability (R) was 0.859 for CBM_{max}, 0.872 for M_{max} and 0.794 for T_{max}; intra- and inter-reader reliability were 0.915 and 0.872, respectively [13].

The normal IMT values are influenced by age, gender and race. Normal values of IMT may be defined in terms of statistical distribution within a healthy population; however, it may be better defined in terms of increased risk. Available data indicate that the relation between carotid IMT and cardiovascular events is continuous; a threshold of 0.9 mm can be taken as a conservative estimate of a significant alteration.

Longitudinal Studies

Traditional risk factors, including male sex, aging, being overweight, elevated blood pressure, diabetes and smoking, are all positively associated with carotid IMT in observational and epidemiological studies [1, 2, 8]. Hypertension and particularly high systolic blood pressure values seem to have the greatest effect on IMT [5, 12–14]. Also, some new risk factors, including various lipoproteins, plasma viscosity, C-reactive protein and hyperhomocysteinemia, have demonstrated an association with increased IMT. Carotid IMT has also been found to be associated with preclinical structural changes in the heart [5], brain, kidney and lower limb arteries.

In the GENIC study that included 510 patients with brain infarction compared with 510 controls, it was observed that common carotid IMT, carotid plaques and the Framingham risk score all significantly correlated with the risk of stroke [15].

Several studies have demonstrated the important prognostic significance of asymptomatic plaque and IMT, as measured by ultrasound.

In patients with asymptomatic carotid atherosclerosis, the annual risk of stroke ranges from 1.3 to 3.3%. The highest risk is observed in patients with the most evident degree of stenosis; Norris et al. [16] observed, in patients with stenosis >75%, a combined annual transient ischemic attack and stroke rate of 10.5%, with 75% of events ipsilateral to the stenosed artery. In the Cardiovascular Health Study (CHS) population [17], 0.5% of subjects had high internal carotid peak velocity (approximately 2.5 m/s, suggesting a stenosis of >70%) and the 5-year risk of an ipsilateral fatal or non-fatal stroke was 5%.

The presence of increased IMT also confers risk for future stroke, as demonstrated by longitudinal prospective studies.

In a large sample of middle-aged (45–65 years) subjects (7,865 women and 6,349 men) enrolled into the ARIC (Atherosclerotic Risk In Communities) study, average IMT, measured by ultrasound at six sites of the carotid arteries, was associated with an increased incidence of stroke [18]. In Cox proportional hazard models, adjusting for age, race and community, the hazard ratio for highest IMT (= or >1 mm) to lowest IMT (<0.6 mm) was 8.5 (95% confidence interval (CI) 3.5–20.7) for women and 3.6 (95% CI 1.5–9.2) for men.

In the Rotterdam study [19] the common carotid IMT was measured in 1,373 control subjects who remained free of cardiovascular diseases, in 98 patients who had an acute myocardial infarction and in 95 patients with a stroke, during a mean follow-up period of 2.7 years. When cases and controls were compared, after adjustment for age and sex, the odds ratio (OR) for stroke per 1 standard deviation (SD) increase of IMT (0.163 mm) was 1.41 (95% CI 1.25–1.82). In men, the OR per SD increase (0.172 mm) was 1.81 (95% CI 1.30–2.51) and in women, an OR of 1.33 (95% CI 1.03–1.71) per 0.155-mm SD increase was observed. When subjects with a previous history of myocardial infarction or stroke were excluded, the ORs were 1.57 (1.27–1.94) for all subjects, 1.89 (95% CI 1.29–2.77) for men, and 1.37 (95% CI 1.02–1.83) for women. Additional adjustment for several cardiovascular risk factors attenuated these associations and the OR per 1 SD increase resulted: 1.34 (95% CI 1.08–1.67), 1.47

Table 1. Outline of the Rotterdam, ARIC and CHS studies

Study	Subjects	Age, years	Follow-up years	Events	Relative risk (95% CI)
Rotterdam study	7,983	>55 (men & women)	3	Acute myocardial infarction and stroke	1.4 (1.2–1.8) 1.4 (1.3–1.8)
ARIC	15,792	45–64 (men & women)	6–9	Stroke	5.5 (3.5–20.7), women 3.6 (1.5–9.2), men
CHS	5,858	>65 (men & women)	6	Acute myocardial infarction and stroke	2.9 (2–4)

(95% CI 1.08–2.02), and 1.14 (95% CI 0.85–1.54), in all subjects, in men and in women, respectively.

A further analysis of the Rotterdam study, comparing the predictive value of several measures of atherosclerosis (carotid IMT and plaques, ankle-arm index, and aortic calcifications) in relation to stroke, has shown that carotid IMT and aortic calcifications were related most strongly to the risk of stroke; the relative risks were 2.23 (95% CI 1.48–3.36) and 1.89 (95% CI 1.28–2.80) for highest versus lowest tertile, respectively. IMT and aortic calcifications were related to the risk of stroke independently of each other [19].

The CHS [20] has prospectively evaluated 4,476 subjects aged >65 years for a follow-up period of 6 years; the annual incidence of stroke increased in the highest quintiles of IMT measured in the common and the internal carotid arteries. The increase of 1 SD in maximal common carotid IMT or maximal combined (common carotid and internal carotid arteries) IMT was associated with a 33–43% increase in risk of stroke after adjustment for age and sex and a 25–33% increase in risk of stroke after adjustment for additional factors ($p < 0.001$ for all comparisons).

The CHS and the Rotterdam study showed that the combined measure of IMT was a stronger predictor than the individual measures, possibly suggesting that the mean maximum IMT may give a more precise estimate of the risk associated to the extent of the atherosclerotic process (table 1).

According to these observations, there is growing evidence that morphological changes of carotid arteries walls may represent a marker of stroke, and as a consequence, an intermediate endpoint for therapeutic intervention in patients at risk for cerebrovascular events. However, it remains to be demonstrated that IMT regression is associated with a reduction in clinical events.

Table 2. Randomized clinical studies evaluating the effect of the treatment with antihypertensive drugs on carotid intima media thickness (IMT) changes

Treatment	Study	IMT	Follow-up, years	IMT progression IMT, mm/year	
				drug	control
Isradipine vs. hydrochlorothiazide	MIDAS	IMT M_{max} 12 walls	3	0.04 (0.002)	0.05 (0.002)
Verapamil vs. chlorthalidone	VHAS	IMT M_{max} 6 walls IM thickening Plaque	4	0.015 (0.005) 0.024 (0.05) −0.06 (0.095)*	0.016 (0.005) 0.021 (0.04) 0.011 (0.09)
Lacidipine vs. atenolol	ELSA	IMT M_{max} 4 walls (CB_{max})	4	0.0057*	0.0146
Nifedipine vs. hydro-chlorothiazide + amiloride	INSIGHT IMT	Common carotid, mean IMT	4	−0.007 (0.002)*	0.0077 (0.002)

MIDAS = Multicenter isradipine diuretic atherosclerotic study; VHAS = verapamil in hypertension and atherosclerosis study; ELSA = European lacidipine study on atherosclerosis; INSIGHT IMT = international nifedipine GITS study: intervention as a goal in hypertension treatment.

* Statistically significant difference vs. control drug.

Effect of Drug Treatment

Therapeutic double-blind trials have assessed the long-term effect mainly of antihypertensive (table 2), and of lipid-lowering drugs on carotid IMT progression.

In hypertensive patients the results indicate a greater effect of calcium antagonists over diuretics and β-blockers on IMT progression [12, 21–23]. In the ELSA [22] a greater effect of lacidipine in plaque progression and regression was shown; the study did not have statistical power to detect differences in clinical events between the two treatment groups. In a small study the effect of a calcium antagonist and of an ACE inhibitor was similar [24].

The effect of angiotensin II antagonists needs to be evaluated in larger studies; available data from small studies indicate that this class of drugs is more effective than β-blockers and similar to ACE inhibitors. As ultrasound methodology is continuously improving, the measurement of plaque volume by three-dimensional reconstruction will be possible, in addition to IMT, for a more precise evaluation of atherosclerotic changes; IMT and plaque volume changes are the endpoint of an ongoing European study comparing an angiotensin II antagonist to a β-blocker [25].

Plaque tissue composition and its changes may be indirectly evaluated by radiofrequency signal or videodensitometric analyses, differentiating the relative amount of lipid-rich macrophages or fibrous tissue. A recent analysis of the plaque composition in the ELSA study has pointed out that in about 70% of patients included in the study plaques are fibrolipidic. After 4 years of treatment with either lacidipine or atenolol, no significant changes in plaque composition were observed, suggesting that treatment with a calcium antagonist may slow IMT progression, without influencing the characteristics of plaque tissue [26].

ACE inhibitors reduce the progression of IMT as compared with placebo or diuretic, in hypertensive hypercholesterolemic patients [27].

In high-risk patients, treatment with an ACE inhibitor, or with a calcium antagonist or a β-blocker, is more effective than administration of placebo (over a conventional treatment) in delaying the progression of IMT [28–30].

A recent meta-regression analysis, including 22 randomized controlled trials, has evaluated the effects of an antihypertensive drug versus placebo or another antihypertensive agent of a different class on carotid IMT. The results have shown that, compared with no treatment, diuretics/β-blockers or ACE inhibitors, CCBs attenuate the rate of progression of carotid intima-media thickening. In the prevention of carotid intima-media thickening, calcium antagonists are more effective than ACE inhibitors, which in turn are more effective than placebo or no treatment, but not more active than diuretics/β-blockers. Among all studies, 9 trials inadequately powered for hard outcomes, reported morbidity and mortality results and the odds ratio for all fatal and non-fatal cardiovascular events in trials comparing active treatment with placebo reached statistical significance (p = 0.007). Therefore, it remains to be demonstrated whether IMT changes may have implications for the long-term prevention of cardiovascular complications such as stroke [31].

In patients with hypercholesterolemia, long-term treatment with a statin may reduce the progression of carotid IMT and favor plaque regression. The changes induced on IMT by statin treatment have about twice the effect observed with antihypertensive drugs. A recent analysis of nine studies, aimed to assess the efficacy of statin treatment on common carotid wall thickness, has demonstrated that carotid IMT reduction was strongly related with LDL decrease. It has been calculated that a 10% reduction in LDL cholesterol concentration is associated with a 0.73% per year decrease in IMT. In the LIPID study and in smaller studies, the occurrence of stroke was significantly lower in the group of patients treated with the active drug in respect to the control group. No correlation between changes in IMT and incidence of stroke is reported [32].

In a recent, randomized, controlled study, the effects of pioglitazone (45 mg/day) and glimepiride (2.7 ± 1.6 mg/day) were compared on carotid

IMT in a large group of 173 patients with type 2 diabetes; despite similar gly-cemic control, an improvement in insulin resistance and a decrease in carotid IMT were observed only in patients treated with pioglitazone [33].

In perimenopausal women [34] the use of hormone replacement therapy was associated with a delayed progression of IMT in the common carotid ar-tery.

Arterial Stiffness

Methodology

Basically, three main methods are used in clinical practice to assess non-invasive measures of arterial stiffness [35].

Aortic stiffness may be obtained by measurement of pulse wave velocity (PWV) along the thoracic and abdominal aorta. Wave forms of the right com-mon carotid artery and the right femoral artery can be detected by applanation tonometry or pressure-sensitive transducers, and the time delay between the feet of the two waveforms is measured. The distance traveled by the pulse wave is measured over the body surface, and the PWV is calculated as the ratio of distance over time (m/s).

In addition, carotid stiffness can be measured directly from the ratio of local pulse pressure (measured by applanation tonometry) to relative stroke change in diameter (measured by ultrasound scan).

Aortic stiffness can be estimated from the augmentation index, i.e. the ad-ditional increase in pressure caused by the pressure wave reflected back from the periphery.

Other parameters and indices of arterial mechanics can also be calculated: (1) the cross-sectional compliance, i.e. the relationship between decline in pressure and decline in volume in the arterial tree during the diastolic pressure decay, which takes into account the volume of the artery, and mainly the age-induced enlargement; (2) the cross-sectional distensibility, i.e. the relative change in vessel diameter (or area) for a given change in pressure, which is re-lated to the mechanical behaviour of the artery as a whole; (3) the Peterson elastic modulus, which is the pressure change required for 100% (theoretical) stretch from resting diameter, and is inversely related to cross-sectional dis-tensibility; (4) the Young's incremental elastic modulus (E_{inc}), which corre-sponds to the elastic modulus per unit area, requires measurement of wall thickness and may give insights on the mechanical behaviour of the wall mate-rial, and (5) the β stiffness index, which corresponds to the ratio of natural logarithm of systolic/diastolic blood pressure to the relative change in diame-ter, and is supposed to be independent of distending pressure.

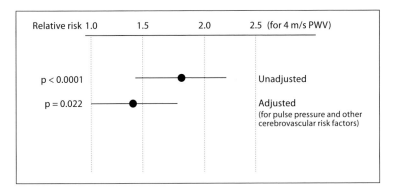

Fig. 1. Predictive value for fatal stroke of pulse wave velocity (PWV) in essential hypertensive patients [from 36].

Brachial pulse pressure (instead of carotid pulse pressure) is used for the calculation of all these parameters and this may reduce their precision. Despite this limitation, all these parameters are well accepted as indices of arterial stiffness [35].

Cross-sectional studies have shown a significant correlation between arterial stiffness and CV risk factors for atherosclerotic lesions, such as aging, hypertension, hypercholesterolemia, type 2 diabetes mellitus or glucose intolerance, metabolic syndrome, and several inflammation parameters, suggesting that arterial stiffness may be considered a marker of CV risk [3].

In addition, longitudinal studies have evaluated the incidence of cardiovascular events, including stroke, during follow-up, and have demonstrated the predictive value of arterial stiffness as an intermediate endpoint.

Longitudinal Studies
Longitudinal studies directly demonstrated that arterial stiffness, measured through carotid-femoral PWV, was an independent predictor of stroke [36] in patients with uncomplicated essential hypertension. In a population of 1,715 essential hypertensive patients, Laurent et al. [36] have found that after a mean follow-up of 7.9 years, for each SD increase in PWV (4 m/s) the relative risk for fatal stroke increased by 1.72 (95% CI 1.48–1.96; $p > 0.0001$). The predictive value of PWV remained significant (RR = 1.39; 95% CI 1.08–1.72; $p > 0.02$) after full adjustment for classic cardiovascular risk factors, including age, cholesterol, diabetes, smoking, mean arterial pressure, and pulse pressure (fig. 1).

Additional evidence of the predictive value of aortic stiffness was provided in patients with end-stage renal disease, although cardiovascular events, i.e. stroke or coronary disease, were not analyzed separately [37].

In 2,488 older subjects participating into the Health, Aging and Body Composition (Health ABC) study [38], aortic PWV was measured at baseline and during the follow-up (over 4.6 years) and 94 stroke events were recorded. The higher quartiles of aortic PWV were significantly associated with an increased risk of stroke, and the association remained statistically significant also after adjustment for age, gender, race, systolic blood pressure, known CV disease, and other variables related to events.

In summary, a significant association between the increase in aortic stiffness and the incidence of cerebrovascular (and cardiovascular) events has been demonstrated, independently from other traditional risk factors. In patients with end-stage renal disease it has also been reported that the lack of decrease in PWV during antihypertensive treatment was associated with a higher cardiovascular mortality, while the improvement of PWV was associated with a lower incidence of cardiovascular events [39].

In addition to aortic stiffness, it may be also important to assess the prognostic significance of carotid stiffness. In stiff carotid arteries the local pulse pressure is increased, and this may influence structural and functional changes of intracranial vessels. Higher local pulse pressure may increase the carotid wall thickness and favor the development of plaques and stenosis, as well as the rupture of unstable plaque.

In patients with end-stage renal disease and with kidney transplantation [38, 40], but not in patients at elevated cardiovascular risk [41], carotid stiffness had a high predictive power for future cardiovascular fatal events, and for ischemic stroke as well.

The pathophysiological mechanisms relating aortic and carotid stiffness to stroke include the association with similar risk factors [42], and the alterations in the vascular wall of aorta that may reflect those in cerebral vessels; in addition, both the carotid arteries and the aorta may be exposed to other pathological mechanisms, such as thrombosis and inflammation [43].

Future trials should provide measurements of both aortic and carotid stiffness in low or moderate CV risk populations, in order to better evaluate their relative prognostic value for cerebrovascular and coronary events.

Effect of Drug Treatment

It is conceivable that the reduction of arterial stiffness may become a therapeutic goal in treating patients at high risk of CV complications [44, 45]. In this regard, an important issue is represented by the ability of different drugs to prevent cardiovascular events by improving arterial distensibility, even independently of the effect on other risk factors.

Organic nitrates, and in particular nitroglycerin, reduce systolic blood pressure, pulse pressure and augmentation index, but have a small effect on peripheral arterial resistance, or on aortic PWV. In fact, organic nitrates may improve symptoms, without modifying mortality or cardiovascular events.

It is generally accepted that ACE inhibitors, calcium antagonists and diuretics may similarly affect large artery stiffness in hypertensive patients, while β-blockers are less effective in this regard [46]. β-Blockers do not reduce central arterial waveform reflection amplitude, while a reduction of the augmentation index has been documented during treatment with β- and α-blockers. The effect of drugs that interfere with the renin-angiotensin system (ACE inhibitors, aldosterone antagonists and angiotensin II antagonists) seems to be, at least in part, independent of blood pressure reduction, since they modify the composition of the vascular wall, including the spatial arrangement of wall material and the collagen content [46–51].

The augmentation index can be reduced by vasodilating drugs and by angiotensin-converting enzyme (ACE) inhibitors in both essential hypertensive patients and in patients with end-stage renal failure. The low-dose combination of the ACE inhibitor perindopril and the diuretic indapamide, in comparison with atenolol, induced a more pronounced effect on central arterial pressure and was associated to a greater decrease in LV mass [50].

The observed effect of ACE inhibitors (and possibly of angiotensin II antagonists) is to some degree influenced by genetic factors [52, 53], since ACE ID and A1166C angiotensin II type 1 receptor polymorphisms are related to carotid-femoral PWV, while M235T angiotensinogen gene and ACE ID polymorphisms are related to carotid stiffness.

In patients with familiar hypercholesterolemia, pravastatin was able to improve arterial stiffness after 13 months of treatment [54], while atorvastatin had no significant effect on carotid stiffness. In non-familiar hypercholesterolemia, short-term treatment with simvastatin did not change aorto-femoral PWV.

In addition, treatment for 2 months with a new compound, that acts as an advanced glycation product cross-link breaker, has been beneficial in ameliorating PWV [55].

Conclusions

Carotid atherosclerosis and arterial stiffness are both related to risk factors associated with the occurrence of stroke. These two markers of 'preclinical' vascular disease are related to the occurrence of stroke independently of other cardiovascular risk factors. Assessment of IMT or of measures of large arteries compliance may therefore identify patients at increased risk for stroke.

Interventional studies have demonstrated that treatment with statins, calcium antagonists, ACE inhibitors, and insulin sensitizers may be particularly effective on slowing the progression or favoring the regression of atherosclerotic changes, and may reduce large artery stiffness. It remains to be demonstrated in large prospective studies whether the regression of increased arterial stiffness or of carotid IMT and plaque have a prognostic significance, i.e. are associated with a reduction of the risk of cerebrovascular events.

References

1   Mancini JGB, Dahlof B, Díéz J: Surrogate markers for cardiovascular disease. Structural markers. Circulation 2004;109(suppl IV):IV-22–IV-30.
2   Simon A, Gariepy J, Chironi G, Megnien JL, Levenson J: Intima-media thickness: a new tool for diagnosis and treatment of cardiovascular risk. J Hypertens 2002;20:159–169.
3   Laurent S: Arterial stiffness intermediate or surrogate endpoint for cardiovascular events. Eur Heart J 2005;26:1152–1154.
4   Oliver J, Webb DJ: Non-invasive assessment of arterial stiffness and the risk of atherosclerotic events. Arterioscler Thromb Vasc Biol 2003;23:554–566.
5   Muiesan ML, Pasini GF, Salvetti M, Calebich S, Zulli R, Castellano M, Rizzoni D, et al: Cardiac and vascular structural changes: prevalence and relation to ambulatory blood pressure in a middle-aged general population in northern Italy: the Vobarno Study. Hypertension 1996;27:1046–1053.
6   Poli A, Tremoli E, Colombo A, Sirtori M, Pignoli P, Paoletti R: Ultrasonographic measurement of the common carotid artery wall thickness in hypercholesterolemic patients: A new model for the quantitation and follow-up of preclinical atherosclerosis in living human subjects. Atherosclerosis 1988;70:253–261.
7   Bots M, Evans GW, Riley WA, Grobbee DE: Carotid intima-media thickness measurements in intervention studies design options, progression rates, and sample size considerations: a point of view. Stroke 2003;34:2985–2994.
8   Baldassarre D, Amato M, Bondioli A, Sirtori C, Tremoli E: Carotid intima-media thickness measured by ultrasonography in normal clinical practice correlates well with atherosclerotic risk factors. Stroke 2000;31:2426–2430.
9   Zureik M, Ducimetiere P, Touboul PJ, Courbon D, Bonithon-Kopp C, Berr C, Magne C: Common carotid predicts occurrence of carotid atherosclerotic plaques: longitudinal results from the Aging Vascular Study (EVA) study. Arterioscler Thromb Vasc Biol 2000;20:1622–1629.
10 Salonen R, Haapanen A, Salonen JT: Measurement of intima-media thickness of common carotid arteries with high resolution B-mode ultrasonography: inter- and intra-observer variability. Ultrasound Med Biol 1991;17:225–230.
11 Furberg CD, Adams HP Jr, Applegate WB, Byington RB, Espeland MA, Hartwell T, et al: Effect of lovastatin on early carotid atherosclerosis and cardiovascular events. Asymptomatic Carotid Artery Progression Study (ACAPS) Research Group. Circulation 1994;90:1679–1687.
12 Borhani NO, Mercuri M, Borhani PA, Buckalow VM, et al: Final outcome results of the Multicenter Isradipine Diuretic Atherosclerosis Study (MIDAS). JAMA 1996;276:785–791.
13 Tang R, Henning M, Thomasson B; Scherz R, Ravinetto R, Cattalini R, et al: Baseline reproducibility of B-mode ultrasonic measurement of carotid artery intima-media thickness: the European Lacidipine Study on Atherosclerosis (ELSA). J Hypertens 2000;18:197–201.
14 Zanchetti A, Bond G, Hennig M, Neiss A, Mancia G, Dal Palù C, Hansson L, Magnani B, Rahn KH, Reid J, Rodicio J, Safar M, Eckes L, Ravinetto R on behalf of the ELSA Investigators: Risk factors associated with alterations in carotid intima-media thickness in hypertension: baseline data from the European Lacidipine Study on Atherosclerosis. J Hypertens 1998;16:949–961.
15 Touboul P, Labreuche J, Vicaeut E, Amarenco P, on behalf of the GENIC Investigators: Carotid intima-media thickness, plaque and Framingham risk score are independent determinants of stroke risk. Stroke 2005;36:1741–1745.

16   Norris JW, Zhu CZ, Bornstein NM, Chambers BR: Vascular risks of asymptomatic carotid stenosis. Stroke 1991;22:1485–1490.

17   Longstreth WT Jr, Shemanski L, Lefkowitz D, O'Leary DH, Polak JF, Wolfson SK Jr: Asymptomatic internal carotid artery stenosis defined by ultrasound and the risk of subsequent stroke in the elderly. The Cardiovascular Health Study. Stroke 1998;29:2371–2376.

18   Chambeless LE, Folsom AR, Clegg LX, Sharret AR, Shahar E, Nieto FJ, Rosamond W, Evans G: Carotid wall thickness is predictive of incident clinical stroke: the Atherosclerosis Risk in Communities (ARIC) Study. Am J Epidemiol 2000;151:478–487.

19   Bots ML, Hoes AW, Koudstaal PJ, Hofman A, Grobbee DE: Common carotid intima-media thickness and risk of stroke and myocardial infarction the Rotterdam study. Circulation 1997;6:1432–1437.

20   O'Leary DH, Polak JF, Kronmal RA, Manolio TA, Burke GL, Wolfson SK for the Cardiovascular Health Study Collaborative Research Group: Carotid intima and media thickness as a risk factor for myocardial infarction and stroke in older adults. N Engl J Med 1999;340:14–22.

21   Zanchetti A, Agabiti-Rosei E, Dal Palù' C, Leonetti G, Magnani B, Pessina A, for the Verapamil in Hypertension and Atherosclerosis Study (VHAS) Investigators: The VHAS: results of long-term randomized treatment with either verapamil or chlortalidone on carotid intima-media thickness. J Hypertens 1998;16:1667–1676.

22   Zanchetti A, Bond MG, Hennig M, Neiss A, Mancia G, Dal Palù C, et al: Calcium antagonist lacidipine slows down progression of asymptomatic carotid atherosclerosis: principal results of the European Lacidipine Study on Atherosclerosis (ELSA), a randomized, double-blind, long-term trial. Circulation 2002;106:2422–2427.

23   Simon A, Gariepy J, Moyse D, Levenson J: Differential effects of nifedipine and co-amilozide on the progression of early carotid atherosclerosis. A four-year randomised, controlled clinical study of intima-media thickness measured by ultrasound. Circulation 2001;103:2949–2954.

24   Stanton AV, Chapman JN, Mayet J, Sever PS, Poulter NR, Hughes AD, Thom SA: Effects of blood pressure lowering with amlodipine or lisinopril on vascular structure of the common carotid artery. Clin Sci 2001;101:455–464.

25   Stumpe KO, Ludwig M: Antihypertensive efficacy of olmesartan compared with other antihypertensive drugs. J Hum Hypertens 2002;16, S24–S28.

26   Paliotti R, Ciulla M, Hennig M, Tang R, Bond G, Mancia G, Magrini F, Zanchetti A: Carotid wall composition in hypertensive patients after 4-year treatment with lacidipine or atenolol: an echoreflectivity study J Hypertens 2005;23:1203–1209.

27   Zanchetti A, Crepaldi G, Bond G, Gallus G, Veglia F, Mancia G, Ventura S, Baggio G, Sampietri L, Rubba P, Sperti G, Magni A on behalf of PHYLLIS Investigators: Different effects of antihypertensive regimens based on fosinopril or hydrochlorothiazide with or without lipid lowering by pravastatin on progression of asymptomatic carotid atherosclerosis principal results of PHYLLIS – a randomized double-blind trial. Stroke 2004;35:2807–2812.

28   Pitt B, Byington RP, Furberg CD, Hunninghake DB, Mancini GB, Miller ME, Riley W (for The PREVENT Investigators): Effect of amlodipine on the progression of atherosclerosis and the occurrence of clinical events. Circulation 2000;102:1503–1510.

29   Lonn EM, Yusuf S, Dzivik V, Doris CI, Yi Q, Smith S, et al: Effect of ramipril and vitamin E on atherosclerosis. The study to evaluate ultrasound changes in patients treated with ramipril and vitamin E (SECURE). Circulation 2001;103:919–925.

30   Hedblad B, Wikstrand J, Janzon L, Wedel H, Berglund G: Low-dose metoprolol CR/XL and fluvastatin slow progression of carotid intima-media thickness: main results from the Beta-Blocker Cholesterol-Lowering Asymptomatic Plaque Study (BCAPS). Circulation 2001;103:1721–1726.

31   Wang JG, Staessen JA, Li Y, Van Bortel LM, Nawrot T, Fagard R, Messerli FH, Safar M: Carotid intima-media thickness and antihypertensive treatment: a meta-analysis of randomized controlled trials. Stroke 2006;37:1933–1940.

32   Amarenco P, Labreuche J, Lavallee P, Touboul PJ: Statins in stroke prevention and carotid atherosclerosis. Systematic review and up-to-date meta-analysis. Stroke 2004;35:2902–2909.

33   Langenfeld MR, Forst T, Hohberg C, Kann P, Lubben G, Konrad T, Fullert SD, Sachara C, Pfutzner A: Pioglitazone decreases carotid intima-media thickness independently of glycemic control in patients with type 2 diabetes mellitus: results from a controlled randomized study. Circulation 2005;111:2525–2531.

34   De Kleijn MJ, Bots ML, Bak AA, Westendorp IC, Planellas J, Coelingh Bennink HJ, et al: Hormone replacement therapy in perimenopausal women and 2-year change of carotid intima-media thickness. Maturitas 1999;32:195–204.

35   Pannier BM, Avolio AP, Hoeks A, Mancia G, Takazawa K: Methods and devices for measuring arterial compliance in humans. Am J Hypertens 2002;15:743–753.

36   Laurent S, Katsahian S, Fassot C, Tropeano AI, Gautier I, Laloux B, Boutouyrie P: Aortic stiffness is an independent predictor of fatal stroke in essential hypertension. Stroke 2003;34:1203–1206.

37   Blacher J, Pannier B, Guerin A, Marchais SJ, Safar ME, London GM: Carotid arterial stiffness as a predictor of cardiovascular and all-cause mortality in end-stage renal disease. Hypertension 1998;32:570–574.

38   Sutton-Tyrrell K, Najjar S, Boudreau R, Venkitachalam L, Kupelian V, Simonsick E, Havlik R, Lakatta E, Spurgeon H, Kritchevsky S, Pahor M, Bauer D, Newman A, for the Health ABC Study: Elevated aortic pulse wave velocity, a marker of arterial stiffness, predicts cardiovascular events in well-functioning older adults. Circulation 2005;111:3384–3390.

39   Guerin AP, Blacher J, Pannier B, Marchais SJ, Safar ME, London GM: Impact of aortic stiffness attenuation on survival of patients in end-stage renal failure. Circulation 2001;20:987–992.

40   Barenbrock M, Kosh M, Joster E, Kisters K, Rhan KH, Hausberg M: Reduced arterial distensibility is a predictor of cardiovascular disease in patients after renal transplantation. J Hypertens 2002;20:79–84.

41   Dijk JM, Algra A, van der Graaf Y, Grobbee DE, Bots ML, on behalf of the SMART Study Group: Carotid stiffness and the risk of new vascular events in patients with manifest cardiovascular disease. The SMART study. Eur Heart J doi:10.1093/eurheartj/ehi254.

42   Dijk JM, van der Graaf Y, Grobbee DE, Bots ML, on behalf of the SMART Study Group: Carotid stiffness indicates risk of ischemic stroke and TIA in patients with internal carotid artery stenosis. The SMART study. Stroke 2004;35:2258–2262.

43   Mahmud A, Feely J: Arterial stiffness is related to systemic inflammation in essential hypertension. Hypertension 2005;46:1118–1122.

44   Laurent S, Boutouyrie P: Arterial stiffness and stroke in hypertension: therapeutic implications for stroke prevention. CNS Drugs 2005;19:1–11.

45   Laurent S, Kingwell B, Bank A, et al: Clinical applications of arterial stiffness: Therapeutic and pharmacology. Am J Hypertens 2002;15:453–458.

46   Safar ME, Van Bortel LMAB, Struijker Boudier HAJ: Resistance and conduit arteries following converting enzyme inhibition in hypertension. J Vasc Res 1997;34:67–81.

47   Benetos A, Lacolley P, Safar M: Prevention of aortic fibrosis by spironolactone in spontaneously hypertensive rats. J Hypertens 1995;13:839–848.

48   Blacher J, Amah G, Girerd X, et al: Association between effects of antihypertensive drugs on arterial reflections, compliance and impedance. Hypertension 1995;26:524–530.

49   Lacolley P, Labat C, Pujol A, et al: Increased carotid wall compliance after long-term antihypertensive treatment: The effects of eplerenone. Circulation 2002;106:2848–2853.

50   Asmar RG, London GM, O'Rourke ME, et al: Improvement in blood pressure, arterial stiffness and wave reflections with a very-low-dose perindopril/indapamide combination in hypertensive patient: a comparison with atenolol. Hypertension 2001;38:922–926.

51   Morgan T, Lauri J, Bertram D, Anderson A: Effect of different antihypertensive drug classes on central aortic pressure. Am J Hypertens 2004;17:118–123.

52   Laurent S, Boutouyrie P, Lacolley P: Structural and genetic bases of arterial stiffness. Hypertension 2005;45:1050–1055.

53   Manolio TA, Boerwinkle E, O'Donnel CJ, Wilson A: Genetics of ultrasonographic carotid atherosclerosis. Arterioscler Thromb Vasc Biol 2004;24:1567–1577.

54   Giannattasio C, Mangoni AA, Failla M, et al: Impaired radial artery compliance in normotensive subjects with familial hypercholesterolemia. Atherosclerosis 1996;124:249–260.

55   Kass DA, Shapiro EP, Kawaguchi M, et al: Improved arterial compliance by a novel advanced glycation end-product cross-link breaker. Circulation 2001;104:1464–1470.

Prof. Enrico Agabiti-Rosei, Chair of Internal Medicine
Department of Medical and Surgical Sciences, University of Brescia
c/o 2ª Medicina Spedali Civili di Brescia, Piazza Spedali Civili 1, IT–25100 Brescia (Italy)
Tel. +39 030 396 044, Fax +39 030 338 8147, E-Mail agabiti@med.unibs.it

Safar ME, Frohlich ED (eds): Atherosclerosis, Large Arteries and Cardiovascular Risk.
Adv Cardiol. Basel, Karger, 2007, vol 44, pp 187–198

. . . .

Atherosclerosis versus Arterial Stiffness in Advanced Renal Failure

A. Guerin   B. Pannier   G. London

Service de Néphrologie, Centre Hospitalier Manhes, Fleury Mérogis, France

Abstract

Epidemiological as well as clinical studies have shown that regardless of the severity
of renal impairment the cardiovascular mortality in renal disease patients is very high
compared to the general population. In uremia, cardiovascular disease is a combination
of atherosclerosis, characterized by the presence of highly calcified plaques, and arteriosclerosis, an arterial wall alteration in response to both hemodynamic changes and humoral modifications such as inflammation or calcium-phosphate imbalance. Vascular
endothelium, recognized as a large and complex endocrine organ strategically located
between the wall of the blood vessel and the blood stream, could be the link between these
two processes evolving during the same course.

Epidemiological and clinical studies have shown that end-stage renal disease (ESRD) patients die from cardiovascular disease much younger than people in the general population. Age-adjusted cardiovascular mortality is about
30 times higher in ESRD than in the general population. In the National Insti-
tutes of Health Hemodialysis Study, prevalence of cerebrovascular disease, peripheral arterial disease or coronary heart disease was respectively 19, 23 and
40% [1]. However, cardiovascular complications are also a cause of mortality
in patients during the course of chronic renal failure before dialysis. It is only
recently that mild renal insufficiency was associated with an increased cardiovascular risk, as some proatherogenic factors are present in early or mild renal
insufficiency. It is important to keep in mind that regardless of how renal disease severity is classified (degree of urine albuminuria or proteinuria, glomer-

ular filtration rate, or presence of ESRD), 10-year mortality for severe renal abnormality is extraordinarily high (107 per 1,000 person-years) compared with that predicted by Framingham data with multiple risk factors (25 per 1,000 person-years) [2].

Moreover, cardiovascular disease in uremia is a combination of atherosclerosis and arteriosclerosis leading to uremic cardiomyopathy. Atherosclerosis, a primary intimal disease characterized by the presence of plaques and occlusive lesions, is the most frequent cause of cardiovascular complications. However, many of these complications occur in the absence of clinically significant atherosclerotic disease [3]. Arterial wall alteration is not only the response to direct injury or to the presence of atherogenic factors, it is also involved in the response to hemodynamic burden modifications [4]. The structural modifications induced by hemodynamic alterations are changes in arterial lumen and/or arterial wall thickness [5].

Atherosclerosis

Atherosclerosis is characterized by the presence of plaques, focal and patchy in its distribution. It occurs preferentially in medium-sized conduit arteries, coronary, iliac, femoral arteries and less often in muscular arteries in the arm or internal mammary. In ESRD, these plaques are characterized by the intensity of calcifications.

There is growing evidence that inflammation probably plays a key role in the initiation and progression of the atherosclerotic process, and atherosclerosis has been consequently defined as an inflammatory disease [6]. A high percentage of chronic kidney disease (CKD) patients have serological evidence of an activated inflammatory response [7, 8]. Serum levels of C-reactive protein appear to reflect the generation of proinflammatory cytokines such as interleukin (IL)-1, IL-6, tumor necrosis factor-α (TNF-α), all of which have been reported to be markedly elevated in ESRD patients and also to predict mortality [8–11]. The causes of this phenomenon are multifactorial, including the decreased renal clearance and increased synthesis of proinflammatory cytokines, comorbidities such as diabetes or chronic heart failure and the atherosclerotic process per se [6], the accumulation of advanced glycation end-products [12] and other factors related to the dialytic procedure such as vascular access infections, membrane bioincompatibility, and contaminated dialysate. However, it is very difficult to distinguish whether chronic inflammation is a cause or a consequence of cardiovascular disease and it is still an open question. Currently, no treatments for the management of chronic inflammation in CKD are recognized, but attention has been paid to all of the factors that can maintain or enhance inflammation in CKD.

Hyperhomocysteinemia, which is now recognized as a proatherogenic factor and as an independent predictor of cardiovascular disease in the general population, is present from the earliest stage of CKD and increases inversely with the reduction in renal function [13]. Hyperhomocysteinemia has many causes in CKD including decreased activity of the remethylation cycle, decreased serum folate and vitamin B intake and decreased renal clearance of homocysteine. Homocysteine may increase oxidative stress, decrease nitric oxide (NO) availability and produce endothelial dysfunction [14]. The intravenous administration of acetylcysteine, a thiol-containing antioxidant, reduces the plasma homocysteine level and probably improves endothelial function in ESRD patients [15]. Although an association between hyperhomocysteine levels and cardiovascular events has been proven, particularly in CKD, the cause has not yet been demonstrated.

Numerous data suggest that CKD is a prooxidant state as shown by the increase in a number of oxidative stress markers in CKD patients [16]. In renal failure, oxidative stress imposes damage on DNA (8-oxo-OH-deoxyguanosine), proteins (carbonyl compounds, advanced oxidation protein products), carbohydrates (advanced glycation end-products) and lipids (oxidized LDL). Oxidative stress involves the increased production of free radicals which can exhaust endogenous antioxidant and lead to vascular injury. The activity of multiple oxidases, including Nox oxidases, nitric oxide synthase, xanthine oxidase, cytochrome P_{450}, cyclooxygenase and mitochondria can contribute to the generation of oxidant species in the vessel wall [17]. On the other hand, in hemodialysis patients oxidative stress is commonly attributed to the recurrent activation of polymorphonuclear neutrophils and monocytes, closely related to membrane biocompatibility, generating the cascade of highly reactive oxygen species (ROS) [18] (fig. 1). The repetitive enhancement of ROS production associated with complement activation and overexpression of adhesive molecules in circulating leukocytes could promote endothelial cell membrane lipid peroxidation leading to endothelial dysfunction. Moreover, activity of the glutathione system has been shown to be significantly decreased in hemodialysis patients. This diminution begins early in the course of chronic renal failure and steadily progresses as renal function decreases [19]. The data concerning other oxidant-scavenging molecules such as superoxide dismutase, ceruloplasmin or transferrin appear less clear. The role of vitamin C is still a matter of debate and vitamin E concentration is normal in the plasma and decreased in erythrocytes and mononuclear cells [20].

The imbalance between free radical formation and neutralization which deteriorate over time may be the causative factor for the activation of an in-

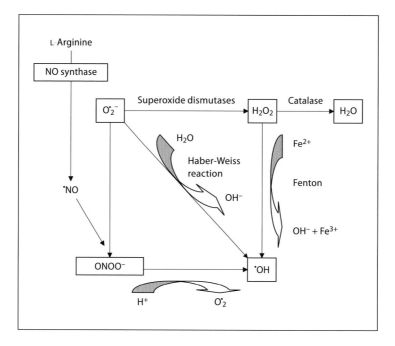

Fig. 1. ROS such as hydrogen peroxide (H_2O_2) or free radical such as superoxide (O_2^-), hydroxyl radical (OH), and nitric oxide (NO) are continuously and physiologically formed in vivo. It is the imbalance between formation of ROS and defense mechanisms, such as superoxide dismutase, that creates oxidative stress [18].

flammatory cascade by a variety of potential stimulators in uremia and dialysis. A common signaling occurs via the generation of oxygen free radicals, activation of the transcription factor nuclear factor-κB (NF-κB) and induction of a number of genes such as adhesion molecules, cytokines, chemokines and matrix proteins [21]. NF-κB is also involved in the proliferation of vascular smooth muscle cells which is a crucial event in the formation of atherosclerosis tissue [22]. Moreover, recent studies indicate that proinflammatory cytokines may also have direct atherogenic properties. IL-6 is a stimulant of adhesion molecule-1 but also contributes to the development of atherosclerosis through various mechanisms reviewed recently by Yudkin et al. [23]. TNF-α has been shown to promote in vitro calcification of vascular cells [24] or to cause endothelial dysfunction [25].

Hypertension appears to promote vascular dysfunction associated with increased scavenging of NO by superoxide anion that seems to originate from an initial activation of Nox oxidases through increased pressure and angiotensin II [26]. There is strong experimental evidence of a role for angiotensin II in increasing oxidative stress, particularly in hypertension [27]. Accordingly, in transgenic rat harboring human renin and angiotensinogen genes, Mervaala et al. [28] showed that experimentally induced oxidative stress was normalized by treatment with valsartan.

Markers of oxidative stress have been correlated with impaired endothelial function or the presence of carotid plaques and intima-media thickness in some studies [29–31]. Recent studies suggested that carotid intima-media thickness is an independent predictor of cardiovascular mortality in the hemodialysis population [32, 33] but the arterial changes could occur early in the course of renal disease [34]. The Secondary Prevention with Antioxidants of Cardiovascular Disease in End-Stage Renal Disease (SPACE) trial has demonstrated positive results on the improvement in cardiovascular outcomes in hemodialysis patients with a history of cardiovascular disease with oral vitamin E supplementation [35]. The prospective study with acetylcysteine administered as an antioxidant in 134 hemodialysis patients showed reduced composite cardiovascular endpoints [36]. Despite these results, there is currently no evidence that increased oxidative stress contributes to the increased cardiovascular morbidity and mortality in CKD patients.

Other targets of ROS are lipids, the oxidation of which is associated with increased cardiovascular risks. First, the process of lipid peroxidation itself generates more free radical and ROS which increase the potential to do harm. Second, the lipid peroxidation is the first step in the generation of oxidized LDL (ox-LDL) which is implicated in atherogenesis. These modified lipids can induce the expression of adhesion molecules, chemokines, proinflammatory cytokines and other mediators of inflammation in macrophages and vascular wall cells. Some studies showed that ESRD patients had a higher level of anti ox-LDL antibody than healthy subjects [37].

More recently, Shoji et al. [38] were able to demonstrate, for the first time, that the serum level of antibody to ox-LDL was an independent predictor of cardiovascular mortality in ESRD patients. On the contrary, the same team showed an inverse association between intima-media thickness of carotid and femoral arteries suggesting an antiatherogenic role of antibody to ox-LDL [39]. ox-LDL and antibodies to ox-LDL play a pivotal but still controversial role in the development of atherosclerosis. Atherogenic ox-LDL increases progressively during the development of renal failure, suggesting that the oxidation of LDL may be associated with endothelial injury and atherogenesis in these patients [40]. Therefore, van den Akker et al. [41] studied the effect of statins on the level of these drugs in a small group of hemodialysis patients. They showed a significant decrease of ox-LDL, but there was no significant change of IgG and IgM autoantibodies to ox-LDL.

Arteriosclerosis and Arterial Remodeling

During the same course, and not independently of the atherosclerosis process, arterial remodeling accompanies the growing hemodynamic burden and humoral abnormalities associated to chronic uremia [42]. Evidence that enhanced tensile stress is relevant to the pathogenesis of atherosclerosis comes from the observation that atherosclerotic plaques are virtually confined to systemic arteries where tensile stress is high. Moreover, the role of shear stress is demonstrated by the predilection of atherosclerosis for sites, characterized by flow pattern and shear stress disturbances, like bending or branching.

The mechanical signals for arterial remodeling associated with hemodynamic overload are the cyclic tensile stress or shear stress [43, 44]. This includes the chronic alterations of mechanical forces which lead to the changes in the geometry and the composition of the vessel wall; changes which may be considered as an adaptative response to long-lasting changes in blood flow and pressure. The quality of the responsiveness of the arterial wall to mechanical stimuli is tightly dependent on the presence of an intact endothelium [45, 46].

Experimental and clinical data indicate that acute and chronic augmentations of arterial blood flow induce proportional increases in the vessel lumen diameter, whereas decreasing flow reduces arterial inner diameter [47]. It is activation of the endothelium, strategically situated at the blood vessel-wall interface, which transforms physical forces into biochemical signals through the generation of vasoactive substances.

Arterial Functions

The conduit function of arteries is to supply an adequate blood flow to peripheral organs. Their physiological adaptability is highly efficient and acute diameter changes are dependent on the endothelium which responds to alterations in shear stress. In chronic overload, the arterial diameters are enlarged and baseline arterial conductance is increased [48].

The role of arteries is also to dampen the pressure and flow oscillations resulting from intermittent ventricular ejection and to transform the pulsatile flow of arteries into a steady flow required in peripheral tissue. The efficiency of the conduit function depends on the viscoelastic properties of the arterial wall as well as the diameter and length of the arteries. The viscoelastic property is best described in term of stiffness (S) [49]. Arterial stiffness can be evaluated by ultrasonography or by measuring the pulse wave velocity (PWV) over a given arterial segment. PWV increases with arterial stiffness [49].

Arterial Stiffness and Blood Pressure Changes: Cardiovascular Consequences

In uremic patients, the arterial system of CKD and ESRD patients undergoes remodeling that is characterized by dilatation and to a lesser degree arterial intima-media hypertrophy of central elastic type, capacitive arteries and wall hypertrophy of peripheral muscular type conduit arteries [34, 48, 50]. Large arteries, like the aorta or common carotid artery, are enlarged in CKD before the onset of dialysis and ESRD patients in comparison with age-, sex- and pressure-matched control subjects [51, 52]. In ESRD patients, this remodeling is associated with arterial stiffening related to alterations of the intrinsic properties of the arterial wall materials including those free of atherosclerosis [48, 53, 54]. Nevertheless, according to Laplace's law [5], the wall-to-lumen ratio should increase in order to normalize tensile stress. This increase was not observed in ESRD patients whose wall-to-lumen ratio in large conduit arteries was not related to pressure changes. This observation suggests that conduit arteries could have limited capacity to hypertrophy in response to a combined flow and pressure load.

Functional Consequences

In ESRD patients, the arterial remodeling is associated with arterial stiffening due to the alterations of the intrinsic properties of arterial wall material. Contrary to the arterial distensibility measurements in essential hypertensive patients in whom distensibility is increased, in ESRD arterial hypertrophy is accompanied by alteration in the intrinsic elastic properties of the vessel wall (incremental modulus, E_{inc}). The observation that the incremental modulus of elasticity is increased in ESRD patients, i.e. a decrease distensibility, strongly favors altered intrinsic elastic properties or major architectural abnormalities like those seen in experimental uremia and the arteries of uremic patients, namely fibroelastic intimal thickening, increased extracellular matrix and high calcium content with extensive medial calcifications [54–56]. Recent data indicate that mediacalcosis and extensive calcifications of the arterial tree are an important factor accounting for the increased of arterial stiffening [55, 56]. Phosphate retention and poorly controlled calcium phosphate balance play an important role in the pathogenesis of these arterial changes. And aortic PWV was found to be associated with an increased serum phosphorus, high calcium phosphate product and the total dose of calcium-based phosphate binder [57]. Arterial calcifications and arterial stiffening in ESRD patients are associated with the presence of systemic microinflammation, as evaluated by serum C-reactive protein levels. The association of dyslipidemia and arterial calcification in CKD is controversial, being found negative or positive [57].

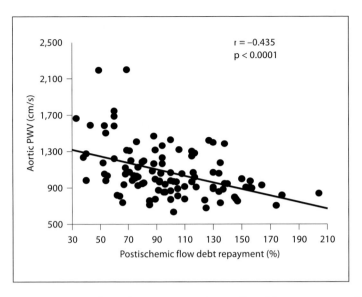

Fig. 2. Correlation between postischemic flow debt repayment and aortic PWV (personal data).

An association between arterial alterations and lipid abnormalities was found only irregularly. An inverse relationship between PWV and HDL cholesterol was shown [53, 58] and a positive relationship was described between carotid intima-media thickness and IDL or LDL cholesterol.

Arterial stiffening in CKD and ESRD patients is associated with an increase in systolic pressure and/or pulse pressure. The mechanism responsible for the alterations of the arterial pressure has been depicted by London et al. [59]. Epidemiological studies have shown that pulse pressure is associated with risk of death in patients undergoing hemodialysis [60]. A recent study demonstrated that arterial stiffening and increased wave reflections are per se independent predictors of all-cause and cardiovascular death in ESRD patients [61].

Endothelial Dysfunction

In recent years the vascular endothelium has been recognized as a large and complex endocrine organ. Endothelium-derived NO is critically involved in the regulation of a wide variety of vascular functions: vasodilatory, antiproliferative and antithrombogenic. Nevertheless, under conditions of increased oxidative stress, as in ESRD, NO may be involved in vascular damage atherosclerosis and probably arteriosclerosis [62], but the results on the vasodilatory effects of NO in ESRD remain controversial. As shown experimentally, the endothelium influences the mechanical and geometric properties of large arteries [63]. Some studies measuring flow-mediated vasodilatation, a surrogate marker in the evaluation of endothelial function, found an impaired endothelial function in CKD and ESRD [64, 65]. The altered hyperemic response is correlated to arterial remodeling parameters and to aortic stiffness (fig. 2, also personal data). Moreover, endothelial cell dysfunction is associated to all-cause mortality [65]. Aside many other causes, circulating endothelial derived microparticles are tightly associated with endothelial dysfunction and arterial dysfunction in ESRD [66].

Conclusion

The vascular complications in ESRD are ascribed to two different but associated mechanisms, namely atherosclerosis and arteriosclerosis. Endothelium, the body's largest organ strategically located between the wall of blood vessels and the bloodstream, could be the link between the two faces of the arterial alteration underlying many common physiological molecules and reactions.

References

1 Cheug AK, Sarnak MJ, Yan G: Atherosclerotic cardiovascular disease risks in chronic hemodialysis patients. Kidney Int 2000;58:353–362.
2 McCullough PA: Cardiorenal risk: an important clinical intersection. Rev Cardiovasc Med 2002; 3:71–76.
3 Rostand RG, Kirk KA, Rutsky EA: Dialysis ischemic heart disease: insight from coronary angiography. Kidney Int 1984;25:653–659.
4 Gibbons GH, Dzau VJ: The emerging concept of vascular remodeling. N Engl J Med 1994;330: 1431–1438.
5 London GM, Marchais SJ, Guerin AP, Metivier F, Adda H: Arterial structure and function in end-stage renal disease. Nephrol Dial Transplant 2002;17:1713–1724.
6 Ross R: Atherosclerosis – an inflammatory disease. N Engl J Med 1999;340:115–126.
7 Zimmerman J, Herlinger S, Pruy A, Metzger T, Wanner C: Inflammation enhances cardiovascular risk and mortality in hemodialysis patients. Kidney Int 1999;55:648–658.
8 Yeun JY, Levine RA, Mantadilok V, Kayssen GA: C-reactive protein predicts all-cause and cardiovascular mortality in hemodialysis patients. Am J Kidney Dis 2000;35:469–476.
9 Pecolts-Filho R, Barany P, Linholm B, Heimburger G, Stenvinkel P: Interleukin-6 is an independent predictor of mortality in patients starting dialysis treatment. Nephrol Dial Transplant 2002; 17:1684–1688.
10 Menon V, Wang X, Greene T, Beck GJ, Kusek JW, Marcovina SM, et al: Relationship between C-reactive protein, albumin and cardiovascular disease in patients with chronic kidney disease. Am J Kidney Dis 2003;42:44–52.

11 Iseki K, Tozawa M, Yoshi S, Fukiyama K: Serum C-reactive protein and risk of death in chronic dialysis patients. Nephrol Dial Transplant 1999;14:1956–1960.

12 Heidland A, Sebekov K, Schinkel R: Advanced glycation end products and the progressive course of renal disease. Am J Kidney Dis 2001;38(suppl 1):S100–S106.

13 Bostom AG, Culleton BF: Hyperhomocysteinemia in chronic renal disease. J Am Soc Nephrol 1999;10:236–244.

14 Kanani PM, Sinkey CA, Browning RL, et al: Role of the oxidant stress in endothelial dysfunction produced by experimental hyperhomocyst(e)inemia in humans. Circulation 1999;100:1161–1168.

15 Scholze A, Rinder C, Beige J, Riezler R, Zidek W, Tepel M: Acetylcysteine reduces plasma homocysteine concentration and improves pulse pressure and endothelial function in patients with end-stage renal failure. Circulation 2004;109:369–374.

16 Massy ZA, Nguyen-Khoa T: Oxidative stress and chronic renal failure: markers and management. J Nephrol 2001;12:2742–2752.

17 Wolin MS, Ahmad M, Gupte SA: The sources of oxidative stress in the vessel wall. Kidney Int 2005;67:1659–1661.

18 Galle J: Oxidative stress in chronic renal failure. Nephrol Dial Transplant 2001;16:2135–2137.

19 Ceballos-Picot I, Witko-Sarsta V, Merad-Boudia M, et al: Glutathione antioxidant system as a marker of oxidative stress in chronic renal failure. Free Radic Biol Med 1996;21:845–853.

20 Peuchant E, Delmas-Beauvieux MC, Dubourg L, et al: Antioxidant effects of a supplemented very low protein diet in chronic renal failure. Free Radic Biol Med 1997;22:313–320.

21 Barnes PJ, Karin M: Nuclear factor-κB: a pivotal transcription factor in chronic inflammation disease. N Engl J Med 1997;336:1066–1071.

22 Hoshi S, Goto M, Kyoama N, Nomoto K, Tanaka H: Regulation of vascular smooth muscle cell proliferation by nuclear factor-κB and its inhibitor, I-κB. J Biol Chem 2000;2:883–889.

23 Yudkin JS, Kumari M, Humpfries SE, Mohamed-Ali V: Inflammation obesity stress and coronary heart disease: is interleukin-6 the link? Atherosclerosis 2000;14:209–214.

24 Tintut Y, Patel J, Parhami F, Demer LL: Tumor necrosis factor-α promotes in vitro calcification of vascular cells via the camp pathway. Circulation 2000;102:2636–2642.

25 Bhagat K, Valance P: Inflammatory cytokines impair endothelium-dependent dilatation in human veins in vivo. Circulation 1997;96:3042–3047.

26 Ungvari Z Csizar A, Kaminski PM: Chronic high pressure induced arterial oxidative stress: involvement of protein kinase C-dependent NAD(P)H oxidase and local renin-angiotension system. Am J Pathol 2004;165:219–226.

27 Barton CH, Ni Z, Vazari ND: Enhanced nitric oxide inactivation an aortic coarctation-induced hypertension. Kidney Int 2001;60:1083–1087.

28 Mervaala EM, Cheng ZJ, Tikkanen I, Lapatto R, Nurminen K, Vapaato H, Tuiler DN, Fiebeler A, Ganten K, Ganten D, Luft FC: Endothelial dysfunction and xanthine oxidoreductase activity in rats with human renin and angiotensinogen genes. Hypertension 2001;37:414–418.

29 Annuk M, Zilmer M, Lind L, Linde T, Fellstrom B: Oxidative stress and endothelial function in chronic renal failure. Am J Soc Nephrol 2001;12:2747–2752.

30 Stenvinkel P, Heimburger O, Paultre F, et al: Strong association between malnutrition, inflammation and atherosclerosis in chronic renal failure. Kidney Int 1999;55:1899–1911.

31 Drueke T, Vitko-Sarsat V, Massy Z, et al: Iron therapy, advanced oxidation protein products and carotid artery intima-media thickness in end-stage renal disease. Circulation 2002;106:2212–2217.

32 Kato A, Takita T, Maruyama Y, Kumagai H, Hishida A: Impact of carotid atherosclerosis on long-term mortality in chronic hemodialysis patients. Kidney Int 2003;64:1472–1479.

33 Blacher J, Pannier B, Guerin AP, Marchais SJ, Safar ME, London GM: Carotid arterial stiffness as a predictor of cardiovascular and all-cause mortality in end-stage renal disease. Hypertension 1998;32:570–574.

34 Preston E, Ellis MR, Kulinskaya E, Davies AH, Brown EA: Association between carotid intima-media thickness and cardiovascular risk factors in CKD. Am J Kidney Dis 2005;46:856–862.

35 Boaz M, Smetana S, Weinstein T, et al: Secondary prevention with antioxidants of cardiovascular disease in end-stage renal disease (SPACE): randomised placebo-control trial. Lancet 2000;356:1213–1218.

36 Tepel M, van der Giet M, Statz M, Jankovski J, Zidek W: The antioxidant acetylcysteine reduces cardiovascular events in patients with end-stage renal failure. A randomized, controlled trial. Circulation 2003;107:992–995.

37 Maggi E, Bellagi R, Gazo A, et al: Autoantibodies against oxidatively-modified LDL in uremic patients undergoing dialysis. Kidney Int 1994;46:869–876.

38 Shoji T, Fukumoto M, Kimoto E, Shinohara K, Emoto M, Tahara H, Koyama H, Ishimura E, Nakatani T, Miki T, Tsujimoto Y, Tabata T, Nishizawa Y: Antibody to oxidized low-density lipoprotein and cardiovascular mortality in end-stage renal disease. Kidney Int 2002;62:2230–2237.

39 Shoji T, Kimoto E, Shinohara K, Emoto M, Ishimura E, Miki T, Tsujimoto Y, Tabata T, Nishizawa Y: The association of antibodies against oxidized low-density lipoprotein with atherosclerosis in hemodialysis patients Kidney Int 2003;63(suppl 84):S128–S130.

40 Holvoet P, Donk J, Landeloos M, Brouwers E, Luijtens K, Arnout J, Lasaffre E, Vanrenterghem Y, Collen D: Correlation between oxidized low-density lipoproteins and von Willebrand factor in chronic renal failure. Thromb Haemost 1996;76:663–669.

41 Van den Akker J, Bredie SJH, Diepenveen SHA, van Tits LJH, Stalenhoer AFH, Van Leusen R: Atorvastatin and simvastatin in patients on hemodialysis: effects on lipoprotein, C-reactive protein and in vivo oxidizes LDL. J Nephrol 2003;16:238–244.

42 London GM, Guerin AP, Marchais SJ, Pannier B, Safar ME, Day M, et al: Cardiac and arterial interactions in end-stage renal failure. Kidney Int 1996;50:600–608.

43 Davies PF, Tripathi SC: Mechanical stress mechanism and the stress to flow change in the canine carotid artery. Circ Res 1993;235–239.

44 Pohl U, Holtz J, Busse R, Bassenge E: Crucial role of endothelium in the vasodilator response to increased flow in vivo. Hypertension 1986;8:37–44.

45 Tronc F, Wassef M, Esposito B, Henrion D, Glagov S, Tedgui A: Role of NO in flow-induced remodelling of the rabbit common carotid artery. Arterioscler Thromb Vasc Biol 1996;16:1256–1262.

46 Langille BL, O'Donnell F: Reduction in arterial diameters produced by chronic decrease in blood flow are endothelium-dependent. Science 1986;231:405–407.

47 Girerd X, London GM, Boutouyrie P, Mourad JJ, Laurent S, Safar M: Remodelling of radial artery and chronic increase in shear stress. Hypertension 1996;27:799–803.

48 Nichols WW, O'Rourke MF: Vascular impedance; in McDonald's Blood Flow in Arteries: Theoretical, Experimental and Clinical Principles, ed 4. London, Arnold, 1998.

49 London GM, Yaginuma T: Wave reflection: clinical and therapeutic aspect; in Safar ME, O'Rourke MF (eds): The Arterial System in Hypertension. Dordrecht, Kluwer Academic, 1993, pp 221–237.

50 Mourad JJ, Pannier B, Blacher J, Rudnichi A, Benetos A, London GM, et al: Creatinine clearance, pulse wave velocity, carotid compliance in essential hypertension. Kidney Int 2001;59:1834–1841.

51 Shinohara K, Shoji T, Tsujimoto Y, Kimoto I, Tahara H, Komana H, et al: Arterial stiffness in predialysis patients with uremia. Kidney Int 2004;65:936–943.

52 Luik AJ, Spek JJ, Charra B, van Bortel L, Laurent G, Leunissen K: Arterial compliance in patients on long-time dialysis. Nephrol Dial Transplant 1997;12:2629–2632.

53 Guerin AP, Pannier B, Marchais S, Metivier F, London GM: Arterial remodelling and cardiovascular function in end-stage renal disease; in Grünfeld JP, Bach JF, Kreiss H, Maxwell MH (eds): Advances in Nephrology. St Louis, Mosby Yearbooks, 1998, vol 27, pp 105–109.

54 Amann K, Neusüa R, Ritz E, Irzyniec T, Wiest G, Mall G: Changes of vascular architecture independent of blood pressure in experimental uremia. Am J Hypertens 1995;8:409–417.

55 Blacher J, Guerin AP, Pannier B, Marchais SJ, London GM: Arterial calcifications, arterial stiffness, and cardiovascular risk in end-stage renal disease. Hypertension 2001;38:938–942.

56 London GM, Guerin AP, Marchais SJ, Metivier F, Pannier B, Adda H: Arterial medial calcification in end-stage renal disease impact on all-cause and cardiovascular mortality. Nephrol Dial Transplant 2003;18:1731–1740.

57 London GM, Marchais SJ, Guerin AP, Metivier F: Arteriosclerosis, vascular calcifications and cardiovascular disease in uremia. Curr Opin Nephrol Hypertens 2005;14:525–531.

58   Saito Y, Shirai K Uchino J, Okazawa M, Hattori Y, Yoshida T, et al: Effect of nifedipine adminis-
     tration on pulse wave velocity of chronic hemodialysis patients – two-year trial. Cardiovasc Drug
     Ther 1990;4:987–990.
59   London GM, Guerin AP, Pannier B, Marchais SJ, Bentos A, Safar ME: Increased systolic pressure
     in chronic uremia: role of arterial wave reflections. Hypertension 1992;20:10–19.
60   Klassen PS, Lowrie EG, Reddan DN, DeLong ER, Colodanoto JA, et al: Association between
     pulse pressure and mortality in patients undergoing hemodialysis. JAMA 2002;287:1548–1555.
61   Blacher J, Guerin AP, Pannier B, Marchais SJ, Safar ME, London GM: Impact of aortic stiffness
     on survival in end-stage renal disease. Circulation 1999,99:2434–2439
62   Wever RM, Luscher TF, Cosentino F, Rabelink TJ: Atherosclerosis and the two faces of endothe-
     lial nitric oxide synthetase. Circulation 1998;97:108–112.
63   Levy BI, Elfertak L, Pieddeloup C, Barouki F, Safar ME: Role of the endothelium in the mechan-
     ical response of the carotid arterial wall to calcium blockade in spontaneously hypertensive and
     Wistar-Kyoto rats. J Hypertens 1993;11:57–63.
64   Nakanishi T, Ishigami Y, Otaki Y, Izumi M, Hiraoka K, Inoue T, Takamitsu Y: Impairment of
     vascular response to reactive hyperemia and nitric oxide in chronic renal failure. Nephron 2002;
     93:529–535.
65   London GM, Pannier B, Agharazii M, Guerin AP, Verbeke FH, Marchais SJ: Forearm reactive
     hyperemia and mortality in end-stage renal disease. Kidney Int 2004;65:700–704.
66   Amabile N, Guerin AP, Leroyer A, Mallat Z, Nguyen C, Boddaert J, London GM, Tedgui A, Bou-
     langer CM: Circulating endothelial microparticles are associated with vascular dysfunction in
     patients with end-stage renal failure. J Am Soc Nephrol 2005;16:3381–3388.

Alain Guerin
Service de Néphrologie, Centre Hospitalier F-H Manhes
8 Grande Rue, FR–91712 Fleury Mérogis (France)
Tel. +33 1 6925 6458/+33 06 0325 3079
Fax +33 1 6925 6525, E-Mail alguerin@club-internet.fr

Safar ME, Frohlich ED (eds): Atherosclerosis, Large Arteries and Cardiovascular Risk.
Adv Cardiol. Basel, Karger, 2007, vol 44, pp 199–211

··························

Arterial Stiffness and Peripheral Arterial Disease

Michel E. Safar

The Diagnosis Center, Hôtel-Dieu Hospital, Paris, France

Abstract

Of the atherosclerotic diseases, peripheral arterial disease is the most characterized
by its association with systolic hypertension, increased arterial stiffness and disturbed
wave reflection. This disease raises the question to which extent sclerosis in 'atherosclerosis' is necessary per se to cause an increase in systolic blood pressure.

Arteriosclerosis obliterans or peripheral arterial disease (PAD) usually
denotes a degenerative arteriopathy affecting the abdominal aorta and mostly
the upper and lower limbs [1]. This vascular disease is characterized by occlusive lesions, primarily of atherosclerotic origin, but often accompanied by fibrosis and calcification of the tunica media. A varying degree of thrombosis is
frequently associated. In the past, arteriosclerosis obliterans has been considered to be an occlusive arterial disease, exclusively or predominantly affecting
the lower limbs.

In this report, the abnormalities of circulatory homeostasis in patients
with PAD are studied with particular reference to the modifications in systolic blood pressure (SBP), arterial stiffness, and wave reflections. Consequences with regard to diseased atherosclerotic limbs and the relationship
with cardiovascular (CV) morbidity and mortality are also taken into account.

Ankle-Brachial Index

Intermittent claudication, the major symptom of PAD, is absent in the majority of patients. A useful tool for screening patients is known to be ABI, i.e. the ratio of SBP measured at the ankle to SBP at the brachial artery [1–3]. Without an obstruction to blood flow, SBP in the ankle is greater than brachial SBP (ankle-brachial index ≥1.0). This hemodynamic profile is due to wave reflections (see Chapter 1). It is observed because a great amount of reflected waves from the toes merges with the forward wave at the systolic phase of the pressure waveform (due to the small distance between toes and ankle). As the lumen narrows, SBP beyond the obstruction falls and a pressure gradient can be measured between sequential segments of each extremity. The fall in peripheral (ankle) SBP lowers the ABI (table 1). The ABI is further reduced in subjects with systolic hypertension since brachial SBP is augmented. For the diagnosis of peripheral artery disease of the lower limbs, several threshold values have been proposed, but the majority of authors consider values <0.9 to be abnormal, since this value is 95% sensitive to angiographically proven peripheral artery stenosis. High values of ABI (>1.4–1.5) are also considered to be abnormal. The reason is that they reflect increased rigidity of the arteries of the lower limb, which prevents their compression by the cuff, leading to false results, even in the absence of systolic hypertension [4–6].

ABI <0.9 has been recognized as a strong predictor of subsequent CV mortality and stroke [2]. Recently it has been even demonstrated that both high (>1.4) and low (<0.9) ABI similarly predict CV and total mortality [3].

PAD, Blood Pressure and Systemic Hemodynamics

For many years, the incidence of systolic-diastolic hypertension, assessed from non-invasive indirect determinations of BP, has been reported to be consistently higher in patients with PAD than in age-matched control subjects [1]. This finding may be discussed on the basis of the validity of BP measurements in PAD patients. Since the initial description by Osler [4], it has become well accepted that elderly subjects may have inappropriately elevated cuff pressure when compared with intra-arterial pressure, due to excessive atheromatosis and/or medial hypertrophy of the arterial tree [5, 6]. In the elderly, cuff determinations overestimate DBP whereas SBP remains largely accurate [7]. Such results strongly suggest that the incidence of hypertension in PAD patients should have to be reviewed on the basis of intra-arterial BP measurements.

Table 1. Systemic and regional hemodynamic parameters in resting patients with PAD of the lower limbs by comparison with age- and sex-matched controls [8–10]

Parameters	Control subjects	PAD patients
Systolic arterial pressure, mm Hg	140±4	148±6
Diastolic arterial pressure, mm Hg	89±3	81±2
Mean arterial pressure, mm Hg	107±3	104±4
Pulse pressure, mm Hg	50±2	68±6[a]
Heart rate, beats/min	75±2	71±3
Ankle systolic pressure, mm Hg	155±5	73±6[b]
Ankle systolic pressure/brachial systolic pressure, ABI++	1.10±0.01	0.50±0.05[b]
Resting calf blood flow (RCBF) ml/min/100 ml	2.79±0.27	1.96±0.25[c]
Calf peak blood flow (CPBF) ml/min/100 ml	25.96±1.85	5.75±0.35[b]
CPBF/RCBF ×10, arbitrary units	101.0±8.2	34.7±3.7[b]

Values are mean ± 1 SEM. [a] $p < 0.01$; [b] $p < 0.001$; [c] $p < 0.05$.

Intra-arterial determinations of brachial artery BP have been performed after 3 days' hospitalization in patients with PAD (aged between 30 and 70), compared with age- and sex-matched normal subjects [8, 9] (table 1). While DBP remains mostly maintained within the normal range, a significant and sustained increase of SBP was observed, resulting in a substantial elevation of pulse pressure (PP). This finding was observed even in PAD patients with the same mean arterial pressure (MAP) as normal subjects [8–10] (table 1). In the latter case, it was even shown that not only SBP was significantly increased but also that DBP was slightly reduced, thus contributing to the elevated PP [11]. However, it is worth noting that these hemodynamic abnormalities have been recorded at the brachial artery, a site where the PP is usually of higher amplitude than in the central aorta [12]. Although there is some reduction in amplification of the pulse with age, the age-related increase in PP in the central aorta can be considered as probably greater than is apparent from recordings of brachial artery BP [12]. Thus, it seems likely that an elevated incidence of increased SBP and PP does exist in patients with PAD.

In patients with PAD, cardiac output and systemic vascular resistance remain largely within the normal range [8, 9]. Ventricular ejection, assessed from the ratio between stroke volume and left ventricular ejection time [8,

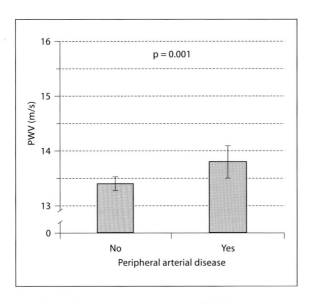

Fig. 1. Mean pulse wave velocity (PWV) in a population of subjects with peripheral disease, adjusted for age, sex, MAP, and heart rate in elderly subjects of the Rotterdam study. Bars indicate 95% confidence interval. Probability value indicates p for difference between the groups (reproduced with permission from van Popele et al. [17]).

9], is comparable to that of age-matched normal subjects. Finally, the increase in PP in patients with PAD seems to be predominantly due to modifications in arterial stiffness or in wave reflections, or to a combination of both factors. In that regard, modifications in the status of large arteries are particularly important to evaluate in patients with PAD. Experimental studies have shown that reduced elasticity of the large arteries is able to cause not only an increase in SBP, but also a reduction in DBP, as observed in PAD patients [12–15].

Arterial Stiffness and Wave Reflections in PAD

Increased aortic pulse wave velocity (PWV) [16, 17] has been observed in PAD patients, denoting an intrinsic increase on the stiffness of the aorta since MAP was similar as in controls (fig. 1). The elastic properties of the femoral artery are also significantly reduced in patients with PAD of the lower limbs as compared to age- and gender-matched controls [18, 19]. Study of the common carotid artery shows the same results [19]. Such results, in combination with the increased intima-media thickness of the carotid and femoral arteries that was also found, imply that interactive relationship between arterial stiffness and atherosclerosis may be observed and are not confined to the lower limbs. Furthermore, coexistence of PAD with abdominal aortic aneurysm is associated with greater carotid stiffness than with aortic aneurysm alone [20]. Finally, in patients with PAD, simultaneous determination of inner brachial artery diameter and PWV in the forearm showed clearly that the slope of the pressure-volume relationship (dV/dP), which represents arterial compliance, is reduced in comparison with controls matched for age, sex and MAP [7]. Thus, elderly patients with PAD and systolic hypertension exhibit intrinsic alterations of the brachial artery wall, unrelated to the level of MAP. Such stiffness changes are observed not only at the site of lower limbs but also at arterial sites where clinical symptoms are absent [7, 21]. Thus the increased arterial stiffness in patients with PAD might reflect generalized modifications of large vessels. Increased stiffness of the overall arterial tree has also been observed in patients with PAD [8, 9, 17], and may be responsible for the increase in SBP. High plasma insulin levels are statistically associated with low ABI and increased indices of femoral artery stiffness [22].

For the mechanism of increased systemic SBP in patients with PAD, another important factor may interfere: the role of wave reflections. In normal human subjects, the region of the terminal abdominal aorta acts as an important reflection site [12–14]. In subjects with PAD, which involves gross arterial lesions of the lower part of the body, the terminal abdominal aorta may be a major site of reflection, the reflected wave returning in the direction of the heart. The pressure waves thus traverse the arterial system more quickly because of smaller dimensions in association with increased arterial stiffness. This causes superimposition of the forward and backward waves during systole, and leads to a marked increase in systemic SBP. Indirect evidence for this mechanism has been provided by the study of subjects with a past story of traumatic amputation of the lower limbs. Such subjects display a high incidence of systolic hypertension over 50 years of age, resulting from an increase in arterial stiffness together with a shorter length of the arterial system due to traumatic amputation of the limbs [23, 24].

Structural and Functional Components of Increased Arterial Stiffness in Patients with PAD

Since increased arterial stiffness in patients with PAD reflects intrinsic alterations of the arterial wall, it seems likely that the increased rigidity could be due to structural modifications of the arterial wall which are possibly in relation with atherosclerosis. Studies in non-human primate models of diffuse atherosclerosis due to high cholesterol diet have shown that aortic PWV reaches 1.5–2.0 times the values seconded in control animals [25–27]. However, no consistent difference in the incremental (Young's) modulus of elasticity was observed between the two populations. In contrast, the in vitro pressure-strain elastic modulus of the atherosclerotic aorta was more than twice that of controls, indicating that the increased aortic stiffness might result from the presence of rigid and calcified atherosclerotic material rather than from the histo-pathological changes classically described by Young's modulus and represented by the collagen/elastin ratio [25–27].

For a long time, it was believed that structural changes of the arterial wall provided the exclusive explanation for increased SBP and PP in elderly patients with PAD. However, it is obvious that foam cells by themselves cannot provide any increase in arterial rigidity. More recently, the role of functional factors was evaluated from studies of endothelial function and of the effects of sodium intake, administration of nitrates, and finally abnormalities in the functioning of the sympathetic or the renin-angiotensin systems.

Endothelial dysfunction has been shown in patients with PAD. Numerous studies that revealed impaired flow-mediated dilatation of the brachial artery [28, 29] and elevated plasma concentration of markers of endothelial dysfunction [30, 31]. Patients with intermittent claudication have lower flow-mediated dilatation compared to asymptomatic patients with abnormal ABI [32]. Flow-mediated dilatation and exercise tolerance are improved after exercise rehabilitation [33], denoting a positive effect of aerobic exercise. Both are also improved after L-arginine administration [34] and autologous bone-marrow cell implantation [35].

Isotonic saline infusion causes a higher increase in brachial SBP in patients with PAD and systolic hypertension than in age-matched controls [21]. The increase in SBP is mainly due to an increase in arterial stiffness following saline administration, whereas DBP is marginally modified. The findings suggest that sodium may act on the arterial wall either directly, or through associated modifications of the autonomic nervous system, or by a combination of both factors [21]. In the literature [36, 37], the observation in elderly subjects of an increase in PWV with sodium intake, and a decrease with salt restriction, is consistent with the effects of saline infusion in patients with PAD.

While sodium intake acts to increase brachial SBP in patients with PAD, nitrate compounds have an opposite effect on systemic hemodynamics [38]. Following acute administration, nitroglycerine has been shown to decrease SBP selectively in such patients [9]. This reduction in SBP is associated to a reduction in arterial stiffness. No significant change in ventricular ejection and

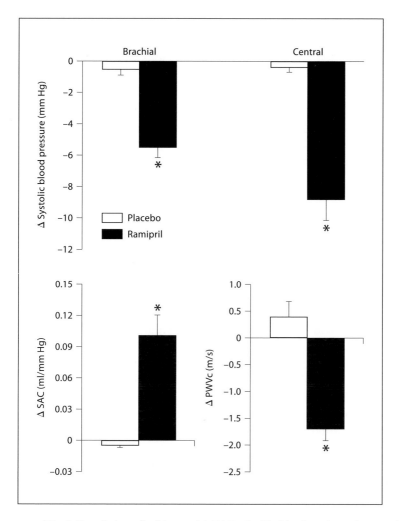

Fig. 2. Population of subjects with PAD: double-blind study evaluating the effect of the converting enzyme inhibitor ramipril vs. placebo. Change in brachial and central SBP (upper panel) and systemic arterial compliance (SAC lower left) and central pulse wave velocity (PWVc, lower right) in the placebo (white bars) and ramipril groups (black bars). The two populations had the same MAP [41]. Data are presented as mean ± SEM. * p < 0.001 compared with control.

vascular resistance is observed [38]. Similar effects on SBP reduction have been observed in elderly subjects with isolated systolic hypertension, and confirm that nitrate compounds improve arterial stiffness in such patients in conjunction with delayed wave reflections [13, 24].

Several lines of evidence suggest that the autonomic nervous system is affected in patients with PAD. A slight but significant decrease in baseline heart rate has been reported [8, 9, 21]. Since age or previous treatment could not explain this relative bradycardia, two possible mechanisms have been explored: an alteration in the intrinsic pacing function of the heart and a baroreflex-mediated mechanism related to the increased arterial stiffness. To test this latter hypothesis, baroreflex mechanisms were evaluated according to the method of Smyth et al. [39]. The curve relating SBP to the RR interval of EKG after phenylephrine was clearly reset, so that a higher stretch was required in patients with PAD to obtain the same heart rate as in controls [21]. Furthermore, the expected enhancement of baroreflex sensitivity usually observed in normal subjects following administration of cardiotonic substances [40] was not observed in patients with PAD [21]. This latter result suggests a complex disturbance of baroreflex mechanisms involving sodium pumps. Finally, acute administration of propranolol in patients with PAD showed that the abnormalities of the autonomic nervous system affected not only the heart but also blood vessels [8]. Indeed, following propranolol administration, arterial stiffness was significantly increased despite the lack of BP change. On the opposite, in subjects with PAD, converting enzyme inhibition reduces arterial stiffness and delays wave reflections independently of MAP [41] (fig. 2).

The alterations of the autonomic nervous system in patients with PAD are difficult to interpret. They may be involved in the development of the overall atherosclerotic process, or take place within the context of disease of the lower limbs. In a previous study in patients with PAD and unilateral intermittent claudication, Lorensten [42] observed that both systemic SBP and DBP increased to significantly higher levels during exercise with the diseased limb than during exercise with the healthy limb. Furthermore, after the first minutes of recovery following exercise, the systemic SBP (but not the DBP) in the diseased limb stayed higher than the pressure measured at rest immediately before exercise. Such results suggested that active contraction of muscle cells under ischemic conditions might cause stimulation of local receptors involving generalized circulatory pressor reflexes, with a predominant influence on SBP [43].

Relevance of Systolic Hypertension and Systemic Hemodynamics for the Interpretation of Intermittent Claudication

The hemodynamic changes of the diseased lower limbs of patients with PAD are usually analyzed in terms of a linear mathematical model resulting from the association of two major resistances coupled in series (the stenotic and the arteriolar resistances), rather than predominantly in terms of the downstream arteriolar resistance as it is normally the case [44]. Under these conditions, mean blood flow is determined by the driving pressure across these two resistances, the mean systemic BP being an important component. However, studies of human atherosclerotic femoral arteries have shown that non-linear models are more relevant to describe the hemodynamic changes. In that condition, vascular impedance is a more reliable index of the severity of large vessel atherosclerotic stenosis than is resistance [45]. Therefore, the oscillatory component of blood flow and BP is important to consider with regard to the mechanisms of the disease of the lower limbs. In clinical studies, both MAP and PP should be considered separately in evaluating the role of systemic hemodynamics in the severity of intermittent claudication.

Under resting conditions, calf blood flow is known to remain within the normal range in patients with PAD [46, 47]. Furthermore, calf blood flow is positively correlated with BP in patients with PAD, but not in normal subjects [10]. The results suggest that systemic BP in patients with PAD contributes to maintain an adequate perfusion of the lower limbs. Interestingly, in such patients, baseline calf blood flow is positively correlated with both systemic MAP and PP [10]. Despite the interest of hemodynamic determinations at rest, it is clear that the limiting influence of the PAD disease will occur rather at elevated flow rates, i.e. during exercise and post-occlusive reactive hyperemia. Indeed the pressure drop caused by the stenosis increases with increasing flow [45–48]. Under such conditions, it is interesting to observe that walking distance and post-occlusive reactive hyperemia are strongly correlated with baseline PP, and not with baseline MAP: the higher the PP, the greater the reduction in walking distance and the greater the alteration in vascular reserve, as evaluated from post-occlusive reactive hyperemia [10]. Such results emphasize the role of the oscillatory component of BP (i.e. PP) in the mechanism of the intermittent claudication. In that regard, it is important to note that exercise in man produces not only arteriolar vasodilatation, but also increase in PWV and arterial stiffness [49]. This observation is important to consider in patients with increased baseline arterial stiffness, as those with PAD, and suggests that stiffness abnormalities may play a major role in the severity of intermittent claudication.

Concluding Remarks

For the study of contribution of PAD in CV risk, several previous reports have drawn attention to the strong association between PAD and stenosis of the internal carotid artery, PAD and coronary heart disease [50]. Given such associations, the value of the symptomatic expression of PAD, intermittent claudication, as a predictive factor of CV mortality has been widely investigated. It has been suggested that claudication is not an independent marker of mortality, once adjustments have been made for other risk factors, and mainly signs and symptoms of coexisting coronary heart disease [51]. On the other hand, more recent studies using highly reliable non-invasive hemodynamic tests of large vessel disease have indicated a more than fourfold excess risk of subjects with PAD, independent of other CV risk factors or disease [52]. In our opinion, discrepancies in assessment of the validity of intermittent claudication as a CV risk factor may be better understood in the light of the pathophysiological mechanisms of PAD as described in this chapter. Indeed, SBP and PP are the most important CV risk factor in individuals of around 50 years of age [53], and increased SBP is also an important feature in patients with PAD, in whom it plays a significant part in the systemic hemodynamic modifications.

Accepting the hemodynamic changes observed in patients with PAD, the possible links between PAD and mortality due to coronary heart disease may be better understood. As far as the cardiac muscle is concerned, it is known that the metabolic needs of the left ventricle are greatly influenced by the level of SBP, and therefore by the increase in systemic arterial stiffness and the modification of the timing and amplitude of reflected waves initiated and/or favored by PAD [12, 23]. On the other hand, the coronary circulation is primarily dependent on mean DBP, due to the predominant diastolic perfusion of coronary arteries [12]. Since DBP tends to be reduced in patients with PAD, the supply/demand ratio may be altered under various circumstances, such as the development of cardiac hypertrophy, or exercise, or both. For these reasons alone, the alterations of systemic hemodynamics which characterize patients with PAD (i.e. increase SBP and decrease in DBP due to increased arterial stiffness) may by themselves be detrimental to the heart. Clearly, these are important fields for further clinical research in patients with PAD and atherosclerotic disease.

References

1   Juergens JL, Baker NW, Hines EA: Arteriosclerosis obliterans: review of 520 cases with special reference to pathogenic and prognostic factors. Circulation 1960;21:188–195.
2   Tsai AW, Folsom AR, Rosamond WD, Jones DW: Ankle-brachial index and 7-year ischemic stroke incidence: the ARIC study. Stroke 2001;32:1721–1724.
3   Resnick HE, Lindsay RS, McDermott MM, Devereux RB, Jones KL, Fabsitz RR, Howard BV: Relationship of high and low ankle-brachial index to all-cause and cardiovascular disease mortality: the Strong Heart Study. Circulation 2004;109–733–739.
4   Osler W: The Principles and Practices of Medicine. New York, Appleton, 1982.

5   Spence JD, Sibbald WJ, Cape RD: Pseudohypertension in the elderly. Clin Sci Mol Med 1978;55: 399s–402s.

6   Messerli FH, Ventura HO, Amodeo C: Osler's maneuver and pseudohypertension. N Engl J Med 1985;312:1348–1351.

7   Safar ME, Laurent S, Amar RA, Safavian A, London GM: Systolic hypertension in patients with arteriosclerosis obliterans of the lower limbs. Angiology 1987;38:287–295.

8   Levenson JA, Simon AC, Fiessinger JN, Safar ME, London GM, Housset EM: Systemic arterial compliance in patients with arteriosclerosis obliterans of the lower limbs: observations on the effect of intravenous propranolol. Arteriosclerosis 1982;2:266–271.

9   Levenson JA, Simon AC, Safar ME, Fiessinger JN, Housset EM: Systolic hypertension in arteriosclerosis obliterans of the lower limbs. Clin Exp Hypertens A 1982;4:1059–1072.

10 Safar ME, Totomoukouo JJ, Asmar RA, Laurent SM: Increased pulse pressure in patients with arteriosclerosis obliterans of the lower limbs. Arteriosclerosis 1987;7:232–237.

11 Safar ME, Totomoukouo JJ, Bouthier JA, Asmar RA, Levenson JA, Simon AC, London GM: Arterial dynamics, cardiac hypertrophy and antihypertensive treatment. Circulation 1987;(suppl I):156–161.

12 O'Rourke MF: Arterial Function in Health and Disease. Melbourne, Churchill Livingstone, 1982, pp 68–71.

13 Noordergraaf A: The arterial tree: in Circulatory System Dynamics. New York, Academic Press, 1978, pp 137–139.

14 Milnor WR: Hemodynamics. London, William & Wilkins, 1982, pp 56–91.

15 O'Rourke MF: Pulsatile arterial hemodynamics in hypertension. Aust NZ J Med 1976;6(suppl 2):40–46.

16 Maarek B, Simon AC, Levenson J, Pithois-Merli I, Bouthier J: Heterogeneity of the atherosclerotic process in systemic hypertension poorly controlled by drug treatment. Am J Cardiol 1987; 59:414–417.

17 Van Popele NM, Grobbee DE, Bots ML, Asmar R, Topouchian J, Reneman RS, Hoeks AP, van der Kuip DA, Hofman A, Witteman JC: Association between arterial stiffness and atherosclerosis: the Rotterdam study. Stroke 2001;32:454–460.

18 Tai NR, Giudiceandrea A, Salacinski HJ, Seifalian AM, Hamilton G: In vivo femoropopliteal arterial wall compliance in subjects with and without lower limb vascular disease. J Vasc Surg 1999;30:936–945.

19 Cheng KS, Tiwari A, Baker CR, Morris R, Hamilton G, Seifalian AM: Impaired carotid and femoral viscoelastic properties and elevated intima thickness in peripheral vascular disease. Atherosclerosis 2002;164–113–120.

20 Cheng KS, Tiwari A, Morris R, Hamilton G, Seifalian AM: The influence of peripheral vascular disease on the carotid and femoral wall mechanics in subjects with abdominal aortic aneurysm. J Vasc Surg 2003;37:403–409.

21 Levenson JA, Simon AC, Maarek BE, Gitelman RJ, Fiessinger JN, Safar ME: Regional compliance of brachial artery and saline infusion in patients with arteriosclerosis obliterans. Arteriosclerosis 1985;5:80–87.

22 Achimastos A, Brahimi M, Raison J, Billaud E, Ayache M, Moatti N, Safar ME: Plasma insulin, plasminogen activator inhibitor, and ankle-brachial systolic blood pressure ratio in overweight hypertensive subjects. J Hum Hypertens 1999;13:329–335.

23 Labouret G, Achimastos A, Benetos A, Safar M, Housset E: L'hypertension artérielle systolique des amputés traumatiques. Presse Méd 1983;12:1349–1350.

24 Safar ME, Simon AC: Hemodynamics in systolic hypertension; in Zanchetti A, Tarazi RC (eds): Handbook of Hypertension, vol 7: Pathophysiology of Hypertension; Cardiovascular Aspects. Amsterdam, Elsevier Science, 1986.

25 Farrar DJ, Green HD, Bond MG, Wagner WD, Grobbee RA: Aortic pulse wave velocity, elasticity, and composition in a nonhuman primate model of atherosclerosis. Atherosclerosis 1978;43: 52–62.

26 Farrar DJ, Bond MG, Sawyer JK, Green HD: Pulse wave velocity and morphological changes associated with early atherosclerosis progression in the aortas of cynomolgus monkeys. Cardiovasc Res 1984;18:107–118.

27 Farrar DJ, Green HD, Wagner WD, Bond MG: Reduction in pulse wave velocity and improvement of aortic distensibility accompanying regression of atherosclerosis in the rhesus monkey. Circ Res 1980;47:425–432.

28 Yataco AR, Corretti MC, Gardner AW, Womack CJ, Katzel LI: Endothelial reactivity and cardiac risk factors in older patients with peripheral arterial disease. Am J Cardiol 1999;83:754–758.

29 Poredos P, Golob M, Jensterle M: Interrelationship between peripheral arterial occlusive disease, carotid atherosclerosis and flow mediated dilation of the brachial artery. Int Angiol 2003;22:83–87.

30 Brevetti G, Martone VD, de Cristofaro T, Corrado S, Silvestro A, Di Donato AM, Bucur R, Scopacasa F: High levels of adhesion molecules are associated with impaired endothelium-dependent vasodilation in patients with peripheral arterial disease. Thromb Haemost 2001;85:63–66.

31 Makin AJ, Chung NA, Silverman SH, Lip GY: Thrombogenesis and endothelial damage/dysfunction in peripheral artery disease. Relationship to ethnicity and disease severity. Thromb Res 2003;111:221–226.

32 Silvestro A, Scopacasa F, Ruocco A, Oliva G, Schiano V, Zincarelli C, Brevetti G: Inflammatory status and endothelial function in asymptomatic and symptomatic peripheral arterial disease. Vasc Med 2003;8:225–232.

33 Brendle DC, Joseph LJ, Corretti MC, Gardner AW, Katzel LI: Effects of exercise rehabilitation on endothelial reactivity in older patients with peripheral arterial disease. Am J Cardiol 2001;87:324–329.

34 Boger RH, Bode-Boger SM, Thiele W, Creutzig A, Alexander K, Frolich JC: Restoring vascular nitric oxide formation by L-arginine improves the symptoms of intermittent claudication in patients with peripheral arterial occlusive disease. J Am Coll Cardiol 1998;32:1336–1344.

35 Higashi Y, Kimura M, Hara K, Noma K, Jitsuiki D, Nakagawa K, Oshima T, Chayama K, Sueda T, Goto C, Matsubara H, Murohara T, Yoshizumi M: Autologous bone-marrow mononuclear cell implantation improves endothelium-dependent vasodilation in patients with limb ischemia. Circulation 2004;109:1215–1218.

36 Avolio AP, Deng FQ, Li WQ, Luo YF, Huang ZD, Xing LF, O'Rourke MF: Effects of aging on arterial distensibility in populations with high and low prevalence of hypertension: comparison between urban and rural communities in China. Circulation 1985;71:202–210.

37 Avolio AP, Clyde CM, Beard TC, Cooke HM, Kenneth KL, O'Rourke MF: Improved arterial distensibility in normotensive subjects on a low salt diet. Arteriosclerosis 1986;6:166–169.

38 Simon AC, Levenson JA, Levy BI, Bouthier JE, Perroneau PP, Safar ME: Effect of nitroglycerin on peripheral large arteries in hypertension. Br J Clin Pharmacol 1982;14:241–245.

39 Smyth HS, Sleight P, Pickering GW: The reflex regulation of arterial pressure during sleep in man: a quantitative method of assessing baroreflex sensitivity. Circ Res 1969;24:109–115.

40 Ferrari A, Gregorini L, Ferrari MC, Preti L, Mancia G: Digitals and baroreceptor reflexes in man. Circulation 1981;61:279–285.

41 Ahismastos AA, Natoli AK, Lawlaer A, Blolbery PA, Kingwell BA: Ramipril increases large-artery stiffness in peripheral arterial disease and promotes elastogenic remodeling in cell culture. Hypertension 2005;45:1201–1206.

42 Lorensten E: Systematic arterial blood pressure during exercise in patients with atherosclerosis obliterans of the lower limbs. Circulation 1972;46:257–263.

43 Rowell LB, Freund PR, Hobbs SF: Cardiovascular responses to muscle ischemia in humans. Circ Res 1981;48:37–47.

44 Young DF, Cholvin NR, Roth AC: Pressure drop across artificially induced stenosis in the femoral arteries of dogs. Circ Res 1978;36:735–743.

45 Farrar DJ, Malindzak GS, Johnson G: Large vessel impedance in peripheral atherosclerosis. Cardiovascular Surg 1977;II-56:170–178.

46 Strandness DE, Bell JW: An evaluation of the hemodynamic response of the claudication extremity to exercise. Surg Gynecol Obstet 1964;119:1237–1245.

47 Yao VST, Hobbs JT, Irvine WI: Ankle systolic pressure measurements in arterial disease affecting the lower extremities. Br J Surg 1969;56:676–687.

48   Skinner JS, Strandness DE: Exercise and intermittent claudication. I. Effect of repetition and intensity of exercises. Circulation 1964;36:15–22.
49   Murgo JP, Westerhof N, Giolma JP, Altobelli SA: Effects of exercise on aortic input: impedance and pressure wave forms in normal humans. Circ Res 1981;48:334–343.
50   Friedman SA, Pandya M, Greif E: Peripheral arterial occlusion in patients with acute coronary heart disease. Am Heart J 1973;86:415–421.
51   Reunanen A, Takkunen H, Aromaa A: Prevalence of intermittent claudication and its effect on mortality. Acta Med Scand 1982;211:249–256.
52   Criqui MH, Coughlin SS, Fronek A: Noninvasively diagnosed peripheral arterial disease as a predictor of mortality: results from a prospective study. Circulation 1985;72:768–773.

Prof. Michel Safar
Centre de Diagnostic, Hôtel-Dieu, 1, place du Parvis Notre-Dame
FR–75181 Paris Cedex 04 (France)
Tel. +33 1 4234 8025, Fax +33 1 4234 8632
E-Mail michel.safar@htd.ap-hop-paris.fr

Safar ME, Frohlich ED (eds): Atherosclerosis, Large Arteries and Cardiovascular Risk.
Adv Cardiol. Basel, Karger, 2007, vol 44, pp 212–222

·····················

Cardiovascular Risk Factors, Atherosclerosis and Pulse Pressure

Jacques Amar   Bernard Chamontin

Service de Médecine Interne et d'hypertension artérielle, CHU Toulouse, France

Abstract

Blood pressure is a complex phenomenon that can be divided into two components: a steady and a pulsatile component. The pulsatile component is estimated by the pulse pressure which is mainly influenced by the large artery stiffness. The purpose of this review was to describe the relation between pulse pressure, cardiovascular risk factors and atherosclerosis. Epidemiological studies have shown positive correlations between pulse pressure and smoking or glucose metabolism impairment. More controversial data have been reported on the relation between blood lipids and large artery stiffness or pulse pressure. In cross-sectional studies, carotid, aortic and coronary plaques were associated with aortic stiffness, particularly echogenic or ulcerative plaques, and in a longitudinal study, the progression of atherosclerosis is accompanied by an increase in pulse pressure. From a pathophysiological point of view, the deleterious influence of most risk factors on endothelial function and the development of atheroma are likely to contribute to these relations. Furthermore, with respect to the connections observed between C-reactive protein, most cardiovascular risk factors, atherosclerotic diseases and pulse pressure, subclinical inflammation might also underlie these relations.

There is impressive body of evidence of relationships between blood pressure, other cardiovascular risk factors and atherosclerosis: numerous studies have indicated that hypertensive subjects have an atherogenic lipoprotein profile [1] and impaired glucose metabolism [2] and elevated blood pressure is an established risk factor for atherosclerotic diseases. Blood pressure is a complex phenomenon that can be divided into two components: a steady and a pulsatile component [3]. The steady component is determined exclusively by cardiac output and vascular resistance. The pulsatile component represents the varia-

Table 1. Stepwise multiple regression analysis between pulse pressure and clinical and lipid variables [from 9]

	Coefficient $\pm$ SEM	F	p
Mean blood pressure	0.226 ± 0.078	8.53	0.004
Apoprotein B	5.824 ± 2.346	6.16	0.014

tion of the pressure curve around the steady component, and it is mainly influenced by the large artery stiffness. The pulsatile component is estimated by the pulse pressure which is the difference between systolic and diastolic blood pressure. The purpose of this review was to describe the relation between pulse pressure, cardiovascular risk factors and atherosclerosis.

Epidemiological Aspects

Relation between Pulse Pressure and Cardiovascular Risk Factors

Lipids
Numerous studies have examined the relation between cholesterol and large arteries stiffness in various populations. Divergent results have been reported. In asymptomatic normotensive patients, no relation [4], reduced [5] and increased arterial stiffness [6] with elevated total or LDL cholesterol have been successively described. In asymptomatic men with elevated cholesterol [7], no significant correlation was observed between carotid femoral pulse wave velocity – a surrogate marker of aortic stiffness – and total or LDL cholesterol. However, a positive link was observed in this population between HDL3 subfraction and aortic stiffness. In hypertensive patients with a low prevalence of known symptomatic atheromatous disease, Dart et al. [8] failed to find any significant correlation between total cholesterol and large arteries stiffness in older subjects (65–84 years).

Fewer studies have assessed the relation between pulse pressure and blood lipids. A weak but significant association has been reported between pulse pressure and apoprotein B in a population-based study conducted in Haute Garonne, a French region with a low cardiovascular risk (table 1) [9]. Furthermore, this association remained significant after adjustment for mean blood pressure. In agreement with these data, a correlation between cholesterol and pulse pressure have been reported in 18,336 men aged 40–69 years, who were followed up for a mean period of 9.5 years in a French cohort [10] and in 2,207

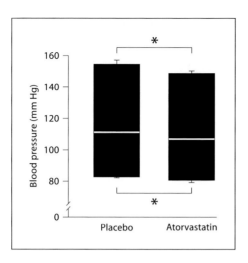

Fig. 1. Rest blood pressure of the brachial artery after placebo administration and after atorvastatin treatment. The top portion of each bar represents systolic blood pressure; the white band in the middle represents mean arterial pressure, and the base portion of each bar represents diastolic blood pressure. Values are mean ± SEM. * p < 0.05 for systolic, diastolic and mean blood pressure [from 13].

treated hypertensive patients in the USA [11]. However, no significant link with total cholesterol was observed in apparently healthy subjects in epidemiological studies conducted in Chicago in apparently healthy subjects [12]. Interestingly, in a randomized, cross-over design, controlled trial [13] comparing the effect of atorvastatin to placebo, it was found that intensive cholesterol reduction with atorvastatin over 3 months reduced large artery stiffness and blood pressure (fig. 1) in normocholesterolemic patients with stage I isolated systolic hypertension. However, blood pressure reduction does not occur with statin treatment in hypercholesterolemic normotensive patients [14]. In patients with controlled hypertension who were also hypercholesterolemic, divergent results have been reported: two studies [15, 16] found no change in blood pressure under statin therapy whereas others [17] demonstrated that additional statin therapy led to greater reduction in blood pressure.

In summary, divergent results have been reported on the relation between both pulse pressure and aortic stiffness and lipids. It is possible that in the older population, subjects with elevated cholesterol and large artery stiffness are underrepresented because of such subjects having died contributing to these discrepancies. Also, the major determinants of artery stiffness, namely older age and hypertension, when present, may reduce the potential role of other factors. However, beyond these hypotheses, these discrepancies suggest

Table 2. Cross-sectional associations of pulse pressure, systolic pressure, and diastolic pressure with HbA1c and Amadori albumin [from 21]

Early glycation products	Pulse pressure mm Hg			Systolic pressure mm Hg			Diastolic pressure mm Hg		
	β	SE	p value	β	SE	p value	β	SE	p value
HbA1c, %									
Crude	0.85	0.45	0.06	0.96	0.54	0.08	0.11	0.31	0.73
Model 1	0.50	0.36	0.16	0.33	0.24	0.16	−0.17	0.12	0.16
Amadori albumin, U/ml									
Crude	0.16	0.05	0.003	0.14	0.07	0.03	−0.02	0.04	0.66
Model 1	0.07	0.04	0.12	0.05	0.03	0.12	−0.02	0.01	0.12

Model 1 was adjusted for age, sex, mean arterial pressure, and duration of diabetes. A regression coefficient (β) of 0.85 (top left) indicates that per 1% increase in HbA1c, pulse pressure increases with 0.85 mm Hg. SE indicates standard error of the regression coefficient.

that appropriate genetic or environmental factors are required to observe an association between blood lipids and pulse pressure. In this respect, an interaction was found [18] between angiotensin II type I receptor genotype and the ratio total to HDL cholesterol in terms of the development of aortic stiffness in hypertensive patients who have never been treated.

Glucose Metabolism

The Hoorn study [19] has convincingly shown that arterial stiffness increases with deteriorating glucose tolerance status. Interestingly, an important part of the increased stiffness occurs before the onset of diabetes mellitus type 2. Also, compared with changes in peripheral artery stiffness, the changes in central artery stiffness with deteriorating glucose tolerance status are relatively small. In peripheral arteries, stiffness decreases by 19–31% from normal glucose metabolism to diabetes mellitus compared with a 2 to 11% decrease in estimates of central artery stiffness. Furthermore, it has been shown in a population-based study [20] that an important part of the increased stiffness was explained neither by fasting hyperglycemia nor by fasting hyperinsulinemia. In line with this result, a case-control study [21] conducted in type 1 diabetes found that arterial stiffness is strongly associated with advanced glycation end products such as Amadori albumin but not with HBA1c (table 2), suggesting that the formation of advanced glycation end products is an important pathway in the development of arterial stiffness in type 1 diabetic individuals. Conversely, early glycation products such HBA1c, which is highly reversible, are thought [21] to be relatively unimportant with respect to arterial stiffening. However, longitudinal studies or interventional trials designed to explore the influence of glucose metabolism on arterial stiffness are lacking.

Smokers and Coffee Consumers

Studies have shown that smoking has an unfavorable effect on arterial stiffness and pulse pressure [22]. Smoking causes immediate constriction of arteries that may be related to activation of the sympathetic nervous system. Other pharmacologic effects of smoking that may affect aortic tone include inhibition of prostacyclin production by endothelial cells, activation of platelets and release of vasopressin. Also, it has been shown that active or passive smoking affects endothelium-mediated vascular control in clinically healthy persons. Therefore, active stiffening of the vessels caused by elevated muscular tone may account for the deleterious effect of smoking on pulse pressure.

Interestingly, since in contemporary lifestyles, smoking is very frequently combined with coffee drinking, the negative effect of caffeine consumption has also been suggested [22]. Furthermore, it has been shown that when smoking and caffeine consumption are combined, they have both an acute and chronic deleterious effect on arterial stiffness and peripheral and central pulse pressure. This interaction was also present in chronic coffee consumers and chronic smokers. From a pathophysiological viewpoint, the authors [22] suggest as a plausible mechanism underlying this interaction an antagonism of adenosine and/or release of catecholamines.

Relation between Pulse Pressure and Atherosclerosis

Pulse Pressure and Plaques

In cross-sectional studies, carotid, aortic and coronary plaques were associated with aortic stiffness. Moreover, the importance of the morphology of the plaque on this relation has been documented. It has been found by Zureik et al. [23] that echogenic but not echolucent carotid plaques are associated with aortic stiffness. Also, it has been shown by McLeod et al. [24] that pulse wave velocity correlates with the extent of coronary artery plaque volume. Finally, in a large population [25] of patients with recently symptomatic carotid stenosis in the European carotid surgery trial, pulse pressure appeared as the strongest independent predictor of ulceration of the symptomatic carotid plaque. This correlation was weaker for systolic blood pressure and non-significant for diastolic blood pressure and mean blood pressure (fig. 2).

In a landmark longitudinal study, Witteman et al. [26] examined the association between diastolic blood pressure and progression of aortic athero-

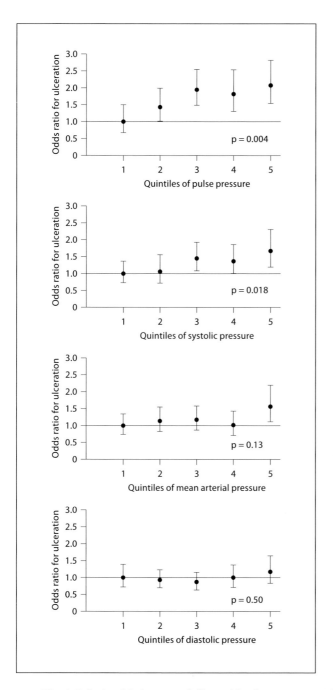

Fig. 2. Relationship between different blood pressure variables and presence of angiographic ulceration at the symptomatic carotid bifurcation [from 25].

sclerosis in a population-based cohort of 855 women. The women were examined radiographically for calcified deposits in the abdominal aorta. The age-adjusted relation risk of substantial atherosclerotic progression in women with a decrease in diastolic blood pressure of $\geq$ 10 mm Hg was 2.5 (95% confidence interval 1.3–3.5) compared with the reference group of women who had a smaller decrease or no change. The excess risk in this group was confined to women whose increase in pulse pressure was above the median. Therefore, this prospective study suggests that the progression of atherosclerosis is accompanied by an increase in pulse pressure.

Atherosclerotic Diseases

Hypertension is a risk factor for the development of atherosclerosis. In this respect, pulse pressure is well established as an important independent predictor of cardiovascular events whereas more recently, large artery stiffness has been linked to total mortality. Of interest to note that in an observational study, brachial pulse pressure is a predictor of coronary heart disease mortality, whereas its predictive value is not significant for cerebrovascular mortality [27]. In line with these observations, in therapeutic trials, coronary morbidity is more substantially reduced in populations of subjects with isolated systolic hypertension (i.e. in patients with high pulse pressure) than in populations involving subjects with systolic-diastolic hypertension [28] whereas it was consistently shown that antihypertensive drug therapy prevented 40% of strokes both in patients with isolated systolic hypertension and systolic-diastolic hypertension.

Pathophysiological Aspects

Relation between Pulse Pressure and Other Cardiovascular Risk Factors

It is unlikely that pulse pressure per se influences glucose or lipid metabolism. Conversely, there are several lines of evidence suggesting that glucose or lipid metabolism impairment results in changes in pulse pressure via changes in endothelial function and the development of atheroma. Also, the role of inflammation as a link between pulse pressure, glucose and lipid metabolisms may be evoked.

Endothelial Dysfunction

Major mechanisms by which cholesterol, glucose metabolism and smoking impairment might affect via arterial stiffness pulse pressure are through alteration in endothelial function and the development of atheroma. Many of the traditional coronary risk factors that enhance the development of atherosclerosis, such as hypercholesterolemia, hypertension, smoking, diabetes are also associated with endothelial dysfunction [29]. The total number of risk factors in a given patient has been found to be a potent independent predictor of endothelial dysfunction as measured by the acetylcholine test.

Effects of circulating lipoproteins on endothelial function are well recognized. There is evidence that the presence of high serum LDL levels impairs endothelium-dependent vasodilation possibly reversed by short-term removal of LDL particles. Also, endothelium-derived relaxing factor is rapidly inactivated by oxidized LDL particles. Improvement in endothelium-dependent vasodilation has been achieved with cholestyramine and LDL apheresis, implicating LDL cholesterol reduction as an important mechanism.

Several molecular mechanisms have been implicated [30] in hyperglycemia-induced endothelial damage: activation of protein kinase C isoforms via de novo synthesis of the lipid second messenger diacylglycerol, increased hexosamine pathway flux, increased advanced glycation end product formation, increased polyol pathway flux, and activation of the proinflammatory nuclear transcription factor nuclear factor-kB. All of these mechanisms are independently associated with overproduction of superoxide by the mitochondrial electron transport chain. As a result, hyperglycemia-induced formation of reactive oxygen species may lead to endothelial dysfunction. Since endothelial function plays a key role on arterial compliance, particularly via the constitutive release of nitric oxide (NO) as shown in young healthy humans [31], it is likely that the deleterious influence of most cardiovascular risk factors on endothelial function may result in increasing pulse pressure. On the other hand, it has been found in spontaneously hypertensive rats [32] that pulse pressure changes disproportionately with age, together with an enhanced isobaric arterial stiffness. The endothelial NO response to norepinephrine is abolished in association with endothelium-dependent heightened norepinephrine reactivity and enhanced accumulation of vessel extracellular matrix. Thus, during aging in spontaneously hypertensive rats, a negative feedback may be observed between NO bioactivity and pulse pressure through changes in arterial structure.

In summary, it is likely that endothelial dysfunction associated with cardiovascular risk factors negatively influences pulse pressure via arterial stiffening and also it could be speculated that increasing pulse pressure in turn may impair endothelial function through changes in arterial structure.

Development of Atheroma

Lipid or glucose metabolism impairment as well as smoking are associated with the development of atheroma. As described above, the development of atheroma results in stiffening of large arteries. Also, the development of plaques may produce reflection sites closer to the heart, as shown in the presence of calcified plaques, particularly at the site of arterial bifurcations (aorta, carotid and femoral arteries, origin of renal arteries). Both the stiffening of large arteries and the development of reflection sites closer to the heart result in increasing pulse pressure, particularly central pulse pressure.

Potential Role of Inflammation
Pulse Pressure

Population-based studies have shown that the C-reactive protein (CRP) level correlates with pulse pressure and predicts the development of hypertension [33]. Supporting a causal relationship leading from pulse pressure to CRP production, it has been reported that perindopril-indapamide combination therapy is more effective than β-blockade in lowering elevated CRP in hypertensive subjects and that this effect is significantly associated with a more effective pulse pressure reduction [34].

Cardiovascular Risk Factors

Subclinical inflammation was associated with most of other cardiovascular risk factors. Indeed, IL-6 plays a key role in the development of the metabolic syndrome [35]. Histologically, there is evidence of significant infiltration of macrophages into white adipose tissue and of the release of IL-6 by the adipose tissue before the development of insulin resistance. In addition, IL-6 is correlated with obesity, glucose intolerance and insulin resistance, and decreases with weight loss. In line with this result, the CRP level where the hepatic synthesis is predominantly controlled by IL-6 levels is also highly correlated with body mass index, waist-hip ratio and insulin resistance. Furthermore, many cross-sectional population-based studies have shown a positive association between CRP and current smoking.

In the light of these data, it could be suggested that pulse pressure and other major traditional risk factors may be linked through inflammation. Also, with respect to the role played by inflammation on cardiovascular events, it is possible that inflammation may contribute to the association between pulse pressure and atherosclerotic diseases.

Conclusion

Pulse pressure is linked with glucose metabolism, smoking and the progression of atherosclerosis. More controversial data have been reported for blood lipids. Collectively, these relations may contribute to the predictive role of pulse pressure on cardiovascular prognosis. The deleterious influence of risk factors on large artery stiffness via endothelial dysfunction and progression of atheroma and the role played by subclinical inflammation are likely to underlie these connections.

References

1   Newman WP 3rd, Freedman DS, Voors AW, Gard PD, Srinivasan SR, Cresanta JL, Williamson GD, Webber LS, Berenson GS: Relation of serum lipoprotein levels and systolic blood pressure to early atherosclerosis. The Bogalusa Heart Study. N Engl J Med 1986;314:138–144.
2   Reaven GM, Lithell H, Landsberg L: Hypertension and associated metabolic abnormalities – the role of insulin resistance and the sympathoadrenal system. N Engl J Med 1996;334:374–381.
3   Safar ME, London GM, Asmar R, Frohlich ED: Recent advances on large arteries in hypertension. Hypertension 1998;32:156–161.
4   Cameron JD, Jennings GL, Dart AM: The relationship between arterial compliance, age, blood pressure and serum lipid levels. J Hypertens 1995;13:1718–1723.
5   Dart AM, Lacombe F, Yeoh JK, Cameron JD, Jennings GL, Laufer E, Esmore DS: Aortic distensibility in patients with isolated hypercholesterolaemia, coronary artery disease, or cardiac transplant. Lancet 1991;338:270–273.
6   Tanaka H, DeSouza CA, Seals DR: Absence of age-related increase in central arterial stiffness in physically active women. Arterioscler Thromb Vasc Biol 1998;18:127–132.
7   Giral P, Atger V, Amar J, Cambillau M, Del Pino M, Megnien JL, Levenson J, Moatti N, Simon A: A relationship between aortic stiffness and serum HDL3 cholesterol concentrations in hypercholesterolaemic, symptom-free men. The PCVMETRA Group (Groupe de Prévention Cardiovasculaire en Médecine du Travail). J Cardiovasc Risk 1994;1:53–58.
8   Dart AM, Gatzka CD, Cameron JD, Kingwell BA, Liang YL, Berry KL, Reid CM, Jennings GL: Large artery stiffness is not related to plasma cholesterol in older subjects with hypertension. Arterioscler Thromb Vasc Biol 2004;24:962–968.
9   Marques-Vidal P, Amar J, Cambou JP, Chamontin B: Relationships between blood pressure components, lipids and lipoproteins in normotensive men. J Hum Hypertens 1996;10:239–244.
10   Darne B, Girerd X, Safar M, Cambien F, Guize L: Pulsatile versus steady component of blood pressure: a cross-sectional analysis and a prospective analysis on cardiovascular mortality. Hypertension 1989;13:392–400.
11   Madhavan S, Ooi WL, Cohen H, Alderman MH: Relation of pulse pressure and blood pressure reduction to the incidence of myocardial infarction. Hypertension 1994;23:395–401.
12   Dyer AR, Stamler J, Shekelle RB, Schoenberger JA, Stamler R, Shekelle S, Berkson DM, Paul O, Lepper MH, Lindberg HA: Pulse pressure. I. Level and associated factors in four Chicago epidemiologic studies. J Chronic Dis 1982;35:259–273.
13   Ferrier KE, Muhlmann MH, Baguet JP, Cameron JD, Jennings GL, Dart AM, Kingwell BA: Intensive cholesterol reduction lowers blood pressure and large artery stiffness in isolated systolic hypertension. J Am Coll Cardiol 2002;39:1020–1025.
14   Matthews PG, Wahlqvist ML, Marks SJ, Myers KA, Hodgson JM: Improvement in arterial stiffness during hypolipidaemic therapy is offset by weight gain. Int J Obes Relat Metab Disord 1993;17:579–583.
15   O'Callaghan CJ, Krum H, Conway EL, Lam W, Skiba MA, Howes LG, Louis WJ: Short-term effects of pravastatin on blood pressure in hypercholesterolaemic hypertensive patients. Blood Press 1994;3:404–406.
16   Foss OP, Graff-Iversen S, Istad H, Soyland E, Tjeldflaat L, Graving B: Treatment of hypertensive and hypercholesterolaemic patients in general practice: The effect of captopril, atenolol and pravastatin combined with lifestyle intervention. Scand J Prim Health Care 1999;17:122–127.
17   Sposito AC, Mansur AP, Coelho OR, Nicolau JC, Ramires JA: Additional reduction in blood pressure after cholesterol-lowering treatment by statins (lovastatin or pravastatin) in hypercholesterolemic patients using angiotensin-converting enzyme inhibitors (enalapril or lisinopril). Am J Cardiol 1999;83:1497–1499, A8.

18   Benetos A, Topouchian J, Ricard S, Gautier S, Bonnardeaux A, Asmar R, Poirier O, Soubrier F, Safar M, Cambien F: Influence of angiotensin II type 1 receptor polymorphism on aortic stiffness in never-treated hypertensive patients. Hypertension 1995;26:44–47.

19   Schram MT, Henry RM, van Dijk RA, Kostense PJ, Dekker JM, Nijpels G, Heine RJ, Bouter LM, Westerhof N, Stehouwer CD: Increased central artery stiffness in impaired glucose metabolism and type 2 diabetes: the Hoorn Study. Hypertension 2004;43:176–181.

20   Amar J, Ruidavets JB, Chamontin B, Drouet L, Ferrieres J: Arterial stiffness and cardiovascular risk factors in a population-based study. J Hypertens 2001;19:381–387.

21   Schram MT, Schalkwijk CG, Bootsma AH, Fuller JH, Chaturvedi N, Stehouwer CD, EURODIAB Prospective Complications Study Group: Advanced glycation end products are associated with pulse pressure in type 1 diabetes: the EURODIAB Prospective Complications Study. Hypertension 2005;46:232–237.

22   Vlachopoulos C, Kosmopoulou F, Panagiotakos D, Ioakeimidis N, Alexopoulos N, Pitsavos C, Stefanadis C: Smoking and caffeine have a synergistic detrimental effect on aortic stiffness and wave reflections. J Am Coll Cardiol 2004;44:1911–1917.

23   Zureik M, Bureau JM, Temmar M, Adamopoulos C, Courbon D, Bean K, Touboul PJ, Benetos A, Ducimetiere P: Echogenic carotid plaques are associated with aortic arterial stiffness in subjects with subclinical carotid atherosclerosis. Hypertension 2003;41:519–527.

24   McLeod AL, Uren NG, Wilkinson IB, Webb DJ, Maxwell SR, Northridge DB, Newby DE: Noninvasive measures of pulse wave velocity correlate with coronary arterial plaque load in humans. J Hypertens 2004;22:363–368.

25   Lovett JK, Howard SC, Rothwell PM: Pulse pressure is independently associated with carotid plaque ulceration. J Hypertens 2003;21:1669–1676.

26   Witteman JC, Grobbee DE, Valkenburg HA, van Hemert AM, Stijnen T, Burger H, Hofman A: J-shaped relation between change in diastolic blood pressure and progression of aortic atherosclerosis. Lancet 1994;343:504–507.

27   Benetos A, Rudnichi A, Safar M, Guize L: Pulse pressure and cardiovascular mortality in normotensive and hypertensive subjects. Hypertension 1998;32:560–564.

28   SHEP Cooperative Research Group: Prevention of stroke by antihypertensive drug treatment in older persons with isolated systolic hypertension: final results of the Systolic Hypertension in the Elderly Program (SHEP). JAMA 1991;265:3255–3326.

29   Davignon J, Ganz P: Role of endothelial dysfunction in atherosclerosis. Circulation 2004; 109(suppl 1):III27–32.

30   Moreno PR, Fuster V: New aspects in the pathogenesis of diabetic atherothrombosis. J Am Coll Cardiol 2004;44:2293–2300.

31   Kinlay S, Creager MA, Fukumoto M, Hikita H, Fang JC, Selwyn AP, Ganz P: Endothelium-derived nitric oxide regulates arterial elasticity in human arteries in vivo. Hypertension 2001;38: 1049–1053.

32   Safar M, Chamiot-Clerc P, Dagher G, Renaud JF: Pulse pressure, endothelium function, and arterial stiffness in spontaneously hypertensive rats. Hypertension 2001;38:1416–1421.

33   Abramson JL, Weintraub WS, Vaccarino V: Association between pulse pressure and C-reactive protein among apparently healthy US adults. Hypertension 2002;39:197–202.

34   Amar J, Ruidavets JB, Peyrieux JC, Mallion JM, Ferrieres J, Safar ME, Chamontin B: C-reactive protein elevation predicts pulse pressure reduction in hypertensive subjects. Hypertension 2005; 46:151–155.

35   Xu H, Barnes GT, Yang Q, Tan G, Yang D, Chou CJ, Sole J, Nichols A, Ross JS, Tartaglia LA, Chen H: Chronic inflammation in fat plays a crucial role in the development of obesity-related insulin resistance. J Clin Invest 2003;112:1821–1830.

Prof. Jacques Amar
Service de Médecine Interne et d'hypertension artérielle
Hôpital Rangueil, Allées Jean Pouilhes
FR– 31059 Toulouse (France)
Tel. +33 5 61 32 30 72, Fax +33 5 61 32 27 10, E-Mail amar.j@chu-toulouse.fr

Safar ME, Frohlich ED (eds): Atherosclerosis, Large Arteries and Cardiovascular Risk.
Adv Cardiol. Basel, Karger, 2007, vol 44, pp 223–233

· ·

Pulse Pressure and Inflammatory Process in Atherosclerosis

Jerome L. Abramson[a]   *Viola Vaccarino*[a, b]

[a]Department of Epidemiology, Rollins School of Public Health, and
[b]Department of Medicine, Division of Cardiology, Emory University
School of Medicine, Emory University, Atlanta, Ga., USA

Abstract

Recent studies have reported positive associations between pulse pressure (PP) and markers of inflammation. These studies are intriguing because they suggest that elevations in PP could induce an inflammatory state and thereby increase the risk of inflammation-related diseases such as atherosclerotic cardiovascular disease. In the present chapter, we review potential mechanisms by which an elevated PP could increase inflammation. We also review human-based studies that have investigated the association between PP and inflammatory biomarkers such as C-reactive protein. The majority of studies support a positive association between PP and inflammatory markers. However, it remains unclear whether the association is truly causal and whether it has relevance in terms of predicting cardiovascular diseases.

Copyright © 2007 S. Karger AG, Basel

Pulse pressure (PP) is defined as the difference between systolic blood pressure (SBP) and diastolic blood pressure (DBP). A number of factors, most notably large artery stiffness [1], can lead to a high PP (i.e. a large or 'wide' difference between SBP and DBP). Recent studies have demonstrated that higher PP values are associated with higher levels of inflammatory markers [2–10]. These studies are of great interest, because they suggest that elevations in PP may induce inflammation, which would help to explain why an elevated PP has been associated with a higher risk of inflammation-dependent atherosclerotic cardiovascular diseases (CVD) [11, 12]. Although the studies of PP and inflammation are intriguing, many issues surrounding the PP/inflammation association remain to be investigated and clarified.

In the present chapter, we will attempt to review current knowledge about the relationship between PP and inflammation. First, we will highlight pathophysiological mechanisms by which an elevated PP might induce inflammations. Second, evidence linking PP to inflammation in humans will be reviewed. Third, a critical assessment of the existing studies of PP and inflammation will be presented.

Pathophysiological Mechanisms Linking PP to Inflammation

In assessing whether a wide PP may lead to higher inflammation, it is important to consider whether there are plausible biological mechanisms by which PP could promote inflammation. Several experimental studies have suggested that such mechanisms may exist. In general, these mechanisms fall under two categories: (1) cyclic strain and (2) non-steady shear stress.

Elevated Cyclic Strain and Inflammation
Higher levels of PP presumably lead to greater degrees of cyclic strain, the repetitive mechanical deformation that is experienced by the arterial wall as it expands and contracts during each cardiac cycle. PP-induced cyclic strain could be a mechanism by which higher PP increases inflammation, because evidence indicates that endothelial cells can detect cyclic strain signals and transmit these signals into pro-inflammatory biochemical responses. For example, studies indicate that cyclic strain is associated with endothelial cell production of superoxide and other reactive oxygen species (ROS) [13,14] that can act as important signaling molecules in inflammation. In addition, cyclic strain induces higher levels of pro-inflammatory factors such as chemokines and adhesion cell molecules. With respect to chemokines, investigators have demonstrated that in endothelial cells, cyclic strain leads to substantial increases in the gene expression of the pro-inflammatory chemokine monocyte chemotactic protein-1 (MCP-1) [14–16]. Similarly, it has been shown that cyclic strain increases endothelial cell gene expression of the pro-inflammatory adhesion molecules intracellular adhesion molecule-1 (ICAM-1) [17, 18], vascular cell adhesion molecule-1 (VCAM-1) [18], and E-selectin [18]. Furthermore, by inducing expression of these pro-inflammatory molecules, cyclic strain leads to greater adhesion of monocytes to endothelial cells [17, 18], an important part of the inflammatory process. In addition to ROS, chemokines, and

adhesion molecules, cyclic strain has also been associated with other factors that appear to be closely linked to inflammatory processes, such as matrix metalloproteinases. For example, production of MMP-2 in endothelial cells exposed to cyclic strain is as much as 4 times greater than MMP-2 production in control cells [19]. Overall, the evidence above tends to suggest that cyclic strain induces endothelial cell responses that could foster inflammation, indicating that cyclic strain may represent a potential biological mechanism by which PP could promote inflammation.

Non-Steady Shear and Inflammation

In addition to cyclic strain, arteries experience a number of other mechanical forces which may be implicated in inflammation. For example, as blood flows through arteries, it creates a frictional force which acts parallel to the lining (endothelium) of the artery. This frictional force is known as shear stress. Although the relationship between PP and shear stress is not entirely clear, it has been suggested that a large PP would result in non-steady shear stress forces. This non-steady shear may actually result in oscillatory (i.e. reversing, or 'back-and-forth') shear stress forces, especially at arterial branch points where blood flow is already non-steady due to the geometry of the branch points [20]. As with cyclic strain, PP-induced non-steady or oscillatory shear may represent a mechanism by which elevated PP could lead to inflammation, because endothelial cells can detect shear stress forces and translate them into inflammatory biochemical responses. For example, Chappel et al. [21] compared the effect of steady and oscillatory shear on the upregulation of pro-inflammatory adhesion molecules in human umbilical vein endothelial cells. They found that, compared to steady shear, oscillatory shear was associated with a much greater (at least 7.5-fold) upregulation of ICAM-1, VCAM-1, and E-selectin. Moreover, they found that this oscillatory shear-induced upregulation of adhesion molecules was associated with a 10-fold increase in the level of monocyte binding. Hsiai et al. [22] examined the effect of oscillatory flow on bovine aortic endothelial cells. They found that oscillatory flow led to significant increases in ICAM-1 and MCP-1 expression, with a concomitant increase in the number of monocytes binding to the endothelial cells. Other investigators have also reported positive associations between oscillatory shear and monocyte adhesion to endothelial cells, and have suggested that such positive association may be mediated by ROS [23]. Overall, this evidence supports the notion that a high PP, by fostering non-steady or oscillatory shear, may promote inflammation.

Studies of PP and Inflammation in Humans

From the preceding discussion, it is apparent that there are plausible mechanisms by which a high PP, in and of itself, could lead to increased inflammation. In recent years, a number of studies have in fact attempted to address whether a high PP is indeed associated with inflammation in humans. In particular, studies have examined whether PP is associated with markers of inflammation that have been linked to an increased risk of CVD in humans, such as C-reactive protein (CRP) and interleukin-6 (IL-6).

Studies of PP and CRP

CRP is the inflammatory biomarker which has shown the most consistent association with increased CVD risk. For this reason, many of the studies looking at PP and inflammation have chosen to look at CRP as the primary marker of inflammation. In general, results from studies of PP and CRP have reported significant, positive associations between PP and CRP. In a study of over 9,000 apparently healthy US adults who participated in the Third National Health and Nutrition Examination Survey (NHANES), we examined the association between peripheral PP (measured at the brachial artery with a standard blood pressure cuff) and CRP levels [2]. We found that a 10 mm Hg increase in PP was associated with a statistically significant 13% increase in the odds of having an elevated CRP (≥ 0.66 mg/dl). This association was observed after adjustment for numerous potential confounding factors, including age, sex, education, lipid levels, body mass index (BMI), smoking status, alcohol consumption, and physical activity. Furthermore, the association between PP and elevated CRP was stronger than the association between SBP and elevated CRP (table 1). In multivariable models including PP and SBP or PP and DBP simultaneously, PP (i.e. increasing SBP at any level of DBP and decreasing DBP at any level of SBP) proved to be the strongest predictor of elevated CRP. Amar et al. [3] also reported a positive, cross-sectional association between peripheral PP and CRP. In particular, they found that a high peripheral PP was associated with elevated CRP (>3.7 mg/l) after adjustment for age, sex, BMI, lipids, glucose, and antihypertensive drugs. Several other studies have also reported significant, positive associations between peripheral PP and CRP [5, 8, 9], though in some studies, the association became fairly weak after adjustment for potential confounding factors. For example, in a study of over 2,000 older British women, investigators found only a small positive association between peripheral PP and CRP after adjustment for age, BMI, smoking and indicators of socio-economic status [5].

Although studies reporting a positive association between peripheral/brachial PP and CRP are of interest, it has been noted that peripheral PP is often

Table 1. Logistic regression models assessing the association between single blood pressure components and the odds of having an elevated CRP level [from 2]

Model[1]	Odds ratio (95% CI) for elevated CRP	p value
Model 1: systolic blood pressure	1.07 (1.00–1.15)	0.05
Model 2: diastolic blood pressure	0.95 (0.84–1.06)	0.33
Model 3: pulse pressure	1.13 (1.04–1.22)	0.004

[1] All three models were adjusted for age, sex, race, education, cholesterol levels, BMI, waist-to-hip ratio, smoking status, alcohol consumption, physical activity, and use of antihypertensive medications. Odds ratios are given per 10 mm Hg increase.

a poor indicator of central PP [1]. Central PP may be the more relevant PP, as this is the PP that is 'seen' by the heart. Thus, some studies have examined the relationship between central PP and CRP. Kampus et al. [7] examined the cross-sectional association between central PP, measured non-invasively with applanation tonometry, and CRP in apparently healthy middle-aged subjects. They found a highly significant positive association between central PP and CRP in a multivariable regression model that was adjusted for age, sex, glucose, and smoking. Similarly, in a sample of 427 healthy persons, Yasmin et al. [10] found that central PP, determined by applanation tonometry, was positively and significantly associated with CRP after adjustment for age and heart rate.

One other intriguing study of PP and CRP comes from Amar et al. [24]. In this study the authors showed that among persons being treated for hypertension, those displaying the greatest reduction in peripheral PP during antihypertensive therapy were also the most likely to show reductions in CRP (table 2). This study is noteworthy because, rather than simply showing that PP and CRP are associated cross-sectionally, it demonstrates that manipulation of PP levels leads to a concomitant change in CRP levels. In demonstrating this, the authors provide even stronger evidence that PP and inflammation may truly be related.

Studies of PP and Other Inflammatory Markers

Although CRP is often the inflammatory marker that receives the most attention in the cardiovascular literature, there are other inflammatory markers which have been linked to CVD risk. PP has also shown associations with

Table 2. Likelihood of CRP decreasing from >3 to ≤3 mg/l with respect to decrease in blood pressure [from 24]

Decrease[1]	Odds ratio	95% CI
Pulse pressure	2.97	1.11–12.03*
Systolic blood pressure	1.92	0.71–5.52
Diastolic blood pressure	1.57	0.57–4.27

Multivariate logistic regression adjusted for baseline CRP and overweight (BMI ≥25 kg/m²). * p = 0.04.
[1] > Median vs. ≤ median decrease (pulse pressure, 7.7 mm Hg; systolic blood pressure, 22.7 mm Hg; diastolic blood pressure, 13.4 mm Hg).

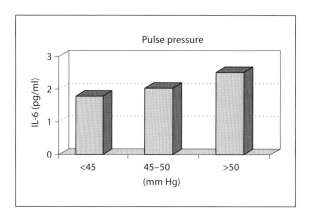

Fig. 1. Relationship between PP (p < 0.001) and plasma level of IL-6 [from 4].

these other inflammatory markers. In a cross-sectional investigation of 508 apparently healthy men, investigators reported that increasing levels of PP were significantly associated with increasing levels of ICAM-1 and IL-6 (fig. 1) [4]. This association was observed after adjustment for age, diabetes, lipids, BMI, smoking, and family history of myocardial infarction. Engstrom et al. [6] investigated the relationship between five inflammation-sensitive plasma proteins (fibrinogen, α_1-glucoprotein, α_1-antitrypsin, haptoglobin and ceruloplasmin) and PP among Swedish men who were not being treated for hypertension. They found that PP was not related to the inflammation-sensitive proteins at baseline. However, they did find that higher levels of inflammation-sensitive proteins at baseline were predictive of greater increases in PP during follow-up. This association was observed after adjustment for numerous confounders such as age, diabetes, baseline blood pressure, plasma lipids, smoking and physical activity. However, the magnitude of the association was not large.

Critical Assessment of the Studies of PP and Inflammation in Humans

Based on the evidence from the studies discussed above, it is tempting to conclude that higher PP is associated with, and may in fact provoke, an inflammatory response. However, before reaching such a conclusion, it is important to critically assess the strengths and weaknesses of the evidence from these studies. On the whole, these studies do have a number of strengths, which tend to bolster one's confidence in the belief in the existence of a real, positive association between PP and inflammation. First, as noted earlier, there are plausible biological mechanisms, such as cyclic strain and non-steady shear, by which a high PP could theoretically promote inflammation. Second, studies have been fairly consistent in reporting positive associations between PP and inflammation in humans. Some studies have reported no association in certain subgroups (e.g. women) [8], have reported that it is only central (and not peripheral) PP that is associated with inflammation [7], or have reported only weak associations after adjustment for confounders [5]. Nevertheless, the vast majority of studies which have examined the association between PP and inflammation have reported a positive association between these two factors. Third, the positive association between PP and inflammation has been observed in a wide variety of populations, including a nationally representative sample of healthy US adults [2], older British women [5], hypertensive persons in a clinical trial [24], and other populations [3, 9]. This fact indicates that the positive association between PP and inflammation may be a general one, and not simply an association that is confined to a selected population. Fourth, PP has been associated with a variety of inflammatory markers, including CRP [2, 3, 5, 7–10, 24], IL-6 [4], ICAM-1 [4], and other markers [6]. Again, this suggests that the positive association between PP and inflammation is valid, being not simply confined to one particular inflammatory marker.

In addition to the strengths just listed, however, the studies of PP and inflammation have a number of weaknesses which raise questions about the nature of the PP/inflammation association. One major limitation is that the studies in humans have primarily been based on observational data [2–8, 10]. As such, these studies have been unable to conclusively prove that PP and inflammation are positively associated, independent of potentially confounding factors. The threat of confounding has been partially addressed through statistical adjustment for potential confounders such as age, sex, race, SBP, lipids, BMI, smoking, physical activity, and socio-economic status. That these studies have observed positive associations between PP and inflammation after adjustment for such confounders helps bolster the notion that the PP/inflammation association is a true, independent association. At the same time, however, these observational studies can never really prove that their results were free of residual confounding or unknown confounders. For example, the study of older British women noted above observed a marked attenuation of the PP/inflammation association after adjustment for potential confounders, raising concern that the small association which remained after adjustment may have simply been due to residual confounding [5]. Of all of the potential confounding factors, perhaps the most problematic is SBP. The correlation between SBP and PP tends to be very strong, and is often as high as 0.80. Due to this high correlation, it is often unclear whether the association between PP and inflammation is really independent of SBP. Regression models which simultaneously include continuous SBP and continuous DBP as predictors of inflammation, can help establish whether it is PP, and not SBP, which is related to inflammation. In such models, if continuous SBP predicts increases in inflammation while DBP predicts decreases in inflammation, it would suggest that it is an increasing difference between SBP and DBP (i.e. an increasing PP), and not simply increasing SBP, which is predictive of increased inflammation. Although some studies have, in effect, adopted this approach [2], others have not [4] and have left open questions about whether their findings of a positive association between PP and inflammation is truly independent of SBP.

A second limitation of studies of PP and inflammation is that almost all of these studies have been cross-sectional in nature (i.e. PP and inflammation were essentially measured at the same time) [2–5, 7–10]. This precludes an understanding of the temporal ordering of the association. In this chapter, we have argued that PP may induce an inflammatory response. However, it is certainly possible that the association is one in which inflammation leads to a higher PP. Indeed, a study of PP and inflammation which was prospective in nature showed that inflammation was predictive of an increase in PP over time [6]. In addition, in a treatment trial of hypertensive patients, a reduction in PP with anti-hypertensive treatment was associated with a decrease in CRP, a relationship not seen with SBP or DBP [24]. Furthermore, several studies seem to show that inflammation is associated with arterial stiffness [7, 10, 25–28], perhaps because inflammation promotes atherosclerosis which then results in stiffening of the arteries. If so, one would expect to see an association between PP and inflammation, not because PP leads to inflammation, but because inflammation leads to arterial stiffness, which then leads to a higher PP. Some studies have argued against this latter possibility, by showing that PP and inflammation are associated, even after accounting for arterial stiffness [3]. Nevertheless, the cross-sectional nature of many studies of PP and inflammation have overall failed to clarify the temporal ordering of the PP/inflammation association, and more data are needed to clarify this issue.

A third limitation is that few studies have assessed the impact of genetic background on the association between PP and inflammation. Data indicate that genetic factors play a role in influencing PP [29]. Genetic factors also influence levels of inflammatory markers such as CRP [30, 31]. Thus, it would seem natural to believe that the association between PP and inflammation may be modified by inherited factors, but few studies have addressed this issue.

A fourth limitation is that the clinical importance of the association between PP and inflammation has not been adequately addressed by existing studies. Although the relationship between PP and inflammation is of scientific interest in the study of the pathophysiology of CVD, an understanding of its clinical significance is also important. Such understanding would require that studies not only analyze the association between PP and inflammation, but assess how this association affects the risk of adverse cardiovascular events. Unfortunately, such analyses have not been conducted.

Summary and Future Research

Overall, the relationship between PP and inflammation remains an intriguing and important area of research. Plausible biological mechanisms exist which suggest that PP may induce inflammation. Additionally, many cross-sectional, observational studies suggest that PP and inflammation are associated with one another in humans. However, due to methodological limitations of existing studies, it remains unclear whether PP and inflammation are truly causally related. Since PP and inflammation have been both associated with CVD risk, any relation between the two factors would also, presumably, have an impact on CVD risk. As such, it would be of considerable importance to conduct further research that would attempt to more definitively establish whether there is a causal relationship between PP and inflammation and, if so, what the precise character of the relationship is. Future studies could focus on establishing more conclusively the independence of the association between PP an inflammation, defining the temporal ordering of this association, and examining the role of genetic factors in the association. Hopefully such studies will improve our understanding of how PP and inflammation are related and, ultimately, how they interact to affect CVD risk.

References

1   Safar ME, Levy BI, Struijker-Boudier H: Current perspectives on arterial stiffness and pulse pressure in hypertension and cardiovascular diseases. Circulation 2003;107:2864–2869.
2   Abramson JL, Weintraub WS, Vaccarino V: Association between pulse pressure and C-reactive protein among apparently healthy US adults. Hypertension 2002;39:197–202.
3   Amar J, Ruidavets JB, Sollier CB, et al: Relationship between C-reactive protein and pulse pressure is not mediated by atherosclerosis or aortic stiffness. J Hypertens 2004;22:349–355.
4   Chae CU, Lee RT, Rifai N, Ridker PM: Blood pressure and inflammation in apparently healthy men. Hypertension 2001;38:399–403.
5   Davey Smith G, Lawlor DA, Harbord R, et al: Association of C-reactive protein with blood pressure and hypertension: life course confounding and mendelian randomization tests of causality. Arterioscler Thromb Vasc Biol 2005;25:1051–1056.
6   Engstrom G, Janzon L, Berglund G, et al: Blood pressure increase and incidence of hypertension in relation to inflammation-sensitive plasma proteins. Arterioscler Thromb Vasc Biol 2002;22:2054–2058.
7   Kampus P, Kals J, Ristimae T, Fischer K, Zilmer M, Teesalu R: High-sensitivity C-reactive protein affects central haemodynamics and augmentation index in apparently healthy persons. J Hypertens 2004;22:1133–1139.
8   Li X, Zhang H, Huang J, et al: Gender-specific association between pulse pressure and C-reactive protein in a Chinese population. J Hum Hypertens 2005;19:293–299.
9   Schillaci G, Pirro M, Gemelli F, et al: Increased C-reactive protein concentrations in never-treated hypertension: the role of systolic and pulse pressures. J Hypertens 2003;21:1841–1846.
10 Yasmin, McEniery CM, Wallace S, Mackenzie IS, Cockcroft JR, Wilkinson IB: C-reactive protein is associated with arterial stiffness in apparently healthy individuals. Arterioscler Thromb Vasc Biol 2004;24:969–974.
11 Benetos A, Rudnichi A, Safar M, Guize L: Pulse pressure and cardiovascular mortality in normotensive and hypertensive subjects. Hypertension 1998;32:560–564.
12 Franklin SS, Khan SA, Wong ND, Larson MG, Levy D: Is pulse pressure useful in predicting risk for coronary heart disease? The Framingham Heart Study. Circulation 1999;100:354–360.
13 Hishikawa K, Luscher TF: Pulsatile stretch stimulates superoxide production in human aortic endothelial cells. Circulation 1997;96:3610–3616.
14 Wung BS, Cheng JJ, Hsieh HJ, Shyy YJ, Wang DL: Cyclic strain-induced monocyte chemotactic protein-1 gene expression in endothelial cells involves reactive oxygen species activation of activator protein 1. Circ Res 1997;81:1–7.
15 Wang DL, Wung BS, Shyy YJ, et al: Mechanical strain induces monocyte chemotactic protein-1 gene expression in endothelial cells. Effects of mechanical strain on monocyte adhesion to endothelial cells. Circ Res 1995;77:294–302.
16 Wung BS, Cheng JJ, Shyue SK, Wang DL: NO modulates monocyte chemotactic protein-1 expression in endothelial cells under cyclic strain. Arterioscler Thromb Vasc Biol 2001;21:1941–1947.
17 Cheng JJ, Wung BS, Chao YJ, Wang DL: Cyclic strain-induced reactive oxygen species involved in ICAM-1 gene induction in endothelial cells. Hypertension 1998;31:125–130.
18 Yun JK, Anderson JM, Ziats NP: Cyclic-strain-induced endothelial cell expression of adhesion molecules and their roles in monocyte-endothelial interaction. J Biomed Mater Res 1999;44:87–97.
19 Von Offenberg Sweeney N, Cummins PM, Birney YA, Cullen JP, Redmond EM, Cahill PA: Cyclic strain-mediated regulation of endothelial matrix metalloproteinase-2 expression and activity. Cardiovasc Res 2004;63:625–634.
20 Barakat A, Lieu D: Differential responsiveness of vascular endothelial cells to different types of fluid mechanical shear stress. Cell Biochem Biophys 2003;38:323–343.
21 Chappell DC, Varner SE, Nerem RM, Medford RM, Alexander RW: Oscillatory shear stress stimulates adhesion molecule expression in cultured human endothelium. Circ Res 1998;82:532–539.
22 Hsiai TK, Cho SK, Wong PK, et al: Micro sensors: linking real-time oscillatory shear stress with vascular inflammatory responses. Ann Biomed Eng 2004;32:189–201.

23   Hwang J, Saha A, Boo YC, et al: Oscillatory shear stress stimulates endothelial production of O_2^- from p47phox-dependent NAD(P)H oxidases, leading to monocyte adhesion. J Biol Chem 2003;278:47291–47298.

24   Amar J, Ruidavets JB, Peyrieux JC, et al: C-reactive protein elevation predicts pulse pressure reduction in hypertensive subjects. Hypertension 2005;46:151–155.

25   Duprez DA, Somasundaram PE, Sigurdsson G, Hoke L, Florea N, Cohn JN: Relationship between C-reactive protein and arterial stiffness in an asymptomatic population. J Hum Hypertens 2005; 19:515–519.

26   Mattace-Raso FU, van der Cammen TJ, van der Meer IM, et al: C-reactive protein and arterial stiffness in older adults: the Rotterdam study. Atherosclerosis 2004;176:111–116.

27   Nagano M, Nakamura M, Sato K, Tanaka F, Segawa T, Hiramori K: Association between serum C-reactive protein levels and pulse wave velocity: A population-based cross-sectional study in a general population. Atherosclerosis 2005;180:189–195.

28   Tomiyama H, Koji Y, Yambe M, et al: Elevated C-reactive protein augments increased arterial stiffness in subjects with the metabolic syndrome. Hypertension 2005;45:997–1003.

29   DeStefano AL, Larson MG, Mitchell GF, et al: Genome-wide scan for pulse pressure in the National Heart, Lung and Blood Institute's Framingham Heart Study. Hypertension 2004;44:152–155.

30   D'Aiuto F, Casas JP, Shah T, Humphries SE, Hingorani AD, Tonetti MS: C-reactive protein (+1444C>T) polymorphism influences CRP response following a moderate inflammatory stimulus. Atherosclerosis 2005;179:413–417.

31   Suk HJ, Ridker PM, Cook NR, Zee RY: Relation of polymorphism within the C-reactive protein gene and plasma CRP levels. Atherosclerosis 2005;178:139–145.

Jerome L. Abramson, PhD
Department of Medicine, Division of Cardiology
Emory University School of Medicine
1365-A Clifton Road, Room 1509, Atlanta, GA 30322 (USA)
Tel. +1 404 778 5542, Fax +1 404 778 5541, E-Mail Jerome.abramson@emory.edu

Safar ME, Frohlich ED (eds): Atherosclerosis, Large Arteries and Cardiovascular Risk.
Adv Cardiol. Basel, Karger, 2007, vol 44, pp 234–244

∙∙∙∙∙∙∙∙∙∙∙∙∙∙∙∙∙∙∙∙∙∙

Calcifications, Arterial Stiffness and Atherosclerosis

Rachel H. Mackey   Lakshmi Venkitachalam   Kim Sutton-Tyrrell

Department of Epidemiology, Graduate School of Public Health, University of
Pittsburgh, Pittsburgh, Pa., USA

Abstract

Vascular calcification can occur in either the intimal or medial layers of the arterial
wall. Intimal calcification is associated with *athero*sclerosis, which is characterized by
lipid accumulation, inflammation, fibrosis and development of focal plaques. Medial calcification is associated with *arterio*sclerosis, i.e. age- and metabolic disease-related structural changes in the arterial wall which are related to increased arterial stiffness. It has
been hypothesized that vascular calcification, either intimal or medial, may directly increase arterial stiffness. Alternatively, arterial stiffness may contribute to the development
of calcification and focal plaque. Ample evidence (i.e. animal data and studies of diabetes
and end-stage renal disease) has demonstrated that medial calcification of elastic fibers
contributes to increased arterial stiffness. Evidence linking intimal calcification with arterial stiffness is less definitive, partly because it is very difficult to differentiate vascular
calcification due to focal plaques (intimal) from medial calcification, and partly because
the number of studies has been small. ***Conclusion:*** Current evidence supports that medial calcification is associated with increases in arterial stiffness. The association between
intimal (atherosclerotic-associated) calcification and arterial stiffness is less definitive.

Introduction

The medium and large arteries are affected by two separate but related
disease processes – *athero*sclerosis, which is characterized by lipid accumulation, inflammation, fibrosis and development of focal plaques, and *arterio*sclerosis, i.e. age- and metabolic disease-related structural changes in the arterial
wall which are related to increased arterial stiffness. Vascular calcification can
occur in the presence or absence of atherosclerosis. In the setting of atheroscle-

rosis, calcification of the intima occurs as a result of an inflammatory response to lipid accumulation and plaque formation. Medial calcification, as seen in arteriosclerosis, is driven by age-related changes in the vascular wall, elevated blood pressure (BP) and inflammation, among other factors. It has been hypothesized that vascular calcification of the medial layer, and possibly of the intimal layer, directly increases arterial stiffness. Conversely, stiffer arteries are less able to buffer the pulsatile blood flow, which increases the strain on arterial walls, contributing to injury and the development or progression of atheroma. These two processes of atherosclerosis (and intimal calcification) and arterial stiffening (arteriosclerosis and medial calcification) likely contribute to each other, accelerating the process of vascular damage. The purpose of this chapter is to review what is known about vascular calcification and its associations with arterial stiffness, to evaluate what conclusions are supported by current evidence.

Vascular Calcifications – Pathophysiology

Historically, vascular calcification was considered to be a passive degenerative process. However, recent human, animal and cell biological studies have demonstrated that vascular calcification is an actively regulated process similar to bone formation. For example, human vascular smooth muscle cells (VSMCs) have been shown to express many bone-regulating proteins, including osteopontin, matrix Gla protein, osteocalcin, osteonectin, collagen I and II, alkaline phosphatase, bone sialoprotein and bone morphogenic proteins [1]. Intense interest in this evolving area has generated several comprehensive reviews [1–4], the details of which are beyond the scope of this chapter.

As previously noted, calcification of the arterial wall can occur either in the intima, as part of a focal atherosclerotic plaque, or in the medial layer in the absence of atherosclerotic plaque. These two forms of arterial calcifications differ in their morphological features and epidemiology and may differ in their clinical significance as discussed below.

Medial Calcification

Calcification of the medial layer of the arteries, which occurs in the absence of atheroma, has been recognized by pathologists for over a century, and has historically been referred to as 'Monckeberg's sclerosis'. Medial calcification typically occurs in lower limb arteries such as the femoral and tibial, but it is also a common finding in the aorta. Medial calcification is non-occlusive, but can occur in the same locations as calcification of focal plaques (intimal calcification.) Medial calcification increases with age, and is widespread in persons with metabolic disorders such as diabetes mellitus and end-stage renal disease (ESRD) [2]. Familial aggregation of medial artery calcification has been reported, suggesting a genetic component. Other risk factors include duration of dialysis, duration of diabetes, and diabetic nephropathy [5].

Medial calcification has a different morphology from that of intimal calcification, appearing first as linear deposits along elastic lamellae, and in more severe cases, forming a thick circumferential sheet of calcium apatite crystals (and even bone tissue) in the center of the medial layer, with VSMCs on both sides [1]. On soft-tissue x-ray of the aorta and lower limbs, the appearance of medial calcification has been described as railroad tracks [2]. Historically, medial artery calcification was believed to be clinically insignificant, but several large studies have now shown that it is associated with increased risk for CVD events, at least among diabetic and ESRD patients [5]. In a recent study of ESRD patients by London et al. [6], patients with predominantly intimal (plaque-associated) calcification had the highest risk of CVD events; patients with only medial arterial calcification had an intermediate risk of events, and patients with no calcifications had the lowest CVD event risk. Those with intimal calcification were older, and had higher levels of calcified common carotid artery (CCA) plaques, smoking, LDL cholesterol and CRP, more prevalent diabetes and atherosclerosis, and longer duration of dialysis. Patients with only medial artery calcification were similar in age to those with no calcifications, but had much longer duration of dialysis. Interestingly, medial artery calcification was less prevalent among black ESRD patients, similar to reported racial differences in coronary artery calcification.

Intimal Calcification

As illustrated by London and colleagues [6], the epidemiology and clinical significance of intimal calcification, or calcification of focal plaques, may differ from that of medial calcification. Intimal calcium deposition in the context of atherosclerosis is mostly seen in the coronaries and large arteries like the aorta and is associated with lipids, macrophages (inflammation) and VSMCs [1]. Intimal calcification occurs in at least two distinct patterns: (1) discrete or punctate in the basal portion of the intima, and (2) diffuse calcification throughout the intima. The discrete pattern is thought to reflect an active, organized and regulated process because hematopoietic marrow, osteoclast-like cells, osteoblasts and other proteins normally associated with bone formation are seen [1]. Histopathological techniques that avoid decalcification have revealed a second, more diffuse pattern of calcification. This type of calcification can be missed by imaging modalities because the overall tissue density is similar to the adjacent, non-calcified tissue. It has been speculated that in intimal calcification, the calcification process begins with a diffuse pattern which undergoes reorganization to form the more discrete pattern [1, 2].

Quantification of intimal calcification in the coronaries has been shown to be a good marker of atherosclerotic burden. To date, the strongest determinants identified are older age, male sex and race/ethnicity, with higher calcification levels among white compared to black individuals [7]. Traditional risk factors such as LDL and total cholesterol have been predictors of coronary calcification burden, with smoking, BP and BMI showing slightly stronger relationships. Coronary calcification scores are much higher in men, but interestingly, this gender difference does not apply to the aorta, where autopsy studies have shown a more similar level of atheroma between men and women [8].

Coronary artery calcification is strongly indicative of atheroma; however, an absence of coronary calcification does not rule out the presence of non-calcified plaques. This has raised the question of whether calcification may be involved in the stabilization of plaques that would otherwise be vulnerable to rupture. The role of calcium deposition in this process is contradictory, depending on the stage of atherosclerosis. When calcium deposition occurs as superficial nodules in early stages of plaque formation, it can protrude, causing rupture [9]. Studies have also shown that plaque rupture is most likely at interfaces between materials of different stiffness; however, as the lesion progresses, deposition of calcium is thought to impart resistance to stress in proportion to its quantity [10].

Imaging of Vascular Calcification

A number of imaging modalities, both invasive and non-invasive, are currently available to detect and quantify vascular calcification. These include plain radiographs (x-ray), ultrasound techniques (intravascular, transthoracic and transesophageal), computed tomography (CT) and magnetic resonance imaging. Of these modalities, x-ray and ultrasound have some ability to distinguish medial and intimal calcification, but provide only semiquantitative assessments [6]; moreover, intravascular ultrasound is invasive and transthoracic and transesophageal methods provide limited or no view of coronary arteries.

Intimal calcification has been studied in the aorta, carotid and femoral arteries using B-mode ultrasound to identify and semiquantify echogenic plaques. Some studies have also used x-rays and plain CT to identify extra-coronary calcification, but with these modalities, authors have usually assumed that they were measuring atherosclerotic calcification and have not always specified that they used a method that would exclude medial calcification from their results. A method of distinguishing between medial and intimal (plaque-associated) calcification on soft-tissue x-ray has been described, but it is user-dependent and provides only semiquantitative assessments [6].

An explosion of interest in calcification of the coronary arteries has been initiated by the recent development of electron-beam CT (EBT). The rapid scanning time (100 ms) of EBT has made it possible to obtain clear images of the coronary arteries without motion artifact. Most of the existing literature on coronary calcification has used EBT, although newer multidetector row spiral CT can also be used. 30–40 adjacent axial images of the heart are typically obtained with a 3- to 6-mm thickness. Trained 'readers' use software to quantify calcium area and density (calcification is detected when pixels >130 Hounsfield units are observed.) Most frequently, summary scores have been calculated using Agatston's method, although more recently some have advocated the determination of volumetric calcification scores [7]. EBT is not currently able to distinguish between medial and intimal calcification. However, coronary calcification is believed to primarily represent intimal calcification of focal plaques, since medial calcification is rare in the coronary arteries [2, 7].

Potential Mechanisms for Association between Arterial Calcification and Stiffness

Medial calcification is believed to directly increase arterial stiffness. The walls of large arteries contain collagen fibers, ensheathing elastic lamellae and VSMCs, all embedded in a non-fibrous matrix. The mechanical properties of the artery are determined mainly by the elastin and collagen components in the media of the artery, with smooth muscle cells also playing a role in vascular tone. With age, structural changes (remodeling) occur in the arterial wall including fragmentation and degeneration of elastin, increases in collagen, dilation of the artery and a thickening of the arterial wall [11]. Animal models have shown that various components of the media, especially elastin, and other components of elastic fibers are prone to calcification [12]. The net effect of these arteriosclerotic changes, including calcification of the elastic components of the medial layer, increases the stiffness of the arterial wall. In contrast, the most intuitive mechanism for a causal relationship between arterial stiffness and intimal calcification is that increased stiffness increases stress on the arterial wall, which makes it more prone to atherosclerosis and calcification.

In summary, when evaluating studies relating arterial stiffness to vascular calcification, it should be recognized that medial calcification is a distinct entity from intimal calcification (calcified atheroma). The current consensus is that coronary calcification represents primarily atherosclerotic intimal calcification. Aortic calcification and calcification of the lower extremities may be medial calcification or a combination of medial and intimal calcification. This is especially true for groups such as the elderly, diabetics, and ESRD patients, who are especially prone to medial calcification. However, current imaging methods generally do not distinguish medial from intimal calcification, and both medial and intimal calcification are associated with increased risk of CVD. In addition, both intimal and medial calcification may be associated with higher arterial stiffness, although for different reasons, as discussed above.

Arterial Stiffness and Vascular Calcification

Ideally, the association between arterial stiffness and vascular calcification would be evaluated separately for medial calcification (arteriosclerosis) versus intimal calcification (atherosclerosis or calcified plaque.) Fortunately, experimental models have the advantage of being able to specifically induce medial calcification in the absence of atheroma. Two different rat models of experimentally induced calcification of the medial elastic fibers of the aorta [13, 14] have demonstrated that an increase in medial calcification increases aortic stiffness, in parallel with an increase in collagen and decrease in elastin. Other evidence that medial calcification stiffens arteries comes from studies of lower limb arteries in diabetic patients, which have demonstrated that calcified arteries are rigid and have reduced blood flow [5]. However, most human studies of arterial stiffness and calcification have not differentiated between medial (arteriosclerosis) and intimal (atherosclerotic) calcification, primarily due to limitations of non-invasive imaging techniques to distinguish between them. Therefore, we will discuss them below according to arterial site (extracoronary vs. coronary), since the current consensus holds that coronary calcification represents primarily intimal calcification, whereas extracoronary calcification may be a combination of medial and intimal calcification. For arterial stiffness, our review includes only well-validated measures of large and medium elastic arterial stiffness, specifically: carotid-femoral pulse wave velocity (cfPWV), pulse pressure (PP), carotid distensibility, and the carotid incremental elastic modulus (E_{inc}).

Arterial Stiffness and Extracoronary Calcification

In the studies which have evaluated the association between arterial stiffness and extracoronary calcification, it is not completely clear whether the calcification measures represent intimal or medial calcification or a combination of the two. In an early paper, Witteman et al. [15] evaluated the 9-year progression of aortic calcification (by x-ray) among women aged 45–64 at baseline. Progression of aortic calcification was associated with a decrease in diastolic BP of 10 mm Hg or more. On further analysis, this was shown to be true only for women above the median in increase in PP. Their longitudinal results support the hypothesis that progression of aortic calcification (which they used as an index of atheroma progression) precedes increases in arterial stiffness. Another study of 116 Japanese men and women (mean age 57.4 ± 8.3, with controlled hyperlipidemia and any aortic calcification at baseline) evaluated the determinants of progression of abdominal aortic calcification (measured by standard CT) during a follow-up of approximately 6 years. After adjustment for age and sex, progression of aortic calcification was significantly associated with BMI, systolic BP, and PP, but PP was the strongest predictor of progression of aortic calcification.

In renal dialysis patients, a strong cross-sectional relationship has been demonstrated between higher number of extracoronary sites with calcifications (carotid, aorta, and femoral) and both lower diastolic BP (i.e. increased PP) [16] and stiffness of both the carotid and aorta [17]. In the second study, arterial stiffness was assessed by CCA incremental elastic modulus, distensibility and cfPWV, and the associations remained after adjustment for age, duration of dialysis, fibrinogen, and the prescribed dose of calcium-based phosphate binders. Extracoronary calcifications were assessed by B-mode ultrasound of the CCA, aorta, and femoral arteries, and x-ray of the abdomen, pelvis and femoral arteries, and analyzed semiquantitatively as a score (0–4) according to the number of arterial sites with calcifications. This definition includes intimal calcification (echogenic plaques), but may also include medial calcification, which is widespread among ESRD patients and would also be visible on x-rays.

In the Rotterdam study (>3,000 participants aged 60–101), higher cfPWV and decreased common carotid distensibility were associated with numerous non-coronary disease measures including higher carotid wall thickness and plaque, calcified aortic plaque, and peripheral vascular disease [18], independent of age, sex, mean arterial pressure, and heart rate. Carotid plaques were evaluated using B-mode ultrasound and summarized as a plaque index, and calcified aortic plaque was evaluated from lateral x-rays of the lumbar spine, and graded from 0 to 5 for severity based on size. Peripheral vascular disease was evaluated by ankle BPs. This large, population-based study of elderly men and women demonstrated a strong association of carotid and aortic stiffness with not only calcified aortic plaques, but also other measures of subclinical atherosclerosis.

Finally, an interesting study has reported differences in arterial stiffness according to carotid plaque morphology (by B-mode ultrasound), among 561 volunteers (mean age 58 ± 10.8 years) without a history of coronary heart disease or stroke [19]. 71.5% had no plaques, 9.1% had echolucent and 19.4% had echogenic plaques. PWV was higher among those with echogenic (calcified) plaques (p < 0.01) compared to those with echolucent or no plaques, and mean PWV was not significantly different between those with echolucent plaques versus those with no plaques. Results remained significant after adjustment for gender, age, BMI, smoking habits, systolic BP, antihypertensive treatment, diabetes, total cholesterol, lipid-lowering medications, serum triglycerides, and CCA-intima-media thickness (IMT). These results are interesting, since they are counter-intuitive to current thinking that echolucent plaques should be more unstable and therefore more high risk than echogenic (calcified) plaques. However, the lack of association with echolucent plaques may be due to survivor bias, since prevalent CVD was an exclusion factor for the study. It is possible that those with both echolucent plaques and high arterial stiffness are at greatest risk of fatal or non-fatal CVD events, thereby excluding them from study and making it impossible to demonstrate an association between high levels of both.

In combination with the animal studies, these few reports suggest that extracoronary calcification, especially in the aorta, is associated with higher levels of large artery stiffness. However, it is unknown what proportion of the extracoronary calcification evaluated in the clinical and epidemiological studies represented medial calcification (arteriosclerosis) versus intimal calcification of focal plaque (atherosclerosis).

Arterial Stiffness and Coronary Artery Calcification

Coronary calcification is thought to represent primarily calcification of atheroma [2, 3]. Evidence of an association between arterial stiffness and coronary calcification has been mixed. Haydar et al. [20] have shown that among 55 men and women with ESRD, cfPWV was positively associated with coronary calcification after adjusting for age, sex, duration of dialysis, CRP, and diastolic BP.

In contrast, Megnien et al. [21] concluded that aortic stiffening (cfPWV) was not associated with coronary or extracoronary atherosclerosis among 190 asymptomatic high-risk men aged 29–62. However, the sample size (n = 190 men) was relatively small, and is a subset of 4,190 subjects who were selected for further evaluation from 16,000 screenees because they had at least one cardiovascular risk factor. Their tables show an increase in cfPWV (unadjusted) across coronary calcium categories (0, 1–9, 10–99) until the highest category (≥100), in which it decreases precipitously. The same pattern was observed across increasing number of sites with any plaque. Since people with fatal or non-fatal CVD events were excluded from the study, it is possible that these results may also reflect a survivor bias, in which men who had both high arterial stiffness and high levels of calcified plaque were unrepresented in the study sample.

Finally, two larger studies (reported as abstracts) have reported strong associations between coronary calcification and cfPWV. First, in a study of 484 older adults (aged 70–96) from the Cardiovascular Health Study, the association between aortic stiffness (cfPWV) and both coronary and aortic calcification was evaluated. Among the older women (mean age 79 years), higher aortic stiffness was associated with higher quartiles of both coronary and aortic calcification after adjustment for age and mean arterial pressure [22]. The absence of an association among these older men may also be due to a survival bias. Second, in a cross-sectional analysis of 477 overweight postmenopausal women (aged 52–62) with no history of coronary heart disease, the prevalence of any coronary calcium was higher among those with higher levels of arterial stiffness (cfPWV) [23]. A 1-SD increase in cfPWV was associated with a 38% increase in odds of coronary calcification. These associations remained significant after adjusting for age, systolic BP, heart rate, waist circumference, weight, fasting glucose and smoking status.

In summary, the few studies which have evaluated the relationship between arterial stiffness and coronary calcification have had mixed results, but the larger studies have shown a positive association between aortic stiffness (as indexed by cfPWV) and coronary calcification. Assuming that coronary calcification represents calcified plaque, an association between coronary calcification and arterial stiffness is supported by evidence that arterial stiffness (cfPWV) is associated with other measures of atheroma such as intravascular ultrasound-detected coronary plaque volume [24]. In an interesting longitudinal study of 304 elderly Japanese men and women, Sawabe et al. [25] found that repeat PWV measures correlated with the overall atherosclerotic burden at autopsy across eight sites of the large arteries. Several studies have also reported that arterial stiffness is associated with thicker carotid IMT, but because IMT may be a marker of both atherosclerosis and arterial remodeling, we have not discussed them here.

Summary and Conclusion

Evidence from animal data and studies of diabetes and ESRD suggests that medial calcification directly increases arterial stiffness. Evidence linking intimal calcification with arterial stiffness is less definitive. The number of studies is small and studies of extracoronary calcification have generally not differentiated between intimal calcification (calcified plaques) versus medial calcification. Other measures of atheroma such as aortic and carotid plaque have also been shown to be associated with higher levels of arterial stiffening, but it is not entirely clear whether or not this is due to shared risk factors or to a causal relationship between arterial stiffness and atheroma development.

As technology allows, future studies should attempt to differentiate between medial, or non-atherosclerotic, calcification versus calcified plaques. Since both arterial stiffness and vascular calcification (both medial and intimal) have been shown to predict cardiovascular risk, further evaluation of the relationship between arterial stiffness and vascular calcification is needed, including investigation into potential differences by race/ethnicity. Also, because atherosclerosis-associated calcification (intimal calcification) is a separate process from arterial stiffening, future studies should also evaluate potential additive effects of arterial stiffness and vascular calcification in predicting CVD risk among various populations, which has already been demonstrated among ESRD patients [16].

References

1 Proudfoot D, Shanahan CM: Biology of calcification in vascular cells: intima versus media. Herz 2001;26:245–251.
2 Doherty TM, Fitzpatrick LA, Inoue D, et al: Molecular, endocrine, and genetic mechanisms of arterial calcification. Endocr Rev 2004;25:629–672.
3 Giachelli CM: Vascular calcification mechanisms. J Am Soc Nephrol 2004;15:2959–2964.
4 Abedin M, Tintut Y, Demer LL: Vascular calcification: mechanisms and clinical ramifications. Arterioscler Thromb Vasc Biol 2004;24:1161–1170.
5 Edmonds ME: Medial arterial calcification and diabetes mellitus. Z Kardiol 2000;89(suppl 2):101–104.
6 London GM, Guerin AP, Marchais SJ, Metivier F, Pannier B, Adda H: Arterial media calcification in end-stage renal disease: impact on all-cause and cardiovascular mortality. Nephrol Dial Transplant 2003;18:1731–1740.
7 O'Rourke RA, Brundage BH, Froelicher VF, et al: American College of Cardiology/American Heart Association Expert Consensus Document on electron-beam computed tomography for the diagnosis and prognosis of coronary artery disease. J Am Coll Cardiol 2000;36:326–340.
8 Tejada C, Strong JP, Montenegro MR, Restrepo C, Solberg LA: Distribution of coronary and aortic atherosclerosis by geographic location, race, and sex. Lab Invest 1968;18:509–526.
9 Naghavi M, Libby P, Falk E, et al: From vulnerable plaque to vulnerable patient: a call for new definitions and risk assessment strategies. I. Circulation 2003;108:1664–1672.
10 Thompson BH, Stanford W: Imaging of coronary calcification by computed tomography. J Magn Reson Imaging 2004;19:720–733.

11   Lakatta EG, Mitchell JH, Pomerance A, Rowe GG: Human aging: changes in structure and function. J Am Coll Cardiol 1987;10:42A–47A.
12   Dao HH, Essalihi R, Bouvet C, Moreau P: Evolution and modulation of age-related medial elastocalcinosis: impact on large artery stiffness and isolated systolic hypertension. Cardiovasc Res 2005;66:307–317.
13   Niederhoffer N, Lartaud-Idjouadiene I, Giummelly P, Duvivier C, Peslin R, Atkinson J: Calcification of medial elastic fibers and aortic elasticity. Hypertension 1997;29:999–1006.
14   Essalihi R, Dao HH, Yamaguchi N, Moreau P: A new model of isolated systolic hypertension induced by chronic warfarin and vitamin K1 treatment. Am J Hypertens 2003;16:103–110.
15   Witteman JC, Grobbee DE, Valkenburg HA, et al: J-shaped relation between change in diastolic blood pressure and progression of aortic atherosclerosis. Lancet 1994;343:504–507.
16   Blacher J, Guerin AP, Pannier B, Marchais SJ, London GM: Arterial calcifications, arterial stiffness, and cardiovascular risk in end-stage renal disease. Hypertension 2001;38:938–942.
17   Guerin AP, London GM, Marchais SJ, Metivier F: Arterial stiffening and vascular calcifications in end-stage renal disease. Nephrol Dial Transplant 2000;15:1014–1021.
18   Van Popele NM, Grobbee DE, Bots ML, et al: Association between arterial stiffness and atherosclerosis: the Rotterdam study. Stroke 2001;32:454–460.
19   Zureik M, Bureau JM, Temmar M, et al: Echogenic carotid plaques are associated with aortic arterial stiffness in subjects with subclinical carotid atherosclerosis. Hypertension 2003;41:519–527.
20   Haydar AA, Hujairi NM, Covic AA, Pereira D, Rubens M, Goldsmith DJ: Coronary artery calcification is related to coronary atherosclerosis in chronic renal disease patients: a study comparing EBCT-generated coronary artery calcium scores and coronary angiography. Nephrol Dial Transplant 2004;19:2307–2312.
21   Megnien JL, Simon A, Denarie N, et al: Aortic stiffening does not predict coronary and extracoronary atherosclerosis in asymptomatic men at risk for cardiovascular disease. Am J Hypertens 1998;11:293–301.
22   Mackey RH, Sutton-Tyrrell K, Kuller LH, Naydeck BL, Newman AB: Aortic stiffness is associated with aortic and coronary calcification in older adults (abstract). Circulation 2001;103:1355.
23   Venkitachalam L, Mackey RH, Patel AS, et al: Pulse wave velocity and coronary calcification in post-menopausal women – The Woman on the Move through Activity and Nutrition (WOMAN) Study (abstract). Circulation 2004;110(suppl III):III-791.
24   McLeod AL, Uren NG, Wilkinson IB, et al: Non invasive measures of pulse wave velocity correlate with coronary arterial plaque load in humans. J Hypertens 2004;22:363–368.
25   Sawabe M, Takahashi R, Matsushita S, et al: Aortic pulse wave velocity and the degree of atherosclerosis in the elderly: a pathological study based on 304 autopsy cases. Atherosclerosis 2005;179:345–351.

Rachel H. Mackey, PhD, MPH
University of Pittsburgh, Graduate School of Public Health
Department of Epidemiology, 130 DeSoto Street
Pittsburgh, PA 15261 (USA)
Tel. +1 412 624 5948, Fax +1 412 624 3775, E-Mail mackey@edc.pitt.edu

Safar ME, Frohlich ED (eds): Atherosclerosis, Large Arteries and Cardiovascular Risk.
Adv Cardiol. Basel, Karger, 2007, vol 44, pp 245–251

· ·

Diabetes and Arterial Stiffening

Nathaniel Winer[a]   *James R. Sowers*[b]

[a]Division of Endocrinology, Diabetes, and Hypertension, SUNY Downstate
Medical Center, New York, N.Y., and [b]University of Missouri School of Medicine
and Harry S. Truman Veterans Affairs Medical Center, Columbia, Mo., USA

Abstract

Type 2 diabetes (DM-2) has become a major global health problem that has been fueled mainly by increasing obesity and aging of the population. Most studies show that arterial stiffening occurs across all age groups in both type 1 diabetes and DM-2, and among those with impaired fasting glucose, impaired glucose tolerance, and the metabolic syndrome. Arterial stiffening in DM-2 results, in part, from the clustering of hyperglycemia, dyslipidemia and hypertension, all of which may promote insulin resistance, oxidative stress, endothelial dysfunction, and the formation of pro-inflammatory cytokines and advanced glycosylation end-products. Likewise, aging may increase arterial stiffening by altering the proportions of elastin and collagen in the aorta. The consequences of arterial stiffening are increased pulse pressure, hypertension, and a greater risk of cardiovascular disease. Treatment strategies to reduce or prevent arterial stiffening include pharmacologic agents that block the renin-angiotensin-aldosterone system, relax vascular smooth muscle, enhance release of nitric oxide from endothelial cells, and break glycosylation end-product cross-links, and fish oil supplementation.

Copyright © 2007 S. Karger AG, Basel

Epidemiology of Diabetes

Diabetes is a growing health problem throughout the world; more than 170 million people are estimated to have diabetes worldwide, the majority of whom have type 2 diabetes (DM-2). Largely unknown early in the 20th century, DM-2 is now the fifth leading cause of death in the USA. Conservative estimates suggest that by 2025 the diabetic population will more than double to over 366 million [1]. From a global perspective, Asia is expected to be the region most heavily impacted by diabetes, with an anticipated 2- to 3-fold increase in prevalence. Factors contributing to the rise in diabetes prevalence are the declining mortality from communicable diseases and infant and maternal mortality in less developed countries, aging and urbanization of the population, and, most importantly, the striking increase in obesity. The parallel rise in the prevalence of obesity and DM-2 has been appropriately labeled 'diabesity' [2].

The complications of diabetes, which include limb amputations, blindness, nerve damage, kidney failure requiring hemodialysis, and cardiovascular disease (CVD), pose the threat of enormous human and economic costs. A prospective study of more than 15,000 persons followed for 25 years confirms that the risk of cardiovascular death in patients with diabetes without previous coronary heart disease (CHD) is equal to that of patients with CHD without diabetes, with the risk in women being higher [3]. Direct healthcare expenditures and the costs of lost productivity attributable to diabetes in the USA were estimated at USD 132 billion in 2002 [4].

Impaired Glucose Metabolism and Metabolic Syndrome

Although numerous past studies show that hyperglycemia is associated with a marked increase in CVD mortality risk [5], recent investigations have focused on the risks posed by impaired glucose metabolism (IGM), i.e., impaired fasting glucose (IFG) and/or impaired glucose tolerance (IGT). In the Hoorn Study, decreased total systemic arterial compliance, increased aortic augmentation index, and decreased carotid-femoral transit time were seen in DM-2 and to a lesser extent in IGM, suggesting that either greater arterial stiffness in DM-2 or increased aortic atherosclerotic plaque reflection sites might increase augmentation index by altering the amplitude and timing of reflected waves [6]. Increased stiffness of the muscular femoral and brachial arteries in IGM may precede elastic carotid artery stiffness in DM-2, because of decreased distension and diameter of the femoral artery coupled with increased pulse pressure. Hyperglycemia and hyperinsulinemia explained about 30% of the arterial changes associated with IGM and DM-2. Other factors included oxidative stress, chronic low-grade inflammation, and endothelial dysfunction, including that caused by the formation of glycosylation end-products (AGEs) [7].

A study of middle-aged Japanese men with IFG, IGT, and DM-2 showed a significant relationship between arterial stiffness, measured by photoplethysmography, and IFG or IGT; stepwise regression analysis showed that IGT is an independent determinant of arterial stiffness that may be more sensitive than FPG in identifying asymptomatic persons with increased arterial stiffness [8].

The metabolic syndrome is characterized by the concurrence of several cardiovascular risk factors: central obesity, dyslipidemia, elevated blood pressure, and high fasting glucose levels. Insulin resistance, a common pathogenetic factor underlying these risk factors, may lead to the development of DM-2 and increased risk of CVD. Intra-abdominal adiposity, sedentary lifestyle, and a genetic predisposition are prime etiologic factors [9].

In the Amsterdam Growth and Health Longitudinal Study the prevalence of the metabolic syndrome among young subjects (mean age 36 years) was 18.3% in men and 3.2% in women. Individuals with the metabolic syndrome showed reduced distensibility and compliance of the carotid and femoral arteries compared to those without risk factors. Stiffness of the muscular femoral artery was greater than that of the elastic carotid artery [9]. Other studies of the metabolic syndrome are in agreement with these findings [10–13]. In middle-aged Japanese men the number of criteria for the diagnosis of the metabolic syndrome was proportional to the pulse wave velocity. In these subjects, pulse wave velocity was higher in those with an elevated C-reactive protein, suggesting that inflammation may aggravate the cardiovascular risk of the metabolic syndrome [14].

Glucose, Insulin, and Potential Mechanisms of Vascular Stiffening
(fig. 1)

Among patients with diabetes [15] or the metabolic syndrome, arterial stiffening is observed across all age groups. In children with severe obesity, arterial wall stiffness and endothelial dysfunction are accompanied by low plasma apolipoprotein A-I levels, insulin resistance, and android fat distribution, changes that may be the main risk factors for the early events leading to atheroma formation [16]. The positive correlation between insulin resistance and central arterial stiffness and the close relationship between the extent of metabolic changes and the degree of arterial stiffness suggest that insulin resistance is a primary underlying factor. In animal models of insulin-resistant diabetes, chronic hyperglycemia and hyperinsulinemia increase local angiotensin II production and expression of vascular Ang II type I receptors via stimulation of TGF-β_1, upregulate plasminogen activator inhibitor-1, and downregulate matrix metalloprotease activity, all of which play a critical role in coronary remodeling and vessel wall hypertrophy and fibrosis. The proliferative effects of insulin occur because insulin resistance impairs PI$_3$-kinase-dependent signaling, while having little effect on the growth-promoting mito-

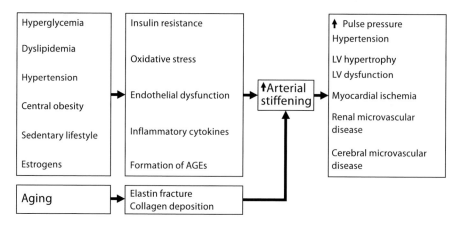

Fig. 1. Increased arterial stiffening is a hallmark of both type 1 and 2 diabetes. The accompanying dyslipidemia, hypertension, visceral obesity and sedentary lifestyle also contribute to structural changes in the arterial wall. Premenopausal women may also have increased arterial stiffening compared to men, suggesting a role for estrogens. Fracture of elastin fibers and increased deposition of collagen associated with aging leads to gradual widening and decreased distensibility of the aorta and the consequent loss of its buffering capacity. These clinical features act through a variety of mechanisms, including insulin resistance, oxidative stress, endothelial dysfunction, and formation of AGEs and pro-inflammatory cytokines, to increase arterial stiffening and increase the risk of CVD.

gen-activated kinase pathways. In addition, insulin resistance enhances non-enzymatic glycation of proteins with covalent cross-linking of collagen (AGEs). Other elements occurring early in the insulin-resistant state, such as elevated levels of LDL cholesterol, free fatty acids, and endothelin-1, or decreased levels of adiponectin and natriuretic peptides, may impair endothelial function and increase arterial stiffness as well. Hyperglycemia in DM-2 causes increased oxidative stress by generating reactive oxygen species, leading to increased glycosylation of functional proteins and glucose autooxidation with activation of the polyol pathway and generation of reactive oxygen species, including superoxide, hydrogen peroxide, and hydroxyl radicals. Elevated glucose levels may also reduce NO synthase activity by enhancing oxidation of tetrahydrobiopterin (BH_4), an essential cofactor for NO synthase. As a result, NO production from arginine and molecular oxygen is reduced and electrons are transferred to molecular oxygen to further increase superoxide and peroxynitrite levels.

Despite lower systolic blood pressure and pulse pressure and more favorable lipid levels, young women have greater small vessel stiffness than age-matched men [17], suggesting that estrogens may lack the vasculoprotective

Table 1. Treatment strategies to reduce arterial stiffening in DM-2

Blockade of renin-angiotensin system (ACEs, ARBs)
Reduced vascular smooth muscle tone (calcium channel blockers)
Aldosterone antagonist treatment (eplerenone)
Increased NO release from endothelial cells (HMG-CoA reductase inhibitors)
Administration of NO synthase cofactor (tetrahydrobiopterin)
Use of antioxidants (vitamin C)
Fish oil supplementation
Regular aerobic exercise
AGE cross-link breakers (alagebrium)

---

effects previously attributed to them. Increased small vessel stiffness in pre-menopausal women may provide a plausible explanation for the failure of post-menopausal estrogen treatment to prevent CHD in recent clinical trials.

Treatment Strategies to Reduce Arterial Stiffening in DM-2 (table 1)

Arterial stiffness increases the risk for cardiovascular events, dementia, renal failure, and death. These adverse outcomes result from decreased compliance of the central vasculature which leads to widened pulse pressure, impaired cardiac performance, and reduced coronary perfusion. In contrast to vascular areas that are protected by vasoconstriction, renal and cerebral vessels are exposed to higher pulsatile circumferential and shear stress, increasing the risk of microvascular disease [18]. Patients with DM-2 are especially vulnerable to small vessel injury of the brain and kidney because renal and cerebral vessels lack the normal resilience to withstand such stresses [19].

Current attempts to reverse arterial stiffening have focused on blocking the renin-angiotensin-aldosterone system with angiotensin-converting enzyme inhibitors (ACEs) or angiotensin II receptor inhibitors (ARBs) and decreasing vascular smooth muscle tone with calcium channel blockers. HMG-CoA reductase inhibitors reduce vascular stiffening by inducing Akt-mediated phosphorylation of NO synthase to increase NO release from endothelial cells [20]. Although administration of BH_4 may not be practical as a therapy for chronic vascular disease states, vitamin C treatment improved NO bioavailability in DM-2 by maintaining normal levels of BH_4 [21]. Fish oil ingestion improved vascular compliance in patients with DM-2 [22], probably by increasing NO production or release [23]. Regular aerobic exercise has been reported to partially restore the loss of central arterial compliance in sedentary middle-aged and older men and would likely improve arterial stiffening in men with diabetes as well [24]. Aldosterone antagonist treatment may also reduce arterial stiffening; in older patients with hypertension and increased pulse pressure, eplerenone lowered systolic blood pressure and pulse wave velocity [25], while in aldosterone-salt-treated rats, eplerenone prevented the increase in carotid wall elastic modulus and fibronectin [26].

AGEs may form stable cross-links with glucose and collagen and elastin; such cross-links, which occur with aging and are accentuated in diabetes, may reduce collagen turnover and increase tissue stiffness. A recent clinical trial found that alagebrium (ALT-711), the first of a new class of thiazolium AGE cross-link breakers, improved arterial compliance in elderly patients with vascular stiffening [27].

References

1   Wild S, Roglic G, Green A, Sicree R, King H: Global prevalence of diabetes: estimates for the year 2000 and projections for 2030. Diabetes Care 2004;27:1047–1053.
2   Ziv E, Shafrir E: *Psammomys obesus*: nutritionally induced NIDDM-like syndrome on a 'thrifty gene' background; in Shafrir E (ed): Lessons from Animal Diabetes. London, Smith-Gordon, 1995, pp 285–300.
3   Whiteley L, Padmanabhan S, Hole D, Isles C: Should diabetes be considered a coronary heart disease risk equivalent? Results from 25 years of follow-up in the Renfrew and Paisley Survey. Diabetes Care 2005;28:1588–1593.
4   Hogan P, Dall T, Nikolov P: Economic costs of diabetes in the US in 2002. Diabetes Care 2003; 26:917–932.
5   Winer N, Sowers JR: Epidemiology of diabetes. J Clin Pharmacol 2004;44:397–405.
6   Schram MT, Henry RM, van Dijk RA, Kostense PJ, Dekker JM, Nijpels G, Heine RJ, Bouter LM, Westerhof N, Stehouwer CD: Increased central artery stiffness in impaired glucose metabolism and type 2 diabetes: the Hoorn Study. Hypertension 2004;43:176–181.
7   Henry RM, Kostense PJ, Spijkerman AM, Dekker JM, Nijpels G, Heine RJ, Kamp O, Westerhof N, Bouter LM, Stehouwer CD: Arterial stiffness increases with deteriorating glucose tolerance status: the Hoorn Study. Circulation 2003;107:2089–2095.
8   Ohshita K, Yamane K, Ishida K, Watanabe H, Okubo M, Kohno N: Post-challenge hyperglycaemia is an independent risk factor for arterial stiffness in Japanese men. Diabet Med 2004;21: 636–639.
9   Grundy SM, Brewer HB Jr, Cleeman JI, Smith SC Jr, Lenfant C, American Heart Association; National Heart, Lung, and Blood Institute: Definition of metabolic syndrome: Report of the National Heart, Lung, and Blood Institute/American Heart Association conference on scientific issues related to definition. Circulation 2004;109:433–438.
10 Ferreira I, Henry RM, Twisk JW, van Mechelen W, Kemper HC, Stehouwer CD: The metabolic syndrome, cardiopulmonary fitness, and subcutaneous trunk fat as independent determinants of arterial stiffness: the Amsterdam Growth and Health Longitudinal Study. Arch Intern Med 2005;165:875–882.
11 Salomaa V, Riley W, Kark JD, Nardo C, Folsom AR: Non-insulin-dependent diabetes mellitus and fasting glucose and insulin concentrations are associated with arterial stiffness: the ARIC study. Circulation 1995;91:1432–1443.
12 Scuteri A, Najjar SS, Muller DC, et al: Metabolic syndrome amplifies the age-associated increases in vascular thickness and thickness. J Am Coll Cardiol 2004;43:1388–1395.

13 Urbina EM, Srinivasan SR, Kieltyka RL, et al: Correlates of carotid artery stiffness in young adults: the Bogalusa Heart Study. Atherosclerosis 2004;176:157–164.

14 Van Popele NM, Westendorp IC, Bots ML, Reneman RS, Hoeks AP, Hofman A, Grobbee DE, Witteman JC: Variables of the insulin resistance syndrome are associated with reduced arterial distensibility in healthy non-diabetic middle-aged women. Diabetologia 2000;43:665–672.

15 Tomiyama H, Koji Y, Yambe M, Motobe K, Shiina K, Gulnisa Z, Yamamoto Y, Yamashina A: Elevated C-reactive protein augments increased arterial stiffness in subjects with the metabolic syndrome. Hypertension 2005;45:997–1003.

16 Winer N, Sowers JR: Vascular compliance in diabetes. Curr Diab Rep 2003;3:230–234.

17 Tounian P, Aggoun Y, Dubern B, Varille V, Guy-Grand B, Sidi D, Girardet JP, Bonnet D: Presence of increased stiffness of the common carotid artery and endothelial dysfunction in severely obese children: a prospective study. Lancet 2001;358:1400–1404.

18 Winer N, Sowers JR, Weber MA: Gender differences in vascular compliance in young, healthy subjects assessed by pulse contour analysis. J Clin Hypertens 2001;3:145–152.

19 O'Rourke MF, Safar ME: Relationship between aortic stiffening and microvascular disease in brain and kidney: cause and logic of therapy. Hypertension 2005;46:200–204.

20 Schram MT, Kostense PJ, Van Dijk RA, Dekker JM, Nijpels G, Bouter LM, Heine RJ, Stehouwer CD: Diabetes, pulse pressure and cardiovascular mortality: the Hoorn Study. J Hypertens 2002; 20:1743–1751.

21 Kureishi Y, Luo Z, Shiojima I, Bialik A, Fulton D, Lefer DJ, Sessa WC, Walsh K: The HMG-CoA reductase inhibitor simvastatin activates the protein kinase Akt and promotes angiogenesis in normocholesterolemic animals. Nat Med 2000;6:1004–1010.

22 Ting HH, Timimi FK, Boles KS, Creager SJ, Ganz P, Creager MA: Vitamin C improves endothelium-dependent vasodilation in patients with non-insulin-dependent diabetes mellitus. J Clin Invest 1996;97:22–28.

23 McVeigh GE, Brennan GM, Cohn JN, Finkelstein SM, Hayes RJ, Johnston GD: Fish oil improves arterial compliance in non-insulin-dependent diabetes mellitus. Arterioscler Thromb 1994;14: 1425–1429.

24 McVeigh GE, Brennan GM, Johnston GD, McDermott BJ, McGrath LT, Henry WR, Andrews JW, Hayes JR: Dietary fish oil augments nitric oxide production or release in patients with type 2 (non-insulin-dependent) diabetes mellitus. Diabetologia 1993;36:33–38.

25 Tanaka H, Dinenno FA, Monahan KD, Clevenger CM, DeSouza CA, Seals DR: Aging, habitual exercise, and dynamic arterial compliance. Circulation 2000;102:1214–1215.

26 White WB, Duprez D, St Hillaire R, Krause S, Roniker B, Kuse-Hamilton J, Weber MA: Effects of the selective aldosterone blocker eplerenone versus the calcium antagonist amlodipine in systolic hypertension. Hypertension 2003;41:1021–1026.

27 Lacolley P, Labat C, Pujol A, Delcayre C, Benetos A, Safar M: Increased carotid wall elastic modulus and fibronectin in aldosterone-salt-treated rats: effects of eplerenone. Circulation 2002;106: 2848–2853.

28 Bakris GL, Bank AJ, Kass DA, Neutel JM, Preston RA, Oparil S: Advanced glycation end-product cross-link breakers: a novel approach to cardiovascular pathologies related to the aging process. Am J Hypertens 2004;17:23S–30S.

Nathaniel Winer
Division of Endocrinology, Diabetes, and Hypertension
SUNY Downstate Medical Center, Box 1205, 450 Clarkson Ave.
Brooklyn, NY 11203-2098 (USA)
Tel. +1 718 270 6320, Fax +1 718 270 2699, E-Mail nwiner@downstate.edu

Safar ME, Frohlich ED (eds): Atherosclerosis, Large Arteries and Cardiovascular Risk.
Adv Cardiol. Basel, Karger, 2007, vol 44, pp 252–260

······················

Insulin Resistance, Arterial Stiffness and Wave Reflection

Hannele Yki-Järvinen   Jukka Westerbacka

Department of Medicine, Division of Diabetes, University of Helsinki,
Helsinki, Finland

Abstract

Insulin resistance is associated with increased cardiovascular morbidity and mortality but the underlying mechanism(s) are incompletely understood. Epidemiological data suggest that insulin resistance and arterial stiffness are interrelated. In insulin sensitive-subjects, insulin acutely decreases the augmentation index as measured using pulse wave analysis. In insulin-resistant subjects, this effect of insulin is blunted implying that insulin resistance involves also large arteries. This may provide one mechanism linking insulin resistance and cardiovascular disease.

The term *insulin resistance* refers to a condition which is characterized by a blunted response to one or several normal biologic actions of insulin [1]. Insulin resistance predicts the development of type 2 diabetes [2] and cardiovascular disease [3, 4]. The mechanism(s) linking insulin resistance to cardiovascular disease are poorly understood. The augmentation index (see chapter by Safar, pp 1–18) is increased by cardiovascular risk factors such as age (see chapter by Izzo and Mitchell, pp 19–34), smoking [5, 6] and hypertension (see chapter by Frohlich and Susic, pp 117–124). It predicts cardiovascular mortality in patients with end-stage renal failure [7] and is an independent marker of severity of coronary artery disease [8]. The following chapter discusses evidence linking arterial stiffness and the augmentation index to insulin resistance.

Epidemiological Data

The possibility that insulin resistance is independently associated with increased arterial stiffness was first suggested by cross-sectional analysis of ARIC (Atherosclerosis Risk in Communities) data. This study explored the relationship between insulin resistance (measured using fasting insulin concentrations) and arterial stiffness measured with ultrasound in 4,701 white and black subjects [9]. In the entire study group, arteries appear to become stiffer at increasing concentrations of fasting glucose and insulin, independent of race or gender. The relationship between glucose and insulin concentrations and stiffness remained significant after adjustment for classic cardiovascular risk factors. This was also true within the non-diabetic subjects, which comprised 95% of the study subjects [9]. In 2,488 adults participating in the Health ABC study, increased serum insulin concentrations and visceral fat volume measured with computed tomography were associated with increased aortic stiffness measured by pulse wave velocity [10]. In the Baltimore Longitudinal Study on Aging, the metabolic syndrome as defined by ATPIII criteria was independently associated with increased arterial stiffness measured using carotid artery ultrasound in 471 subjects [11]. Increased arterial stiffness has been a consistent finding in both type 1 and 2 diabetic patients, both characterized by insulin resistance, in several studies (see chapter by Winer and Sowers, pp 245–251). In a recent cross-sectional study of 228 type 2 diabetic patients, increased central pressure augmentation and central, but not brachial, systolic pressure measured using pulse wave analysis (for methods, see chapter by Safar, pp 1–18) were associated, independent of age, with increased carotid intima-media thickness, an established marker of atherosclerosis [12]. These cross-sectional data do not, however, prove causality and provide no mechanistic insights of the association between insulin resistance and arterial stiffness.

The ability of insulin to stimulate glucose uptake and inhibit endogenous glucose production are the best-known actions of insulin [1]. Insulin has, however, multiple other effects such as regulation of lipid and amino acid metabolism, ion fluxes, platelet function and the activity of the autonomic nervous system. Insulin also has several acute vascular effects such as the ability to decrease the augmentation index. This and other vascular actions of insulin are discussed below.

Vascular Effects of Insulin

Peripheral Vasodilatation
Insulin is a slow vasodilator of peripheral resistance arteries in skeletal muscle [13]. This action of insulin is slow and requires prolonged exposure to supraphysiological doses. In normal subjects, infusion of a high physiological dose of insulin (1 mU/kg · min) increases peripheral blood flow slowly on average by 20% (range 10–90%) within approximately 2 h in normal subjects [13–15]. Factors which contribute to interindividual variation in blood flow responses to insulin include limb muscularity [14], the number of capillaries surrounding muscle fibers [16] and possibly endothelial function [17].

Regarding the mechanism responsible for insulin-induced vasodilatation of resistance vessels in vivo, stimulation of endothelial NO synthesis by insulin seems to be involved. Both Scherrer et al. [18] and Steinberg et al. [19] demonstrated that the insulin-induced increase in blood flow can be abolished by inhibiting NO-dependent vasodilatation with L-NMMA, but not by other vasoconstrictors such as norepinephrine [18]. In vitro studies support these observations. Insulin increases NO production in human vascular endothelial cells in vitro [20], and both removal of the endothelium and inhibition of eNOS using L-NNMA abolish insulin-induced vasodilatation in isolated rat skeletal muscle arterioles [21]. Insulin induces NO-mediated endothelium-dependent vasodilatation in arterioles from red and white gastrocnemius muscles [22]. After removal of functional endothelium in these arteries, insulin paradoxically evokes vasoconstriction. Insulin also increases eNOS gene expression in microvessels in lean but not insulin-resistant obese hyperglycemic rats [23]. Studies in humans have shown that insulin enhances blood flow responses to the endothelium-dependent agonist acetylcholine but not to the endothelium-independent agonist sodium nitroprusside [24–26]. Although these data would suggest that insulin is an endothelium-dependent vasodilator, the time course for insulin action on peripheral blood flow is markedly slower than that of classic endothelium-dependent vasodilators such as acetylcholine, which increases blood flow fivefold within a minute in the human forearm [27]. The reason for the slow vasodilatory effect of insulin on peripheral resistance vessels is unknown. One possibility is that insulin rapidly activates the sympathetic nervous system, and that this counteracts the vasodilatory effects of insulin as discussed below.

Autonomic Nervous Tone
Under normoglycemic conditions, physiological concentrations of insulin increase the activity of the sympathetic nervous system, as determined from increases in plasma norepinephrine but not epinephrine concentrations [28,

29]. Physiological insulin concentrations, lower than those needed for peripheral vasodilatation, also increase muscle sympathetic nerve activity, as measured directly in the peroneal nerve with microneurography [28, 30, 31]. In studies which used power spectral analysis of heart rate variation to assess effects of insulin on autonomic nervous function, insulin has been found to acutely increase the low frequency component of heart rate variation, a measure of predominantly sympathetic nervous system activity in lean insulin-sensitive subjects [32–34] and to decrease the high-frequency component, which reflects vagal control of heart rate variation [32–34]. Insulin-induced sympathetic activation leading to vasoconstriction has been suggested to counteract insulin-induced vasodilatation [28].

Large Arteries

In studies measuring changes in the augmentation index using pulse wave analysis (for methods, see chapter by Safar, pp 1–18) during euglycemic hyperinsulinemic conditions in vivo in normal subjects, insulin decreases central pressure augmentation and the augmentation index [35–37] (fig. 1). This effect is observed within 30–60 min at physiological insulin concentrations in normal lean men [35]. It clearly precedes insulin-induced increases in blood flow (fig. 2) and its magnitude correlates with whole-body insulin sensitivity of glucose uptake [38]. Changes in the augmentation index provide a measure of changes in stiffness, or alternatively of arterial muscular tone, provided both heart rate and peripheral vascular resistance remain unchanged [39, 40]. These conditions were met in the above-mentioned studies during the lower dose insulin infusion.

The discovery that insulin acutely decreases the augmentation index initiated studies examining whether this action is blunted in insulin-resistant subjects. This was the case in both obese men [36], and type 1 [41] and type 2 [37] diabetic patients. In these insulin-resistant groups, in contrast to the normal subjects, the decrease in the augmentation index required supraphysiological insulin concentrations and was not observed until 1.5–2.5 h after start of the insulin infusion. These findings demonstrate that insulin resistance extends to insulin action on large arteries. Consistent with these findings, insulin therapy, which improves insulin sensitivity, has also been shown to decrease the augmentation index in poorly controlled type 2 diabetic patients [42]. In a larger study of 50 non-diabetic men searching for factors associated with insulin action on the augmentation index, none of the most important correlates of the basal augmentation index (age, LDL cholesterol, blood pressure) were significantly associated with insulin action on the augmentation index [38]. The change in the augmentation index was, however, significantly correlated with several features of insulin resistance. These included directly measured

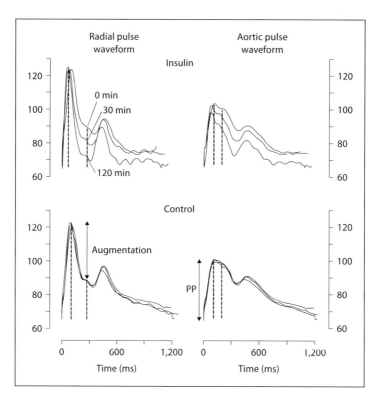

Fig. 1. An example of effects of an acute infusion of insulin (top panels) compared to saline (control, lower panels) on radial and aortic pulse waveforms in insulin-sensitive men [adapted from 35].

whole-body insulin sensitivity by the euglycemic insulin clamp technique, weight, BMI and the waist-to-hip ratio [38]. The finding that insulin action on the augmentation index is blunted in insulin-resistant conditions was recently confirmed in a study involving 20 non-diabetic middle-aged men who were divided into two groups based on their adipocyte IRS-1 protein expression [43]. In this study, low IRS-1 protein was used as a marker of insulin resistance [43].

Regarding the mechanism by which insulin lowers the augmentation index, the acute effect of insulin on wave reflection is similar to that previously described for low doses of glyceryl trinitrate (GTN) [44, 45], which also decreases both augmentation and augmentation index. These doses of GTN have no effect on brachial artery systolic or diastolic pressure or peripheral blood flow [44, 45]. The decrease in the augmentation index does not necessarily im-

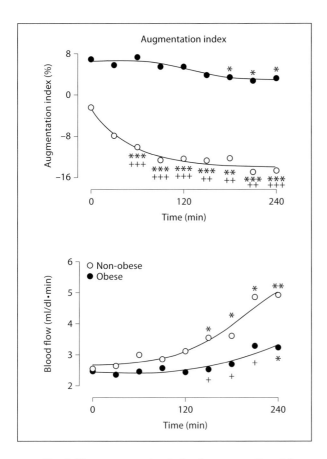

Fig. 2. The augmentation index (upper panel) and forearm blood flow (lower panel) during insulin infusions of 1 (0–120 min) and 2 (120–240 min) mU/kg · min in non-obese insulin-sensitive (○) and obese insulin-resistant (●) subjects. In insulin-sensitive subjects, insulin rapidly decreases the augmentation index whereas in insulin-resistant subjects, a small delayed decrease is observed only after 180 min using supraphysiological insulin dose. Peripheral blood flow increases only at supraphysiological insulin concentration. * $p < 0.05$; ** $p < 0.01$; *** $p < 0.001$ for change vs. 0 min; + $p < 0.05$; ++ $p < 0.01$; +++ $p < 0.001$ for difference between the groups [adapted from 36].

ply a change in stiffness at the level of the aorta [45]. GTN does not alter aortic stiffness despite decreasing wave reflection [45]. This effect of GTN reflects relaxation of muscular conduit arteries [45, 46]. The decreases in the augmentation index by insulin and GTN are closely interrelated [47]. These data raise the possibility that the decrease in the augmentation index reflects acute relaxation of muscular tone in conduit arteries rather than an acute change in the elastic properties of the aorta. A recent study in sheep demonstrated that stiffness of large arteries is locally regulated by NO [48] but whether the effect of insulin on wave reflection is mediated via NO is unknown.

Conclusion

Cross-sectional data from epidemiological studies suggest that arterial stiffness and insulin resistance are interrelated. The augmentation index, as measured by pulse wave analysis, is acutely decreased by insulin in individuals with normal insulin sensitivity. This action of insulin is blunted in insulin-resistant conditions implying that insulin resistance involves large arteries.

References

1   Yki-Järvinen H: The insulin resistance syndrome; in DeFronzo RA, Keen H, Ferrannini E, Zimmet P (eds): International Textbook of Diabetes. Chichester, Wiley, 2004, pp 359–373.
2   Lillioja S, Mott DM, Spraul M, Ferraro R, Foley JE, Ravussin E, Knowler WC, Bennett PH, Bogardus C: Insulin resistance and insulin secretory dysfunction as precursors of non-insulin-dependent diabetes mellitus. N Engl J Med 1993;329:1988–1992.
3   Lakka HM, Laaksonen DE, Lakka TA, Niskanen LK, Kumpusalo E, Tuomilehto J, Salonen JT: The metabolic syndrome and total and cardiovascular disease mortality in middle-aged men. JAMA 2002;288:2709–2716.
4   McNeill AM, Rosamond WD, Girman CJ, Golden SH, Schmidt MI, East HE, Ballantyne CM, Heiss G: The metabolic syndrome and 11-year risk of incident cardiovascular disease in the atherosclerosis risk in communities study. Diabetes Care 2005;28:385–390.
5   Wilkinson IB, Prasad K, Hall IR, Thomas A, MacCallum H, Webb DJ, Frenneaux MP, Cockcroft JR: Increased central pulse pressure and augmentation index in subjects with hypercholesterolemia. J Am Coll Cardiol 2002;39:1005–1011.
6   Vlachopoulos C, Kosmopoulou F, Panagiotakos D, Ioakeimidis N, Alexopoulos N, Pitsavos C, Stefanadis C: Smoking and caffeine have a synergistic detrimental effect on aortic stiffness and wave reflections. J Am Coll Cardiol 2004;44:1911–1917.
7   London GM, Blacher J, Pannier B, Guerin AP, Marchais SJ, Safar ME: Arterial wave reflections and survival in end-stage renal failure. Hypertension 2001;38:434–438.
8   Weber T, Auer J, O'Rourke MF, Kvas E, Lassnig E, Berent R, Eber B: Arterial stiffness, wave reflections, and the risk of coronary artery disease. Circulation 2004;109:184–189.
9   Salomaa V, Riley W, Kark JD, Nardo C, Folsom AR: Non-insulin-dependent diabetes mellitus and fasting glucose and insulin concentrations are associated with arterial stiffness indexes – the ARIC study. Circulation 1995;91:1432–1443.
10 Sutton-Tyrrell K, Newman A, Simonsick EM, Havlik R, Pahor M, Lakatta E, Spurgeon H, Vaitkevicius P: Aortic stiffness is associated with visceral adiposity in older adults enrolled in the study of health, aging, and body composition. Hypertension 2001;38:429–433.
11 Scuteri A, Najjar SS, Muller DC, Andres R, Hougaku H, Metter EJ, Lakatta EG: Metabolic syndrome amplifies the age-associated increases in vascular thickness and stiffness. J Am Coll Cardiol 2004;43:1388–1395.
12 Westerbacka J, Leinonen E, Salonen JT, Salonen R, Hiukka A, Yki-Järvinen H, Taskinen MR: Increased augmentation of central blood pressure is associated with increases in carotid intima-media thickness in type 2 diabetic patients. Diabetologia 2005;48:1654–1662.

13   Yki-Järvinen H, Utriainen T: Insulin-induced vasodilatation: physiology or pharmacology? Diabetologia 1998;41:369–379.

14   Utriainen T, Malmström R, Mäkimattila S, Yki-Järvinen H: Methodological aspects, dose-response characteristics and causes of interindividual variation in insulin stimulation of limb blood flow in normal subjects. Diabetologia 1995;38:555–564.

15   Laakso M, Edelman SV, Brechtel G, Baron AD: Decreased effect of insulin to stimulate skeletal muscle blood flow in obese man. J Clin Invest 1990;85:1844–1882.

16   Utriainen T, Holmäng A, Björntorp P, Mäkimattila S, Sovijärvi A, Lindholm H, Yki-Järvinen H: Physical fitness, muscle morphology, and insulin-stimulated limb blood flow in normal subjects. Am J Physiol 1996;270:E905–E911.

17   Utriainen T, Mäkimattila S, Virkamäki A, Lindholm H, Sovijärvi A, Yki-Järvinen H: Physical fitness and endothelial function (nitric oxide synthesis) are independent determinants of insulin-stimulated blood flow in normal subjects. J Clin Endocrinol Metab 1996;81:4258–4263.

18   Scherrer U, Randin D, Vollenweider P, Vollenweider L, Nicod P: Nitric oxide release accounts for insulin's vascular effects in humans. J Clin Invest 1994;94:2511–2515.

19   Steinberg HO, Brechtel G, Johnson A, Fireberg N, Baron AD: Insulin-mediated skeletal muscle vasodilatation is nitric oxide dependent. A novel action of insulin to increase nitric oxide release. J Clin Invest 1994;94:1172–1179.

20   Zeng G, Quon MJ: Insulin-stimulated production of nitric oxide is inhibited by Wortmannin. Direct measurement in vascular endothelial cells. J Clin Invest 1996;98:894–898.

21   Chen YY, Messina EJ: Dilatation of isolated skeletal muscle arterioles by insulin is endothelium-dependent and nitric oxide mediated. Am J Physiol 1996;270:H2120–H2124.

22   Schroeder CAJ, Chen YL, Messina EJ: Inhibition of NO synthesis or endothelium removal reveals a vasoconstrictor effect of insulin on isolated arterioles. Am J Physiol 1999;276:H815–H820.

23   Kuboki K, Jiang ZY, Takahara N, Ha SW, Igarashi M, Yamauchi T, Feener EP, Herbert TP, Rhodes CJ, King GL: Regulation of endothelial constitutive nitric oxide synthase gene expression in endothelial cells and in vivo: a specific vascular action of insulin. Circulation 2000;101:676–681.

24   Taddei S, Virdis A, Mattei P, Natali A, Ferrannini E, Salvetti A: Effect of insulin on acetylcholine-induced vasodilatation in normotensive subjects and patients with essential hypertension. Circulation 1995;92:2911–2918.

25   Rask-Madsen C, Ihlemann N, Krarup T, Christiansen E, Kober L, Nervil KC, Torp-Pedersen C: Insulin therapy improves insulin-stimulated endothelial function in patients with type 2 diabetes and ischemic heart disease. Diabetes 2001;50:2611–2618.

26   Westerbacka J, Bergholm R, Tiikkainen M, Yki-Järvinen H: Glargine and regular human insulin similarly acutely enhance endothelium-dependent vasodilatation in normal subjects. Arterioscler Thromb Vasc Biol 2004;24:320–324.

27   Makimattila S, Mäntysaari M, Groop PH, Summanen P, Virkamäki A, Schlenzka A, Fagerudd J, Yki-Järvinen H: Hyperreactivity to nitrovasodilators in forearm vasculature is related to autonomic dysfunction in IDDM. Circulation 1997;95:618–625.

28   Anderson EA, Hoffmann RP, Balon TW, Sinkey CA, Mark AL: Hyperinsulinemia produces both sympathetic neural activation and vasodilatation in normal humans. J Clin Invest 1991;87:2246–2252.

29   Randin D, Vollenweider P, Tappy L, Jequier E, Nicod P, Scherrer U: Effects of adrenergic and cholinergic blockade on insulin-induced stimulation of calf blood flow in humans. Am J Physiol 1994;266:R809–R816.

30   Berne C, Fagius J, Pollare T, Hjemdahl P: The sympathetic response to euglycemic hyperinsulinaemia. Diabetologia 1992;35:873–879.

31   Vollenweider P, Tappy L, Randin D, Schneiter P, Jequier E, Nicod P, Scherrer U: Differential effects of hyperinsulinemia and carbohydrate metabolism on sympathetic nerve activity and muscle blood flow in humans. J Clin Invest 1993;92:147–154.

32   Muscelli E, Emdin M, Natali A, Pratali L, Camastra S, Gastaldelli A, Baldi S, Carpeggiani C, Ferrannini E: Autonomic and hemodynamic responses to insulin in lean and obese humans. J Clin Endocrinol Metab 1998;83:2084–2090.

33   Bergholm R, Westerbacka J, Vehkavaara S, Seppälä-Lindroos A, Goto T, Yki-Järvinen H: Insulin sensitivity regulates autonomic control of heart rate variation independent of body weight in normal subjects. J Clin Endocrinol Metab 2001;86:1403–1409.

34   Paolisso G, Manzella D, Rizzo MR, Barbieri M, Varricchio G, Gambardella A, Varricchio M: Effects of insulin on the cardiac autonomic nervous system in insulin-resistant states. Clin Sci (Colch) 2000;98:129–136.

35   Westerbacka J, Wilkinson I, Cockcroft J, Utriainen T, Vehkavaara S, Yki-Järvinen H: Diminished wave reflection in the aorta: a novel physiological action of insulin on large blood vessels. Hypertension 1999;33:1118–1122.

36   Westerbacka J, Vehkavaara S, Bergholm R, Wilkinson I, Cockcroft J, Yki-Järvinen H: Marked resistance of the ability of insulin to decrease arterial stiffness characterizes human obesity. Diabetes 1999;48:821–827.

37   Tamminen M, Westerbacka J, Vehkavaara S, Yki-Järvinen H: Insulin-induced decreases in aortic wave reflection and central systolic pressure are impaired in type 2 diabetes. Diabetes Care 2002;25:2314–2319.

38   Westerbacka J, Seppälä-Lindroos A, Yki-Järvinen H: Resistance to acute insulin-induced decreases in large artery stiffness accompanies the insulin resistance syndrome. J Clin Endocrinol Metab 2001;86:5262–5268.

39   O'Rourke MF, Gallagher DE: Pulse wave analysis. J Hypertens 1996;14:S147–S157.

40   Nichols WW, O'Rourke MF: McDonalds's Blood Flow in Arteries. Theoretical, Experimental and Clinical Principles, ED 4. London, Arnold, 1998.

41   Westerbacka J, Uosukainen A, Makimattila S, Schlenzka A, Yki-Järvinen H: Insulin-induced decrease in large artery stiffness is impaired in uncomplicated type 1 diabetes mellitus. Hypertension 2000;35:1043–1048.

42   Tamminen MK, Westerbacka J, Vehkavaara S, Yki-Järvinen H: Insulin therapy improves insulin actions on glucose metabolism and aortic wave reflection in type 2 diabetic patients. Eur J Clin Invest 2003;33:855–860.

43   Sandqvist M, Nyberg G, Hammarstedt A, Klintland N, Gogg S, Caidahl K, Ahren B, Smith U, Jansson PA: Low adipocyte IRS-1 protein expression is associated with an increased arterial stiffness in non-diabetic males. Atherosclerosis 2005;180:119–125.

44   Kelly RP, Gibbs HH, O'Rourke MF, Daley JE, Mang K, Morgan JJ, Avolio AP: Nitroglycerine has more favourable effects on left ventricular afterload than apparent from measurement of pressure in a peripheral artery. Eur Heart J 1990;11:138–144.

45   Yaginuma T, Avolio A, O'Rourke M, Nichols W, Morgan JJ, Roy P, Baron D, Branson J, Feneley M: Effect of glyceryl trinitrate on peripheral arteries alters left ventricular hydraulic load in man. Cardiovasc Res 1986;20:153–160.

46   Simon AC, Safar ME, Levenson JA, Bouthier JE, Benetos A: Action of vasodilating drugs on small and large arteries of hypertensive patients. J Cardiovasc Pharmacol 1983;5:626–631.

47   Westerbacka J, Tamminen M, Cockcroft J, Yki-Järvinen H: Comparison of in vivo effects of nitroglycerin and insulin on the aortic pressure waveform. Eur J Clin Invest 2004;34:1–8.

48   Wilkinson IB, Qasem A, McEniery CM, Webb DJ, Avolio AP, Cockcroft JR: Nitric oxide regulates local arterial distensibility in vivo. Circulation 2002;105:213–217.

Hannele Yki-Järvinen, MD, FRCP
Department of Medicine, Division of Diabetes, University of Helsinki
PO Box 340, FI–00029 Helsinki (Finland)
Tel. +358 9 471 71991, Fax +358 9 471 71992
E-Mail ykijarvi@cc.helsinki.fi

Safar ME, Frohlich ED (eds): Atherosclerosis, Large Arteries and Cardiovascular Risk.
Adv Cardiol. Basel, Karger, 2007, vol 44, pp 261–277

······················

Cholesterol, Lipids and Arterial Stiffness

Ian Wilkinson[a]   *John R. Cockcroft*[b]

[a]Clinical Pharmacology Unit, University of Cambridge, Addenbrooke's Hospital, Cambridge, and [b]Department of Cardiology, University of Wales College of Medicine, University Hospital, Cardiff, UK

Abstract

Arterial stiffness and pulse pressure are important determinants of cardiovascular risk. Patients with hypercholesterolaemia have a higher central pulse pressure and stiffer blood vessels than matched controls, despite similar peripheral blood pressures. These haemodynamic changes may contribute to the increased risk of cardiovascular disease associated with hypercholesterolaemia and their assessment may improve risk stratification. Lipid-lowering therapy, particularly with statins, generally leads to a reduction in arterial stiffness, re-enforcing the concept that stiffness is a modifiable parameter and risk factor. There are a number of potential mechanisms linking arterial stiffness and plasma lipids, including atherosclerosis, changes in the elastic elements of the arterial wall, endothelial dysfunction and inflammation. This review will focus on the current evidence linking cholesterol to larger artery stiffening, potential therapies and mechanisms.

Copyright © 2007 S. Karger AG, Basel

Introduction

Arterial stiffening is now firmly established as an important, independent predictor of cardiovascular risk [1]. Ageing is associated with aortic stiffening (arteriosclerosis) in both urban and rural populations, even in populations with a low incidence of atherosclerosis [2–5] – reinforcing the distinction between athero- and arteriosclerosis. Although stiffening of the large arteries is often viewed as inevitable – the result of simple 'wear-and-tear' in the large arteries – we now recognize that it is a complex pathological process, which is neither inevitable nor irreversible [6]. Indeed, several indigenous human populations do not show any age-related rise in blood pressure [7, 8], moreover within populations arterial stiffness, and the rate of stiffening, varies considerably [9]. A number of conditions are associated with accelerated arterial stiffening, including renal dysfunction and traditional cardiovascular risk factors such as diabetes and cigarette smoking, leading to so-called 'premature vascular ageing'. The aim of this review is to focus on the relationship between cholesterol, lipids and arterial stiffness. Three main areas will be covered: epidemiological relationships, likely mechanisms and the potential benefits of lipid-lowering.

Epidemiology

Relationship between Cholesterol and Blood Pressure
Several studies have suggested a link between plasma cholesterol and blood pressure. Indeed, pooled epidemiological data suggest a significant, if relatively modest, relationship between peripheral blood pressure and plasma cholesterol [10]. Unfortunately, the majority of studies simply looked at the association between lipids and systolic or diastolic pressure, and data concerning pulse pressure, a frequently used surrogate of arterial stiffness, are lacking. Moreover, as we and others have repeatedly demonstrated, systolic and pulse pressure in the aorta differs significantly from that recorded in the brachial artery. This is important because the heart and brain 'see' aortic, not brachial pressure. Indeed, left ventricular mass and carotid artery remodelling relate more closely to central rather than brachial pressures. Therefore, simply assessing blood pressure in the brachial artery may fail to reveal potentially important differences in differences in aortic pressure or stiffness. Recently, we assessed brachial and ascending aortic pressure – using the technique of pulse wave analysis – in a cohort of 68 subjects with hypercholesterolaemia, and an equal number of age- and sex-matched controls [11]. As shown in figure 1, although there was no significant difference in brachial pulse pressure between the two groups, aortic pulse pressure was 5 mm Hg higher in the hypercholesterolaemic subjects. This was driven mainly by a higher aortic systolic pressure, due to more marked wave reflection – as determined by the augmentation index (28.8 ± 11.3 vs. 15.6 ± 12.1%; $p < 0.001$).

These observations, and the frequent clustering of hypertension and hypercholesterolaemia within individuals, have led some to suggest that one may beget the development of the other. Interestingly, very recent data from the Physicians' Health Study in the USA suggest just this. In a long-term follow-up of 3,110 men enrolled in the Physicians' Health Study in the USA, normotensive men with the highest levels of cholesterol (total, non-high-density lipoprotein (HDL) and total/HDL) had the highest risk of developing hypertension,

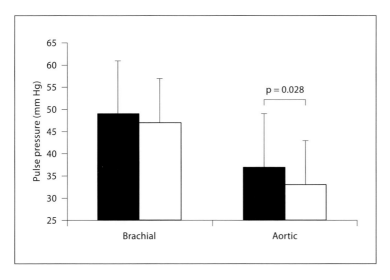

Fig. 1. Brachial artery pressure and ascending aortic pressure in subjects with hyper-cholesterolaemia (□) and matched controls (■). Error bars represent SD; n = 68 per group [data from 11].

independent of other risk factors, over the 14-year follow-up period [12]. Unfortunately, the investigators did not assess the potential mechanisms responsible for the association, but speculated that stiffening of the large arteries may be important. In this respect it would be particularly interesting to know whether individuals with high plasma cholesterol levels are more prone to develop a widened pulse pressure and isolated systolic hypertension than mixed systolic-diastolic hypertension, the latter being largely due to increased resistance and structural changes in small vessels, or vice versa.

Relationship between Cholesterol and Arterial Stiffness per se

In animals, hypercholesterolaemia, induced by a cholesterol-rich diet, leads to an initial reduction in arterial stiffness, followed by a progressive increase over time [13, 14], which can be reversed by lowering serum cholesterol [14, 15]. In humans, a variety of techniques have been used to assess vascular stiffness in vivo [16], and relate this to the serum lipid profile, often with conflicting results (table 1).

Some of the earliest human studies investigating the relationship between cholesterol and arterial stiffness focused on subjects with familial hypercholesterolaemia. This condition is characterized by very high plasma levels of low-density lipoprotein (LDL) cholesterol due to a deficiency in hepatic LDL recep-

Table 1. Familial hypercholesterolaemia and arterial stiffness

Reference	Sample size	Age, years	Measures	Main findings
Lehmann [17]	20 FH heterozygotes 20 controls	15 15	Ultrasound-derived aortic distensibility	FH associated with increased distensibility. Positive association between distensibility and LDL and inverse association with HDL cholesterol
Lehmann [18]	15 FH heterozygotes 15 FH heterozygotes	25–55 20–60	Ultrasound-derived aortic distensibility	FH associated with reduced aortic distensibility. Inverse association between distensibility and LDL and total cholesterol
Pitsavos [21]	60 FH heterozygotes 20 controls	37 34	Ultrasound distensibility	Reduced distensibility in FH subjects. Inverse correlation between LDL cholesterol and distension
Giannattasio [22]	13 FH heterozygotes 10 controls	47 45	Ultrasound-derived radial compliance	Reduced radial artery compliance in FH subjects. Compliance unaltered after dietary and simvastatin treatment
Virkola [19]	23 FH 23 controls	2.7–19 2.7–19	Ultrasound-derived carotid distensibility	Increased stiffness in FH subjects. Inverse relationship between stiffness and HDL-cholesterol
Toikka [23]	10 FH 25 controls	33 34	Ultrasound-derived aortic and carotid compliance	No difference in carotid or aortic compliance between groups. Inverse correlation between oxidized LDL levels and 1compliance
Aggoun [20]	30 FH heterozygotes 27 controls	11 11	Ultrasound-derived carotid distensibility/compliance and elastic modulus	Carotid compliance and distensibility reduced, and incremental elastic modulus increased, in FH subjects

Some of the published studies that have reported indices of large artery stiffness in subjects with familial hypercholesterolaemia (FH).

tors, and is associated with premature, and, severe, coronary disease. Thus it serves as a model of marked cholesterol elevation. Lehmann et al. [17] were amongst the first to investigate large artery haemodynamics in such patients. They reported that children heterozygous for familial hypercholesterolaemia have increased aortic distensibility (i.e. less stiff aortae), suggesting that this may be due to a compensatory dilatation of the aorta in response to the initial acute atherosis phase of atherosclerosis often seen in young individuals. In contrast Lehmann et al. [18] reported reduced aortic distensibility in adults with familial hypercholesterolaemia, and an inverse relationship between aortic distensibility and LDL and total cholesterol. They suggested that this may reflect the change to the 'sclerotic' component of the disease with advancing age.

Virkola et al. [19] and Aggoun et al. [20] both assessed carotid mechanics in young children with familial hypercholesterolaemia, and in contrast to the observations of Lehmann et al. found reduced carotid distensibility and compliance in subjects with familial hypercholesterolaemia, suggesting stiffer carotid arteries. Unfortunately, neither group made measurements of aortic compliance so it is unclear whether the aorta was similarly stiffened, or whether familial hypercholesterolaemia has differential effects on aortic and carotid stiffness in children.

In adults, the results are equally conflicting. In the largest study so far, Pitsavos et al. [21] found aortic distensibility to be reduced in heterozygous young adults with familial hypercholesterolaemia, supporting the observations of Lehmann et al. Giannattasio et al. [22] also demonstrated reduced radial artery compliance in individuals heterozygous for familial hypercholesterolaemia, but Toikka et al. [23] found no difference in carotid or aortic distensibility between subjects with familial hypercholesterolaemia and controls. No doubt, such confusion reflects small sample sizes, the varying indices used to assess arterial stiffness, and different arteries studied. Importantly, data concerning aortic pulse wave velocity, the current 'gold-standard' stiffness measure, in subjects with familial hypercholesterolaemia and its relationship to plasma LDL cholesterol levels are lacking.

Although familial hypercholesterolaemia may provide a useful model to investigate the link between LDL cholesterol and arterial stiffness, it does represent a fairly extreme form of cholesterol elevation. Within the general population the average LDL cholesterol is generally lower – with a slightly skewed normal distribution. Therefore, a number of studies have investigated the relationship between serum lipids and arterial stiffness in subjects without familial hypercholesterolaemia, either treating lipids as a continuous variable, or selecting arbitrary cut-off levels and dichotomizing data. To further complicate matters, a number of different indices of large artery stiffness have been assessed (table 2).

Table 2. Lipids and indices of large artery stiffness in subjects without familial hypercholesterolaemia

Reference	Population	Measures	Main findings
Taquet [24]	429 healthy middle-aged women	Aortic PWV	No independent relationship with cholesterol
Grial [65]	105 hypercholesterolaemic men	Aortic PWV	Independently positive association with HDL3 cholesterol
Pirro	60 hypercholesterolaemics 25 controls	Aortic PWV	Independent negative correlation with LDL cholesterol, disappeared after correction for CRP and waist circumference
Lebrun [26]	385 post-menopausal women	Aortic PWV	Positive relationship with triglycerides, inverse with HDL cholesterol
Czernichow [25]	917 middle-aged subjects	Aortic PWV	No independent association with HDL cholesterol
Wilkinson [11]	68 hypercholesterolaemics and 68 matched controls	Augmentation index	Augmentation index higher in the hypercholesterolaemic subjects and a positive relationship with LDL cholesterol
Alagona [66]	18 low HDL cholesterol subjects 18 matched controls	Augmentation index	No difference between groups
Dart [67]	868 hypertensives age >65	Augmentation index/SAC	No relationship with total or HDL cholesterol
Dart [68]	30 hypercholesterolaemics 24 controls	Aortic distensibility (β index)	Cholesterol positively related to β index
Hopkins [69]	38 healthy adults	Aortic distensibility	Inverse correlation with total and LDL cholesterol, and positive correlation with HDL cholesterol
Toikka [23]	25 healthy men	Aortic and carotid compliance	Carotid but not aortic compliance associated with low HDL:total cholesterol ratio; oxidized LDL correlated with carotid compliance
Urbina [70]	516 random subjects	Carotid elastic modulus	Positive independent association with triglycerides only
Giannattasio [71]	10 controls, 10 hypertensives, 10 hypercholesterolaemics, 10 mixed	Radial artery distensibility	Reduced distensibility in both hypercholesterolaemic groups
Cameron [30]	20 patients with CHD, 20 controls	SAC	Inverse association with LDL cholesterol in CHD patients
Le [72]	223 subjects with CHD risk factors	SAC	Inverse correlation with triglycerides and non-HDL cholesterol

Some of the published studies relating lipids to arterial stiffness. SAC = Systemic arterial compliance; CHD = coronary artery disease; PWV = pulse wave velocity; CRP = C-reactive protein.

Taquet et al. [24] were amongst the first to assess the relationship between cholesterol and aortic pulse wave velocity in 429 healthy middle-aged women. Although they found weak associations between some lipid fractions and pulse wave velocity, they were unable to demonstrate any significant correlation after adjusting for potentially confounding factors such as blood pressure. Similarly, Czernichow et al. [25] failed to find any relationship between pulse wave velocity and HDL cholesterol in a multivariate analysis of 917 middle-aged subjects from a much larger, ongoing, population-based study. In contrast, Lebrun et al. [26] did find an independent, inverse relationship between HDL cholesterol levels and aortic pulse wave velocity in a cohort of healthy postmenopausal women.

The augmentation index provides a measure of the degree to which central systolic pressure is influenced by wave reflection within the arterial tree. As such, it provides a simple composite measure of wave reflection and the stiffness of the large conduit arteries. Both the directly measured carotid augmentation index and the aortic augmentation index, derived from the radial artery using a transfer function, have recently been shown to be independent predictors of cardiovascular risk in selected patient groups. We demonstrated that asymptomatic individuals with hypercholesterolaemia have a higher augmentation index than age- and gender-matched controls, and that there is an independent correlation between LDL cholesterol levels and the augmentation index, but not with HDL cholesterol [11]. In a larger cohort of hypertensive subjects included in a national hypertension trial, Dart et al. [67, 68] found no relationship between the augmentation index or, indeed, systemic artery compliance, and cholesterol levels. This may reflect the confounding influence of hypertension, or the considerably higher average age of the Dart population.

The relationship between serum lipids and a range of other indices of arterial stiffness, including aortic or carotid distensibility/compliance and systemic arterial compliance, have been examined in a number of studies (table 2). The majority of these suggest a positive relationship between large artery stiffness and total or LDL cholesterol, and an inverse relationship with HDL cholesterol, although many have been relatively small, and have included patients with other risk factors or coronary artery disease. The latter makes interpretation of the data difficult since atherosclerosis per se is linked to increased aortic and carotid artery stiffness, and arterial remodelling.

Metabolic Syndrome
Cardiovascular risk factors, including hypercholesterolaemia, rarely occur in isolation. More commonly, two or risk factors co-exist within the same individual. One such clustering of risk factors that has attracted considerable interest is the metabolic syndrome, and lipid abnormalities are central to the

diagnosis of this increasingly common condition. Several groups have demonstrated increased aortic pulse wave velocity in subjects with the metabolic syndrome, and a relationship between the number of features present and aortic stiffness [27, 28]. Urbina et al. [70] assessed the impact of individual component of the metabolic syndrome on carotid wall properties, and found that there was an independent positive correlation between elastic modulus (a measure of stiffness) and triglycerides but not HDL or total cholesterol levels. Nakanishi et al. [29] studied 999 healthy men and women, and related brachial-ankle velocity (a surrogate of aortic stiffness) to various components of the metabolic syndrome. In contrast, they found that stiffness was independently related to HDL cholesterol (inversely), and to triglycerides.

Effect of Acute Changes in Plasma Lipids
Although some lipid fractions are relatively stable in the short term, and are not influenced by eating, others including triglycerides can show marked acute changes, especially after ingestion of fatty food. One recent study examined the effect of a fatty meal on a measure of large artery stiffness termed systemic arterial compliance. Although no outcome data are available for this particular parameter, pervious studies have shown significant correlations with other risk factors, and with cholesterol [30]. Following the meal there was a significant reduction in systemic arterial compliance which correlated with the acute changes in all lipid fractions. These are intriguing data which need to be repeated and allowances made for potential confounders such as postprandial changes in blood pressure, heart rate and also insulin, which we have previously shown to influence arterial stiffness [31].

Summary
Most of the available data suggests that there is probably a positive relationship between arterial stiffness and cholesterol. However, the current studies are far from conclusive and interpretation is hampered by the use of multiple different techniques, indices and small sample sizes. Further, large, well-conducted studies are urgently required to provide more definitive evidence and assess the importance of the various lipid subfractions.

Impact of Lipid Reduction on Arterial Stiffness

In animal models of hypercholesterolaemia, cholesterol-lowering appears to reduce arterial stiffness [14, 15]. In man, a number of studies have addressed the effect of HMG-CoA reductase inhibitors (statins) on large artery stiffness (table 3). Kool et al. [32] failed to find any impact of pravastatin on carotid,

Table 3. Lipid lowering and arterial stiffness

Reference	Population, n	Therapy	Duration	Measures	Main findings
Kool [32]	19 cholesterol 6.5–9.0	Pravastatin 40 mg/placebo	8-week cross-over	Carotid, femoral, brachial compliance/ distensibility	No change in stiffness parameters
Muramatsu [33]	59 cholesterol >5.7	Pravastatin 10 mg	6 months– 5 years	Aortic pulse wave velocity	Stiffness fell most in those with the greatest lowering of cholesterol; maintained for 5 years
Raison [73]	23 hypertensives	Atorvastatin/ placebo	12 weeks	Aortic pulse wave velocity	Increased stiffness in those receiving atorvastatin
Kontopoulos [74]	18 CHD 18 controls	Atorvastatin 20 mg	2 years	Ultrasound-derived aortic stiffness	Reduction following atorvastatin
Ferrier [34]	22 isolated systolic hypertension	Atorvastatin 80 mg/placebo	3-month cross-over	Systemic arterial compliance	Atorvastatin increased compliance and reduced systolic pressure
Matsuo [75]	10 hypercholesterolaemics	Cerivastatin 150 µg	4 weeks	Brachial ankle pulse wave velocity	Reduction in stiffness by 4 weeks

Some of the studies that have investigated the effect of statins on arterial stiffness. CHD = Coronary heart disease.

femoral or brachial distensibility, or compliance, in a short, 8-week, placebo-controlled, cross-over study. In contrast, Muramatsu et al. [33] reported that 6 months' therapy with pravastatin led to a significant reduction in aortic pulse wave velocity, which was sustained for 5 years. However, this was not a controlled or blinded study.

The majority, but not all, of the other available studies, would support the observations of Muramatsu et al. (see table 3). Intriguingly, Ferrier et al. [34] suggest that high-dose statin therapy may provide a useful blood pressure-lowering adjuvant in individuals with isolated systolic hypertension – a condition characterized primarily by increased stiffness of the large arteries. The significant but modest effect of atorvastatin on peripheral systolic pressure was accompanied by an increase in systemic arterial compliance, although the effect of central blood pressure and other more robust measures of aortic stiffness such as aortic pulse wave velocity were not examined.

Pooled data from a number of studies would support the view that cholesterol-lowering can lead to significant, if small, reductions in blood pressure both in normotensive and hypertensive individuals [10]. This view is supported by the recent ASCOT Study – a trial of antihypertensive strategies and lipid-lowering in hypertensive subjects. This study revealed a small but significant reduction in blood pressure following treatment with atorvastatin [35]. Such an effect may help explain the unexpected reductions in stroke seen in most of the secondary prevention statin studies [36], especially since the effect of statins on central pressure may well be larger than the observed effect on peripheral pressure.

Not only are these observations interesting, but together with the data concerning the acute post-prandial effects of a fatty meal, they suggest that any effect of lipids on arterial stiffness may be modifiable. However, the dose of statin required to reduce arterial stiffness, and optimal treatment duration, needs to be further clarified. It is also unclear whether the effects of statins are due to a fall in plasma cholesterol per se, alteration in the lipid profile, or some other pleiotropic effect of statins.

Mechanisms Linking Stiffness and Cholesterol

A number of potential mechanisms may explain the link between serum lipids and arterial stiffness. As already noted, one of the more obvious is the development of atherosclerotic plaques. Atherosclerosis in the coronary arteries, and at other sites, has been consistently associated with increased arterial stiffness (see Section II). This has led some to suggest that stiffening of the large arteries is simply a measure of the amount or degree of atherosclerosis.

However, arterial stiffening occurs in populations with a low prevalence of atherosclerosis, and also affects vessels such as the brachial artery which are not normally a site of plaque development.

Cholesterol and oxidized LDL cholesterol, in particular, have a number of direct, non-atheromatous, effects on the arterial wall, which may lead to arterial stiffening. Oxidized LDL cholesterol also leads to peroxynitrite formation and a generalized state of increased oxidative stress, both of which can damage elastin directly [37, 38]. Oxidized LDL cholesterol is also pro-inflammatory. Several groups, including our own, have recently shown an association between measures of acute inflammation, such as C-reactive protein and arterial stiffness in otherwise healthy individuals [39, 40]. Moreover, Pirro et al. recently found a significant, positive relationship between aortic pulse wave velocity and C-reactive protein in subjects with hypercholesterolaemia. Interestingly, when both C-reactive protein and HDL cholesterol were entered into a multivariate model, only C-reactive protein remained an independent predictor of aortic stiffness.

Systemic and local inflammation may lead to arterial stiffening by a variety of different mechanisms. Cytokines lead to increased expression of a number of inducible enzymes that may damage the structural components of the arterial wall. One enzyme of particular interest is matrix metalloproteinase-9 (MMP-9), which is a gelatinase capable of digesting arterial elastin – the main 'elastic element' of the large arteries. We have recently demonstrated a positive relationship between serum MMP-9 levels and aortic pulse wave velocity in a large cohort of apparently healthy subjects [41]. A pro-inflammatory environment also leads to an influx of inflammatory cells into the arterial wall. This in itself may lead to arterial stiffening possibly due to changes in the ground substance, secretion of destructive enzymes such as MMP-9 and remodelling of the wall. An interesting novel hypothesis is that inflammation, and inflammatory lipids in particular, may promote deposition of calcium within the arterial wall [42]. In animal models, arterial calcification leads to stiffening of the arterial wall [43], and in humans with end-stage renal failure excessive calcification is associated with aortic stiffening and increased mortality [44, 45].

It is unlikely that structural changes in the arterial wall are solely responsible for the relationship between stiffness and cholesterol. As already noted, a fatty meal is associated with an acute increase in arterial stiffness, and statin therapy can lead to a reduction in stiffness with a matter of weeks. These observations suggest that lipid abnormalities may lead to functional arterial stiffening.

Endothelial Function

Mounting evidence suggests that there is a degree of functional regulation of stiffness by the vascular endothelium [46–48]. We and others have recently demonstrated that endothelium-derived nitric oxide, in part, regulates the stiffness of the large arteries [47]. Inhibiting endogenous nitric oxide production leads to arterial stiffening [49, 50].

Hypercholesterolaemia is strongly associated with endothelial dysfunction and reduced nitric oxide bioavailability [51, 52]. Indeed, acute elevation of plasma lipids, achieved by either a fatty meal [53] or intravenous infusion [54], leads to a rapid onset of endothelial dysfunction, which can be equally rapidly corrected by interventions such as plasmapheresis [55]. Hypercholesterolaemia may impair the L-arginine/nitric oxide pathway at a number of sites. Endothelial damage may lead to a decrease in either basal or stimulated release of nitric oxide or, alternatively, there may be an increased breakdown of nitric oxide. The vascular smooth muscle may also exhibit a decreased sensitivity to the actions of nitric oxide. Finally, the buildup of endogenous inhibitors of nitric oxide synthase, such as asymmetric dimethyl arginine (ADMA), may decrease the biological activity of the endothelial isoform of nitric oxide synthase (eNOS) and hence the production of nitric oxide.

Oxidized LDL cholesterol is the major molecule mediating both atherosclerosis and endothelial dysfunction [56]. Indeed, oxidized LDL cholesterol impairs endothelial function to a greater extent than native LDL cholesterol [57]. Furthermore, oxidized LDL cholesterol downregulates eNOS expression [58], and reduces the uptake of L-arginine into endothelial cells [59], both of which lead to decreased nitric oxide production. In addition, LDL cholesterol has recently been shown to increase the synthesis of ADMA [60].

Interestingly, many of the above deleterious effects of LDL cholesterol can be reversed by statins, providing a potential explanation for the beneficial effects of these agents on both endothelial function and arterial stiffness. In addition to decreased nitric oxide production, abnormal vascular function may also be caused by overproduction of constrictors such as endothelin-1 which, in contrast to nitric oxide, is an atherogenic molecule. LDL cholesterol increases production of endothelin-1 [61], an effect that can also be inhibited by statins [62]. We have also recently demonstrated that endothelin-1 is involved in the functional regulation of large artery stiffness [63], providing yet another link between stiffness and hypercholesterolaemia, and one further explanation for the beneficial effects of cholesterol reduction on arterial stiffness. Other agents with therapeutic potential in hypercholesterolaemia include angiotensin-converting enzyme (ACE) inhibitors. These drugs increase the bioavailability of nitric oxide, possibly via increasing circulating levels of bradykinin, upregulating expression of eNOS or decreasing superoxide production. ACE inhibitors improve endothelial function in patients with hypercholesterolaemia, independently of cholesterol reduction [64]. Although ACE inhibition has been shown to decrease arterial stiffness in other disease states, as yet, its effect on arterial stiffness in patients with hypercholesterolaemia has not been studied.

To summarize: The majority of the available evidence suggests a positive relationship between plasma cholesterol and the stiffness of the large arteries. Lipid-lowering agents appear to significantly reduce arterial stiffness. However, a number of important questions remain unanswered. It is unclear which of various lipid subfractions best correlate with arterial stiffness, and the strength, or indeed, pathophysiological importance of any independent associations. It is important to remember that associations, even if independent, do not necessarily imply causality. Stiffening may reflect atherosclerosis rather than a direct effect of cholesterol on the mechanical properties of the large arteries themselves. Likewise, it is unclear whether the beneficial effect of statins results from lipid-lowering per se, or the much talked about pleiotropic effect of this drug class. Greater evidence of causality is likely to come from studying much larger cohorts of younger subjects – free for the confounding effects of atherosclerosis, and other cardiovascular risk factors – and examining the longitudinal relationship between different lipid fractions and arterial stiffening. Longitudinal studies also need to be undertaken in populations with different prevalences of atherosclerosis and average cholesterol levels. Finally, carefully designed studies are required to separate the cholesterol-lowering effect of statins from their potential pleiotropic effects on large arteries.

References

1 Willum Hansen T, Staessen JA, Torp-Pedersen C, Rasmussen S, Thijs L, Ibsen H, Jeppesen J: Prognostic value of aortic pulse wave velocity as index of arterial stiffness in the general population. Circulation 2006;113:664–670.
2 Avolio AP, Chen SG, Wang RP, Zahang CL, Li MF, O'Rourke MF: Effects of ageing on changing arterial compliance and left ventricular load in a northern Chinese urban community. Circulation 1983;68:50–58.
3 Avolio AP, Fa-Quan D, Wei-Qiang L, Yao-Fei L, Zhen-Dong H, Lian-Fen X, O'Rourke MF: Effects of ageing on arterial distensibility in populations with high and low prevalence of hypertension: comparison between urban and rural communities in China. Circulation 1985;71:202–210.
4 Lakatta EG, Levy D: Arterial and cardiac aging: major shareholders in cardiovascular disease enterprises. I. Aging arteries: a 'set up' for vascular disease. Circulation 2003;107:139–146.
5 Mitchell GF, Parise H, Benjamin EJ, Larson MG, Keyes MJ, Vita JA, Vasan RS, Levy D: Changes in arterial stiffness and wave reflection with advancing age in healthy men and women: the Framingham Heart Study. Hypertension 2004;43:1239–1245.
6 Najjar SS, Scuteri A, Lakatta EG: Arterial aging. Is it an immutable cardiovascular risk factor? Hypertension 2005;46:454–462.

7   Truswell AS, Kennelly BM, Hansen JD, Lee RB: Blood pressures of Kung bushmen in northern Botswana. Am Heart J 1972;84:5–12.

8   Poulter NR, Khaw KT, Mugambi M, Peart WS, Rose G, Sever P: Blood pressure patterns in relation to age, weight and urinary electrolytes in three Kenyan communities. Trans R Soc Trop Med Hyg 1985;79:389–392.

9   Benetos A, Adamopoulos C, Bureau JM, Temmar M, Labat C, Bean K, Thomas F, Pannier B, Asmar R, Zureik M, Safar M, Guize L: Determinants of accelerated progression of arterial stiffness in normotensive subjects and in treated hypertensive subjects over a 6-year period. Circulation 2002;105:1202–1207.

10   Goode GK, Miller JP, Heagerty AM: Hyperlipidaemia, hypertension, and coronary heart disease. Lancet 1995;354:362–364.

11   Wilkinson IB, Prasad K, Hall IR, Thomas A, MacCallum H, Webb DJ, Cockcroft JR: Increased central pulse pressure and augmentation index in subjects with hypercholesterolemia. J Am Coll Cardiol 2002;39:1005–1011.

12   Halperin RO, Sesso HD, Ma J, Buring JE, Stampfer MJ, Gaziano JM: Dyslipidemia and the risk of incident hypertension in men. Hypertension 2006;47:45–50.

13   Pynadath TI, Mukherjee DP: Dynamic mechanical properties of atherosclerotic aorta: a correlation between the cholesterol ester content and the viscoelastic properties of atherosclerotic aorta. Atherosclerosis 1977;26:311–318.

14   Farrar DJ, Bond MG, Riley WA, Sawyer JK: Anatomic correlates of aortic pulse wave velocity and carotid artery elasticity during atherosclerosis progression and regression in monkeys. Circulation 1991;83:1754–1763.

15   Farrar DJ, Green HD, Wagner WD, Bond G: Reduction in pulse wave velocity and improvement of aortic distensibility accompanying regression of atherosclerosis in the rhesus monkey. Circ Res 1980;47:425–432.

16   Mackenzie IS, Wilkinson IB, Cockcroft JR: Assessment of arterial stiffness in clinical practice. Q J Med 2002;95:67–74.

17   Lehmann ED, Watts GF, Fatemi-Langroudi B, Gosling RG: Aortic compliance in young patients with heterozygous familial hypercholesterolaemia. Clin Sci 1992;83:717–721.

18   Lehmann ED, Hopkins KD, Gosling RG: Aortic compliance measurements using Doppler ultrasound: in vivo biochemical correlates. Ultrasound Med Biol 1993;19:683–710.

19   Virkola K, Pesonen E, Akerblom HK, Siimes MA: Cholesterol and carotid artery wall in children and adolescents with familial hypercholesterolaemia: a controlled study by ultrasound. Acta Paediatr 1997;86:1203–1207.

20   Aggoun Y, Bonnet D, Sidi D, Girardet JP, Brucker E, Polak M, Safar ME, Levy BI: Arterial mechanical changes in children with familial hypercholesterolemia. Arterioscler Thromb Vasc Biol 2000;20:2070–2075.

21   Pitsavos C, Toutouzas K, Dernellis J, Skoumas J, Skoumbourdis E, Stefanadis C, Toutouzas P: Aortic stiffness in young patients with heterozygous familial hypercholesterolemia. Am Heart J 1998;135:604–608.

22   Giannattasio C, Mangoni AA, Failla M, Carugo S, Stella, ML, Stefanoni P, Grassi G, Vergani C, Mancia G: Impaired radial artery compliance in normotensive subjects with familial hypercholesterolemia. Atherosclerosis 1996;124:249–260.

23   Toikka JO, Niemi P, Ahotupa M, Niinikoski H, Viikari JSA, Ronnemaa T, Hartiala JJ, Raitakari OT: Large-artery elastic properties in young men: relationships to serum lipoproteins and oxidized low-density lipoproteins. Arterioscler Thromb Vasc Biol 1999;19:436–441.

24   Taquet A, Bonithon-Kopp C, Simon A, Levenson J, Scarabin Y, Malmejac A, Ducimetiere P, Guize L: Relations of cardiovascular risk factors to aortic pulse wave velocity in asymptomatic middle-aged women. Eur J Epidemiol 1993;9:298–306.

25   Czernichow S, Bertrais S, Blacher J, Oppert JM, Galan P, Ducimetiere P, Hercberg S, Safar M, Zureik M: Metabolic syndrome in relation to structure and function of large arteries: a predominant effect of blood pressure. A report from the SU.VI.MAX Vascular Study. Am J Hypertens 2005;18:1154–1160.

26   Lebrun CE, van der Schouw YT, Bak AA, de Jong FH, Pols HA, Grobbee DE, Lamberts SW, Bots ML: Arterial stiffness in postmenopausal women: determinants of pulse wave velocity. J Hypertens 2002;20:2165–2172.

27 Nakanishi N, Suzuki K, Tatara K: Clustered features of the metabolic syndrome and the risk for increased aortic pulse wave velocity in middle-aged Japanese men. Angiology 2003;54:551–559.

28 Li S, Chen W, Srinivasan SR, Berenson GS: Influence of metabolic syndrome on arterial stiffness and its age-related change in young adults: the Bogalusa Heart Study. Atherosclerosis 2005;180:349–354.

29 Nakanishi N, Shiraishi T, Wada M: Brachial-ankle pulse wave velocity and metabolic syndrome in a Japanese population: the Minoh study. Hypertens Res 2005;28:125–131.

30 Cameron JD, Jennings GL, Dart AM: The relationship between arterial compliance, age, blood pressure and serum lipid levels. J Hypertens 1995;13:1718–1723.

31 Westerbacka J, Wilkinson I, Utriainen T, Vehkavaar S, Cockcroft J, Yki-Järvinen H: Diminished wave reflection in the aorta: a novel physiological action of insulin. Hypertension 1999;33:1118–1122.

32 Kool M, Lustermans F, Kragten H, Struijker BH, Hoeks A, Reneman R, Rila H, Hoogendam I, Van Bortel L: Does lowering of cholesterol levels influence functional properties of large arteries? Eur J Clin Pharmacol 1995;48:217–223.

33 Muramatsu J, Kobayashi A, Hasegawa N, Yokouchi S: Hemodynamic changes associated with reduction in total cholesterol treatment with the HMG-CoA reductase inhibitor pravastatin. Atherosclerosis 1997;130:179–182.

34 Ferrier KE, Muhlmann MH, Baguet JP, Cameron JD, Jennings GL, Dart AM, Kingwell BA: Intensive cholesterol reduction lowers blood pressure and large artery stiffness in isolated systolic hypertension. J Am Coll Cardiol 2002;39:1020–1025.

35 Poulter NR, Wedel H, Dahlof B, Sever PS, Beevers DG, Caulfield M, Kjeldsen SE, Kristinsson A, McInnes GT, Mehlsen J, Nieminen M, O'Brien E, Ostergren J, Pocock S: Role of blood pressure and other variables in the differential cardiovascular event rates noted in the Anglo-Scandinavian Cardiac Outcomes Trial-Blood Pressure Lowering Arm (ASCOT-BPLA). Lancet 2005;366:907–913.

36 Blauw G, Lagaay A, Smelt A, Westendrop R: Stroke, statins and cholesterol: A meta-analysis of randomized, placebo-controlled, double-blind trials with HMG-CoA reductase inhibitors. Stroke 1997;28:946–950.

37 Ciba Foundation Symposium: The Molecular Biology and Pathology of Elastic Tissues. Chichester, Wiley, 1995.

38 Paik DC, Ramey WG, Dillon J, Tilson MD: The nitrite/elastin reaction: implications for in vivo degenerative effects. Connect Tissue Res 1997;36:241–251.

39 Yasmin, McEniery CM, Wallace S, Mackenzie IS, Cockcroft JR, Wilkinson IB: C-reactive protein is associated with arterial stiffness in apparently healthy individuals. Arterioscler Thromb Vasc Biol 2004;24:969–974.

40 Duprez DA, Somasundaram PE, Sigurdsson G, Hoke L, Florea N, Cohn JN: Relationship between C-reactive protein and arterial stiffness in an asymptomatic population. J Hum Hypertens 2005;19:515–519.

41 Yasmin, Wallace S, McEniery CM, Dakham Z, Pusalkar P, Maki-Petaja K, Ashby MJ, Cockcroft JR, Wilkinson IB: Matrix metalloproteinase-9 (MMP-9), MMP-2, and serum elastase activity are associated with systolic hypertension and arterial stiffness. Arterioscler Thromb Vasc Biol 2005;25:372.

42 Abedin M, Tintut Y, Demer LL: Vascular calcification: mechanisms and clinical ramifications. Arterioscler Thromb Vasc Biol 2004;24:1161–1170.

43 Niederhoffer N, Lartaud-Idjouadiene I, Giummelly P, Duvivier C, Peslin R, Atkinson J: Calcification of medial elastic fibers and aortic elasticity. Hypertension 1997;29:999–1006.

44 Guerin AP, London GM, Marchais SJ, Metivier F: Arterial stiffening and vascular calcifications in end-stage renal disease. Nephrol Dial Transplant 2000;15:1014–1021.

45 London GM, Guerin AP, Marchais SJ, Metivier F, Pannier B, Adda H: Arterial media calcification in end-stage renal disease: impact on all-cause and cardiovascular mortality. Nephrol Dial Transplant 2003;18:1731–1740.

46 Dobrin PB, Rovick AA: Influence of vascular smooth muscle on contractile mechanisms and elasticity of arteries. Am J Physiol 1969;217:1644–1651.

47   Wilkinson IB, Franklin SS, Cockcroft JR: Nitric oxide and the regulation of large artery stiffness. From physiology to pharmacology. Hypertension 2004;44:112–116.
48   Nichols WW, O'Rourke MF: McDonald's Blood Flow in Arteries: Theoretical, Experimental and Clinical Principles, ed 5. London, Arnold, 2005.
49   Wilkinson IB, Qasem A, McEniery CM, Webb DJ, Avolio AP, Cockcroft JR: Nitric oxide regulates local arterial distensibility in vivo. Circulation 2002;105:213–217.
50   Schmitt M, Avolio A, Qasem A, McEniery CM, Butlin M, Wilkinson IB, Cockcroft JR: Basal NO locally modulates human iliac artery function in vivo. Hypertension 2005;46:227–231.
51   Chowienczyk PJ, Watts GF, Cockcroft JR, Ritter JM: Impaired endothelium-dependent vasodilatation of forearm resistance vessels in hypercholesterolaemia. Lancet 1992;340:1430–1432.
52   Wilkinson IB, Cockcroft JR: Cholesterol, endothelial function and arterial stiffness. Curr Opin Lipidol 1998;9:237–442.
53   Ong PJ, Dean TS, Hayward CS, la Monica PL, Sanders TA, Collins P: Effect of fat and carbohydrate consumption on endothelial function. Lancet 1999;354:2134.
54   Steinberg HO, Tarshoby M, Monestel R, Hook G, Cronin J, Johnson A, Bayazeed B, Baron AD: Elevated circulating free fatty acid levels impair endothelium-dependent vasodilation. J Clin Invest 1997;100:1230–1239.
55   Tamai O, Matsuoka H, Itabe H, Wada Y, Kohno K, Imaizumi T: Single LDL apheresis improves endothelium-dependent vasodilatation in hypercholesterolemic humans. Circulation 1997;95: 76–82.
56   Witztum JL, Steinberg D: Role of oxidized low density lipoprotein in atherogenesis. J Clin Invest 1991;88:1785–1792.
57   Jacobs M, Plane F, Bruckdorfer KR: Native and oxidized low-density lipoproteins have different inhibitory effects on endothelium-derived relaxing factor in the rabbit aorta. Br J Pharmacol 1990;100:21–26.
58   Liao JK, Shin WS, Lee WY, Clark SL: Oxidized low-density lipoprotein decreases the expression of endothelial nitric oxide synthase. J Biol Chem 1995;270:319–324.
59   Chen LY, Mehta P, Mehta JL: Oxidized LDL decreases L-arginine uptake and nitric oxide synthase protein expression in human platelets: relevance of the effect of oxidized LDL on platelet function. Circulation 1996;93:1740–1746.
60   Boger RH, Sydow K, Borlak J, Thum T, Lenzen H, Schubert B, Tsikas D, Bode-Boger SM: LDL cholesterol upregulates synthesis of asymmetrical dimethylarginine in human endothelial cells: involvement of S-adenosylmethionine-dependent methyltransferases. Circ Res 2000;87:99–105.
61   Sakurai K, Cominacini L, Garbin U, Fratta PA, Sasaki N, Takuwa Y, Masaki T, Sawamura T: Induction of endothelin-1 production in endothelial cells via cooperative action between CD40 and lectin-like oxidized LDL receptor (LOX-1). J Cardiovasc Pharmacol 2004;44:S173–S180.
62   Hernandez-Perera O, Perez-Sala D, Navarro-Antolin J, Sanchez-Pascuala R, Hernandez G, Diaz C, Lamas S: Effects of the 3-hydroxy-3-methylglutaryl-CoA reductase inhibitors, atorvastatin and simvastatin, on the expression of endothelin-1 and endothelial nitric oxide synthase in vascular endothelial cells. J Clin Invest 1998;101:2711–2719.
63   McEniery CM, Qasem A, Schmitt M, Avolio A, Cockcroft JR, Wilkinson IB: Endothelin-1 regulates arterial pulse wave velocity in vivo. J Am Coll Cardiol 2003;42:1975–1981.
64   Lee AFC, Dick JBC, Bonnar CE, Struthers AD: Lisinopril improves arterial function in hyperlipidaemia. Clin Sci 1999;96:441–448.
65   Giral P, Atger V, Amar J, Cambillau M, Del PM, Megnien JL, Levenson J, Moatti N, Simon A: A relationship between aortic stiffness and serum HDL3 cholesterol concentrations in hypercholesterolaemic, symptom-free men. The PCVMETRA Group (Groupe de Prévention Cardiovasculaire en Médecine du Travail). J Cardiovasc Risk 1994;1:53–58.
66   Alagona C, Soro A, Westerbacka J, Ylitalo K, Salonen JT, Salonen R, Yki-Järvinen H, Taskinen MR: Low HDL cholesterol concentration is associated with increased intima-media thickness independent of arterial stiffness in healthy subjects from families with low HDL cholesterol. Eur J Clin Invest 2003;33:457–463.
67   Dart AM, Gatzka CD, Cameron JD, Kingwell BA, Liang YL, Berry KL, Reid CM, Jennings GL: Large artery stiffness is not related to plasma cholesterol in older subjects with hypertension. Arterioscler Thromb Vasc Biol 2004;24:962–968.

68 Dart AM, Lancombe F, Yeoh JK, Cameron JD, Jennings GL, Laufer E, Esmore DS: Aortic distensibility in patients with isolated hypercholesterolaemia, coronary artery disease, or cardiac transplantation. Lancet 1991;338:270–273.

69 Hopkins KD, Lehmann ED, Gosling RG, Parker JR, Sonksen P: Biochemical correlates of aortic distensibility in vivo in normal subjects. Clin Sci 1993;84:593–597.

70 Urbina EM, Srinivasan SR, Kieltyka RL, Tang R, Bond MG, Chen W, Berenson GS: Correlates of carotid artery stiffness in young adults: the Bogalusa Heart Study. Atherosclerosis 2004;176: 157–164.

71 Giannattasio C, Mangoni AA, Failla M, Stella ML, Carugo S, Bombelli M, Sega R, Mancia G: Combined effects of hypertension and hypercholesterolemia on radial artery function. Hypertension 1997;29:583–586.

72 Le NA, Brown WV, Davis WW, Herrington DM, Mosca L, Homma S, Eggleston B, Willens HJ, Raines JK: Comparison of the relation of triglyceride-rich lipoproteins and muscular artery compliance in healthy women versus healthy men. Am J Cardiol 2005;95:1049–1054.

73 Raison J, Rudnichi A, Safar ME: Effects of atorvastatin on aortic pulse wave velocity in patients with hypertension and hypercholesterolaemia: a preliminary study. J Hum Hypertens 2002;16: 705–710.

74 Kontopoulos AG, Athyros VG, Pehlivanidis AN, Demitriadis DS, Papageorgiou AA, Boudoulas H: Long-term treatment effect of atorvastatin on aortic stiffness in hypercholesterolaemic patients. Curr Med Res Opin 2003;19:22–27.

75 Matsuo T, Iwade K, Hirata N, Yamashita M, Ikegami H, Tanaka N, Aosaki M, Kasanuki H: Improvement of arterial stiffness by the antioxidant and anti-inflammatory effects of short-term statin therapy in patients with hypercholesterolemia. Heart Vessels 2005;20:8–12.

Dr. John R. Cockcroft
Department of Cardiology
University of Wales College of Medicine
University Hospital
Cardiff CF4 4XN (UK)
Tel. +44 29 2074 3489, Fax +44 29 2074 3500, E-Mail cockcroftjr@cf.ac.uk

Safar ME, Frohlich ED (eds): Atherosclerosis, Large Arteries and Cardiovascular Risk.
Adv Cardiol. Basel, Karger, 2007, vol 44, pp 278–301

....

Homocysteine and Large Arteries

Coen van Guldener[a]   *Coen D.A. Stehouwer*[b]

[a]Department of Internal Medicine, Amphia Hospital, Breda, and [b]Department of
Internal Medicine, Academic Hospital Maastricht and Cardiovascular Research
Institute Maastricht, Maastricht University, Maastricht, The Netherlands

Abstract

High plasma concentrations of the amino acid homocysteine have been associated
with atherothrombotic disease, first in individuals with inborn errors of homocysteine
metabolism, who have very high plasma homocysteine concentrations, and later also in
the general population. In general, the cardiovascular risk associated with hyperhomocysteinemia is significant, but modest and probably differs between populations. High
homocysteine concentrations are thought to impair endothelial function, increase oxidative stress, impair methylation reactions, and alter protein structure. Although some studies have shown improvement of vascular surrogate end points, homocysteine-lowering
treatment has not yet been associated with a significant reduction of cardiovascular
events. Studies that have examined the relationship between plasma homocysteine and
arterial stiffness parameters have shown heterogenous results.

Relationship between Atherosclerosis and Hyperhomocysteinemia

Homocysteine Metabolism

Homocysteine is a sulfur-containing amino acid, which in humans can
only be derived from the demethylation of the essential amino acid methionine. S-adenosylmethionine and S-adenosylhomocysteine are intermediates
in this important biochemical pathway, called transmethylation, in which S-
adenosylmethionine donates its methyl group to a variety of acceptors, such
as guanidinoacetic acid, phosphatidylethanolamine, norepinephrine, DNA,
RNA and protein amino acid residues. This reaction is driven towards the generation of homocysteine as long as homocysteine is further metabolized. Ho-

mocysteine can either be remethylated to methionine or be transsulfurated to cysteine. There are two remethylation pathways. The first is catalyzed by methionine synthase (MS) and requires 5-methyltetrahydrofolate as methyl donor and reduced cobalamin as cofactor. 5-Methyltetrahydrofolate is generated by a reaction catalyzed by 5,10-methylenetetrahydrofolate reductase (MTH-FR). The second remethylation reaction is catalyzed by betaine-homocysteine methyltransferase and uses betaine as methyl donor. The transsulfuration pathway is considered irreversible and consists of two reactions. In the first, homocysteine condenses with serine to form cystathionine (facilitated by cystathionine β-synthase (CBS)) and in the second, cystathionine is cleaved into cysteine and α-ketobutyrate (by γ-cystathionase). Both require pyridoxal phosphate as cofactor. Cysteine can be incorporated into protein, used for the synthesis of compounds such as taurine and glutathione, or further metabolized to sulfate, which is excreted in the urine, and to α-ketobutyrate, which is oxidized in the Krebs cycle.

Homocysteine metabolism takes place intracellularly and exhibits tissue-specific activity. In humans, transmethylation and folate-dependent remethylation occurs in all cells. Betaine-dependent remethylation occurs only in the liver and kidney, whereas complete transsulfuration takes place only in the liver, kidney, small intestine and pancreas. Transport of homocysteine from the intra- to the extracellular compartment is enhanced when its intracellular production is increased, and, vice versa, when homocysteine production is inhibited, transmembrane transport decreases, suggesting that the intracellular homocysteine level is controlled and kept within a certain range, and that the extracellular homocysteine level (e.g. in plasma) reflects the intracellular level. In plasma, homocysteine is present in different forms. About 70–80% is protein-bound, mainly to albumin. Non-protein-bound homocysteine is found in 'mixed disulfide' (i.e. the dimer of homocysteine and cysteine), homocystine (the oxidized disulfide of homocysteine) and reduced homocysteine. Reduced homocysteine forms only about 1% of the total plasma homocysteine content. Laboratories usually measure plasma total homocysteine concentration, which is the sum of all homocysteine fractions. The upper limit of normal plasma total homocysteine concentration is generally set at 12 μmol/l.

Homocysteine and Vascular Disease

Homocystinuria was discovered in 1962, when some of the mentally retarded children who were screened for abnormal (patterns of) urinary amino acids showed large amounts of homocystine in their urine. The disease was shown to be caused by a deficiency of the transsulfuration enzyme CBS, the gene for which was later found to be located on chromosome 21. Clinically, CBS deficiency is characterized by skeletal abnormalities, dislocation of the optic lens, mental retardation, thromboembolic processes and premature atherosclerosis. Laboratory abnormalities include elevated plasma methionine levels, strongly elevated plasma homocysteine levels, low plasma cysteine levels, and homocystine excretion in the urine [1].

In 1969, McCully [2] proposed that elevated plasma homocysteine levels can cause atherosclerotic disease. This theory was based on observations that advanced and similar arterial lesions were found at autopsy in two children who had two distinct enzyme abnormalities (a transsulfuration defect in one and a remethylation defect in the other), but shared the biochemical abnormality of a severe hyperhomocysteinemia. This theory, although attractive, was neglected for a long time, which was mainly due to the low prevalence of inborn errors of metabolism that were accompanied by severe hyperhomocysteinemia.

In 1976, hyperhomocysteinemia regained a world-wide interest, when Wilcken and Wilcken [3] observed an abnormal rise in plasma homocysteine after oral methionine loading in 17 of 25 patients who had angiographically documented coronary artery disease, whereas this was the case in only 5 of 22 control subjects. Important messages of this study were that an abnormal methionine-homocysteine metabolism was not as rare as current thinking at that time suggested and that sulfur amino acid abnormalities might be related to premature atherosclerotic disease in a large proportion of patients from the general population.

Since then, a large number of retrospective, cross-sectional and prospective studies have been performed in different patient groups or community-based populations in order to assess the cardiovascular risk that is associated with elevated plasma homocysteine levels.

The first prospective study on the association between plasma homocysteine and coronary heart disease was published in 1992 and described a nested case-control study of the Physicians' Health Study, in which 14,916 male physicians were followed for up to 5 years [4]. Mean plasma homocysteine was higher in the 271 cases who developed myocardial infarction than in the 271 controls (11.1 ± 4.0 vs. 10.5 ± 2.8 μmol/l, p = 0.03) and the relative risk for individuals in the highest 5% of plasma homocysteine level versus the lowest 90% was 3.1 (95% CI 1.3–8.8). Subsequently, several other prospective studies have been carried out in individuals (mainly) without cardiovascular disease [5–29], in patients with coronary heart disease [16, 30–34], stroke [35], diabetes [36–39], renal failure [40–46], and other diseases [47]. In some of these studies, plasma homocysteine was investigated as a predictor of total mortality only [36–38].

The first meta-analysis of homocysteine as a vascular risk factor was published in 1995 and consisted mainly of retrospective studies and studies that used post-methionine-loading homocysteine levels [48]. A 5-μmol/l increase in fasting plasma homocysteine was associated with an odds ratio for coronary artery disease of 1.6 (95% CI 1.4–1.7) in men and 1.8 (95% CI 1.3–1.9) in women, whereas the odds ratio for cerebrovascular disease was 1.5 (95% CI 1.3–1.9). The meta-analysis also showed for the first time that prospective studies found lower risk estimates than retrospective studies.

Prospective studies in patients with established coronary artery disease have consistently shown that higher plasma homocysteine levels are associated with a lower survival [30–33]. In the study by Nygard et al. [30], the mortality during a follow-up of 4.6 years in patients with a plasma homocysteine of >20 μmol/l was 27% compared to 4% in those with a plasma homocysteine of <9 μmol/l. In patients with chronic kidney disease, such as maintenance dialysis patients, the study outcomes are less consistent. Some investigators have linked hyperhomocysteinemia to cardiovascular events in these patients [40–43], whereas others have not, or even found the opposite, i.e. that a low homocysteine concentration is associated with an adverse cardiovascular outcome [44–46].

Controversy as to whether the relationship between homocysteine and vascular disease is causal already arose when some large prospective population-based studies found that plasma homocysteine was not significantly related to vascular disease [6, 9]. The greatest impact had a nested case-control analysis of the Multiple Risk Factor Intervention Trial, an observational study of 12,886 men aged 35–57 years [9]. Plasma homocysteine was measured in 93 individuals who developed a non-fatal myocardial infarction and 186 matched controls, and in 147 individuals who died of coronary heart disease and 286 matched controls. The odds ratio for a coronary event of the highest (>15 μmol/l) versus the lowest (<9.6 μmol/l) quartile of homocysteine level was 0.92 (95% CI 0.6–1.5). The results contrasted with the British United Provident Association study, a prospective study of 21,520 men aged 35–64 years, in which the risk of ischemic heart disease in the quartile with the highest homocysteine level was 2.9 times higher than in the lowest quartile [12].

A second meta-analysis, published in 2002, which included 20 prospective trials, concluded that plasma homocysteine was significantly related to coronary artery disease (odds ratio 1.23 (95% CI 1.14–1.32) for each 5-μmol/l increment in plasma homocysteine) and to cerebrovascular disease (odds ratio 1.42 (95% CI 1.21–1.66)) [49]. As this meta-analysis included individuals with and without vascular disease, it was still unclear whether the relationship between homocysteine and atherosclerotic disease is causal. There are (at least) four different ways to further clarify whether homocysteine is truly a vascular risk factor in humans.

Homocystinuria

The clinical features and natural history of patients with classical homocystinuria, i.e. CBS deficiency, have been described in detail by Mudd et al. [1]. The lack of the enzyme leads to very high plasma concentrations of methionine and of homocysteine (up to 200 μmol/l) with overflow in the urine. Untreated, 50% of affected individuals will have suffered from a vascular event by the age of 29 years. About 50% of these events are arterial (32% cerebrovascular, 4% coronary and 11% peripheral arteries). As McCully pointed out, patients with other inborn errors of metabolism also resulting in very high plasma homocysteine levels, but not hypermethioninemia, may also suffer from enhanced arterial disease [2]. As classical risk factors for atherosclerotic disease are usually absent in these young patients, homocysteine seems to be an important factor in the development of arterial disease. Homocysteine-lowering treatment has led to an enormous reduction of vascular disease in these patients [50].

Prospective Studies in Healthy Individuals

A number of prospective studies have reported the risk estimates of arterial events or vascular and/or total mortality conferred by homocysteine in populations without vascular disease at baseline [4–29]. A careful meta-analysis of relevant studies by the Homocysteine Studies Collaboration focused on the association between homocysteine concentration and risk of ischemic heart disease and stroke in populations without existing cardiovascular disease, diabetes mellitus, renal disease or systemic lupus erythematosus [51]. The meta-analysis showed that a 25% lower plasma homocysteine (about 3 μmol/l) was independently associated with an 11% (95% CI 4–17%) lower risk of ischemic heart disease, and a 19% (95% CI 5–31%) lower risk of stroke (fig. 1). Studies that were published after this report do not substantially differ from these results [16, 18, 26–29]. Overall, plasma homocysteine, therefore, seems to be a modest, but significant independent predictor of arterial occlusive disease in otherwise healthy subjects.

Studies in low-risk populations which reported only on mortality have consistently shown that plasma homocysteine is associated with an increased risk of both cardiovascular and total mortality [19–21, 24]. The magnitude of this risk seems to be similar for total and cardiovascular mortality and amounts to a 50% higher mortality risk per 5 μmol/l increase in plasma homocysteine [20, 24], or to a 50% higher mortality in individuals of the upper 20–25% of plasma homocysteine values [19, 21].

Mendelian Randomization

Plasma homocysteine level is related to different variables, such as age, blood pressure, smoking status, renal function, B-vitamin status, caffeine con-

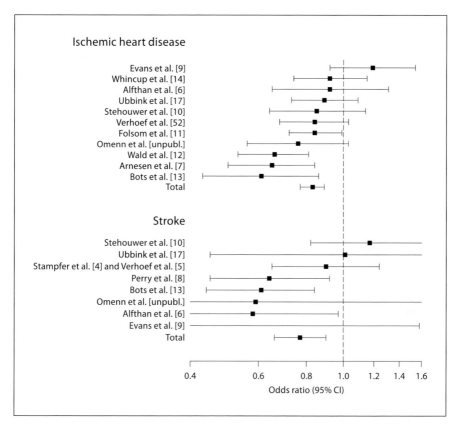

Fig. 1. Odds ratios of ischemic heart disease (upper panel) and stroke (lower panel) for a 25% lower usual homocysteine level in individual studies [modified from 51].

sumption and, possibly, to unknown factors. The relationship between plasma homocysteine and vascular disease may therefore be subject to residual confounding. In addition, observations that patients with vascular disease have higher plasma homocysteine levels than healthy individuals may also be the result of reverse-causality bias.

Mendelian randomization refers to the examination of the consistency between risk assessments based on genotype and phenotype conditions in order to understand the nature of disease determinants more precisely.

A genetic determinant of plasma homocysteine level in the general population is the common C677T polymorphism in the gene encoding for MTHFR. Homozygosity for this mutation (TT) leads to a less active variant of MTFHR and has a mean prevalence of about 10% in various populations. A TT status is associated with higher plasma homocysteine levels, especially when folate status is low [53]. As carriage of this mutation is subject to random parental inheritance according to Mendel's second law, the relationships between MTHFR genotype and homocysteine or vascular disease should not be influenced by other confounding factors that determine plasma homocysteine concentration, or be subject to reverse causality. In addition, if homocysteine is a true vascular risk factor, individuals with the TT polymorphism should have an elevated risk of vascular disease that is proportional to the increase in plasma homocysteine that is associated with this mutation. There are several reports on the relation between MTHFR status and vascular disease (mostly coronary heart disease, stroke and venous thromboembolism), but more precise quantification of such associations have used meta-analyses of the available studies. In a meta-analysis of 72 case-control studies (46 on ischemic heart disease, 26 on VTE and 7 on stroke) comprising 16,849 vascular cases and 16,849 controls, Wald et al. [49] found that the odds ratio of the TT versus the CC genotype was 1.21 (95% CI 1.06–1.39) for ischemic heart disease and 1.31 (0.80–2.15) for stroke. The difference in plasma homocysteine between TT and CC individuals was 2.7 μmol/l, which would amount to an odds ratio for ischemic heart disease of 1.42 (1.11–1.84) for a 5-μmol/l increase in plasma homocysteine. Based on 16 prospective studies, the calculated odds ratio for ischemic heart disease was found to be 1.32 (1.19–1.45) for each 5-μmol/l increase in plasma homocysteine. In a more recent meta-analysis, which focused on homocysteine and stroke, the mean difference in plasma homocysteine between healthy individuals with the TT genotype (n = 1,887) and the CC genotype (n = 7,252) was 1.93 μmol/l (1.38–2.47) [54]. The only other determinant of this difference was serum folate. Using the meta-analysis of Wald et al. [49], the expected odds ratio for stroke of an increase of this 1.93 μmol/l in plasma homocysteine would be 1.20 (1.38–2.47). Based on 30 studies on stroke and MTHFR, the calculated odds ratio was 1.26 (1.14–1.40).

Both meta-analyses conclude that the observed increase in risk of vascular disease conferred by plasma homocysteine in prospective studies is similar to the increase in risk based on Mendelian randomization of the MTHFR TT genotype, and, therefore, that plasma homocysteine is causally related to ischemic heart disease and stroke.

Homocysteine-Lowering Treatment

From our understanding of sulfur amino acid metabolism, it follows that reduction of plasma homocysteine concentration is expected to be achieved by administration of folate, vitamin B_{12}, vitamin B_6, betaine or serine, by enhancement of urinary homocysteine excretion or by reduction of homocysteine synthesis by dietary means (methionine restriction with or without cystine supplementation). Estrogens are also known to decrease plasma homocysteine levels, especially in post-menopausal women, although the mechanism of this reduction is unknown. Of these methods, folate treatment has been shown to be superior in lowering fasting plasma homocysteine levels [55]. In a meta-analysis of 12 randomized trials, which included more than 1,000 (mostly healthy) subjects, the effect of several doses of folic acid, but also the addition of vitamin B_6 and vitamin B_{12}, was investigated [56]. The main findings were that the reduction in plasma homocysteine was highest in subjects with the highest baseline homocysteine level: 16% (95% CI 11–20%) reduction in those with plasma homocysteine levels <8.9 μmol/l and 39% (95% CI 36–43%) reduction in those with a baseline concentration of >18.5 μmol/l (p for trend <0.001). The dose of folic acid had a non-significant effect on the homocysteine reduction. All dose ranges, i.e. <1 mg (mean 0.5 mg/day), 1–3 mg (mean 1.2 mg/day) and >3 mg (mean 5.7 mg/day), were associated with a mean 25% reduction in plasma homocysteine level. The addition of vitamin B_{12} (mean 0.5 mg/day) led to an additional reduction in plasma homocysteine only by about 7%, and the addition of vitamin B_6 (mean 16.5 mg/day) had no significant effect. Folic acid, therefore, is the cornerstone of homocysteine-lowering treatment in general, whereas vitamin B_{12} is usually reserved for cobalamin deficiency. Vitamin B_6 is used in patients with CBS deficiency and to lower the plasma homocysteine concentration after methionine loading.

If effective homocysteine-lowering treatment significantly decreased the occurrence of vascular disease, the evidence that homocysteine is indeed a vasculotoxic amino acid would be stronger. Many years elapsed before prospective placebo-controlled randomized homocysteine-lowering studies were initiated, mostly due to the lack of interest of funding such trials. Eventually, several studies were performed or are still underway. In some studies, surrogate vascular end-points were used [57–64], whereas clinical events were taken as the primary end-point in other, larger studies [65–67]. Most homocysteine-lowering therapies that were used consisted of a combination of folic acid, vitamin B_6 and cobalamin.

The results of the surrogate end-point trials are summarized in table 1. It can be seen that homocysteine-lowering treatment was associated with beneficial vascular effects in some studies (less abnormal exercise ECGs, more patent coronary arteries and less revascularization procedures after angioplasty), but also that other studies reported a lack of significant vascular effects (restenosis after coronary stenting, biochemical markers of endothelial function and inflammation). Differences in study population characteristics, therapies that were used and the types of vascular end-points make it virtually impossible to compare these trials in order to conclude whether homocysteine-lowering therapy in general prevents vascular disease. From the large inter-

Table 1. Randomized, controlled homocysteine-lowering trials with surrogate vascular end-points

Study	Subjects	Sample	Treatment	Outcome
Vermeulen et al. [57]	Healthy siblings of vascular patients	158	FA 5 mg + 250 mg B_6 vs. placebo. F.u. 2 years	OR 0.4 (0.17–0.93). Abnormal exercise ECG OR 0.87 (0.56–1.33). Ankle-brachial index OR 1.02 (0.26–4.05). Carotid stenosis OR 0.86 (0.47–1.59). Peripheral stenosis
Vermeulen et al. [58]	Healthy siblings of vascular patients	158	FA 5 mg + 250 mg B_6 vs. placebo. F.u. 2 years	Decrease in urinary albumin/creatinine ratio No significant effect on E-selectin, VCAM-1, vWF, tPA, PAI-1 and CRP
Vermeulen et al. [59]	Healthy siblings of vascular patients	158	FA 5 mg + 250 mg B_6 vs. placebo. F.u. 2 years	OR 0.48 (0.17–1.41). Cerebrovascular atherosclerosis on MRA OR 0.48 (0.14–1.60). Cerebral microangiopathy on MRI
Schnyder et al. [60]	Post-coronary angioplasty	205	FA 1 mg + B_{12} 0.4 mg + B_6 10 mg vs. placebo for 6 months. F.u. 6 months	RR 0.52 (0.32–0.86). Restenosis
Schnyder et al. [61]	Post-coronary angioplasty	553	FA 1 mg + B_{12} 0.4 mg + B_6 10 mg vs. placebo for 6 months. F.u. 11 months	RR 0.68 (0.48–0.96). Revascularization, myocardial infarction or death
Lange et al. [62]	Post-coronary stenting	636	FA 1.2 mg + B_6 48 mg + B_{12} 0.06 mg vs. placebo. 6 months	RR 1.30 (1.00–1.69). In-stent restenosis
Dusitanond et al. [63]	Stroke/TIA	285	FA 2 mg + B_{12} 0.5 mg + B_6 25 mg vs. placebo. 6 months	No significant effect on C-reactive protein, sCD40L, IL-6, VCAM-1, ICAM-1, vWF, P-selectin, prothrombin fragments 1 and 2, and D-dimer
Durga et al. [64]	Mild hyperhomo-cysteinemia (≥13 μmol/l)	530	FA 0.8 mg vs. placebo. 1 year	No significant effect on C-reactive protein, sICAM-1, oxidized LDL and autoantibodies against oxidized LDL

FA = Folic acid; B_6 = vitamin B_6; B_{12} = vitamin B_{12}; F.u. = follow-up.

vention studies (table 2), only the VISP trial has been published so far [66]. In this study, 3,680 stroke patients with a baseline plasma homocysteine of 13.4 μmol/l were randomized to a high- or low-dose multivitamin B treatment. After 2 years, the primary end-point, recurrent ischemic stroke, was reached in 9.2% in the high-dose vitamin group and in 8.8% in the low-dose group. There was also no significant difference in a composite end-point consisting of stroke, coronary artery disease or death between the two groups (risk ratio 1.0, 95% CI 0.8–1.1). The disappointing results may have been related to the small difference in plasma homocysteine that was achieved. Plasma homocysteine was about 13 μmol/l in the low-dose group and 11 μmol/l in the high-dose group. The small difference was probably due to the dietary folic acid fortification that was instituted in North America in 1998 in order to reduce the risk of neural tube defects in newborns. Inclusion of patients took place from 1997 to 2001 and those who had been randomized to the control group exhibited lower plasma homocysteine levels during follow-up than expected. However, a small beneficial effect of active homocysteine-lowering treatment could not be excluded in this trial. Results of other trials are awaited eagerly, but due to the folic acid fortification, studies taking place in North America may suffer from a similar power shortage.

Pathophysiological Considerations
Several animal models of hyperhomocysteinemia have been used to elucidate the mechanisms behind the atherogenic properties of homocysteine. Hyperhomocysteinemia has been induced in animals by supplementation of methionine or homocysteine, by dietary restriction of folate, choline, cobalamin, and/or pyridoxine, and by disrupting genes encoding for enzymes involved in homocysteine metabolism, such as CBS, MTHFR and MS.

Genetically induced hyperhomocysteinemia does not seem to cause atherosclerosis in animal models [68, 69], whereas dietary-induced hyperhomocysteinemia was shown to be associated with the development and acceleration of atherosclerotic lesions, especially in susceptible animal models, such as the apolipoprotein E (apoE)-deficient mouse [70, 71]. Mice lacking the gene for apoE develop hypercholesterolemia and spontaneous atherosclerotic lesions in the aortic root and branch points, which resemble human atherosclerosis. Interestingly, apoE knockout mice which were also made deficient for CBS (double knockout mice), exhibited larger atherosclerotic lesions than apoE control mice [72].

Endothelial Dysfunction
Normal endothelium is a highly active organ with many vascular functions. These include the regulation of vascular tone, the composition of suben-

Table 2. Randomized, controlled homocysteine-lowering trials with clinical end-points

Study	Subjects	Sample	Treatment	Outcome
Liem et al. [65]	Stable CAD	593	Open label FA 0.5 mg vs. standard care. F.u. 2 years	RR 1.05 (0.63–1.75) All-cause mortality and composite vascular end-point
Cambridge Heart Antioxidant Study (CHAOS-2)	Myocardial infarction or unstable angina	1,882	FA 5 mg vs. placebo Terminated after 1.7 years	RR 1.0 (0.7–1.3) Revascularization, myocardial infarction or cardiac death
Norwegian Study of Homocysteine Lowering with B-vitamins Myocardial Infarction (NORVIT)	Myocardial infarction	3,750	2 × 2 factorial design FA 0.8 mg + B_{12} 0.4 mg vs. placebo with B_6 40 mg vs. placebo	
Western Norway B-vitamin Intervention Trial (WENBIT)	Coronary artery disease on angiography	3,000	2 × 2 factorial design FA 0.8 mg + B_{12} 0.4 mg vs. placebo with B_6 40 mg vs. placebo	
Study of the Effectiveness of Additional Reductions in Cholesterol and Homocysteine (SEARCH)	Myocardial infarction	12,064	2 × 2 factorial design FA 2 mg + B_{12} 0.8 mg vs. placebo with simvastatin 20 mg vs. 80 mg	
Woman's Antioxidant and Cardiovascular Disease Study (WACS)[1]	CVD or high risk	5,442	FA 2.5 mg + B_{12} 1 mg + B_6 50 mg vs. placebo	
Heart Outcomes Prevention Evaluation (HOPE-2)[1]	Arterial disease	5,522	FA 2.5 mg + B_{12} 1 mg + B_6 50 mg vs. placebo	
Su.Fol.Om3	CHD or stroke	(3,000)	FA 0.5 mg + B_{12} 0.02 mg + B_6 3 mg vs. placebo	
Toole et al. [66][1]	Stroke	3,680	FA 2.5 mg + B_{12} 0.4 mg + B_6 25 mg vs. FA 0.02 mg + B_{12} 0.006 mg + B_6 0.2 mg F.u. 2 years	RR 1.0 (0.8–1.3) Recurrent stroke RR 1.0 (0.8–1.1) Composite vascular end-point
VITAmins TO Prevent Stroke Study (VITATOPS)	Stroke	8,000	FA 2 mg + B_{12} 0.5 mg + B_6 25 mg vs. placebo	
Wrone et al. [67][1]	End-stage renal disease	510	FA 1 mg vs. 5 mg vs. 15 mg. F.u. 2 years	No difference in mortality and vascular events, p = 0.47
Folic Acid for Vascular Outcome Reduction in Transplantation (FAVORIT)[1]	Renal transplant recipients	(4,000)	FA 2.5 mg + B_6 20 mg + B_{12} 0.4 mg vs. placebo	
Homocysteine Study (HOST)[1]	Renal disease	2,056	FA 40 mg + B_{12} 2 mg + B_6 100 mg vs. placebo	

FA = Folic acid; B_6 = vitamin B_6; B_{12} = vitamin B_{12}; F.u. = follow-up.
[1] Folic-acid-fortified population.

dothelial matrix, the proliferation of smooth muscle cells, the balance between coagulation and fibrinolysis, the permeability to substances and the adhesion and migration of blood cells. These functions are carried out by the synthesis and release of a variety of substances that are deposited in the subendothelial matrix or have vasoactive or modulating properties, such as nitric oxide (NO), prostacyclin, endothelin, angiotensin II, von Willebrand factor, thrombomodulin, tissue-type plasminogen activator, plasminogen activator inhibitor type 1, vascular cell adhesion molecules, and vascular endothelial growth factor. Many substances have more than one function. For example, NO not only is a vasodilator but also has inhibitory effects on the growth of smooth muscle cells and the adhesion and aggregation of platelets. From the multitude of vascular effects, it is clear that there is no gold standard for the assessment of endothelial function. Normally, the endothelium keeps the vascular tone low, inhibits smooth muscle cell proliferation, and provides an antithrombotic inner vascular surface. Dysfunction of the endothelium is a major and early event in the development of atherothrombosis.

One of the main theories on the atherogenic properties of homocysteine is that homocysteine is toxic to endothelium and causes endothelial dysfunction. Early studies have shown that intravenous infusion of homocysteine in baboons resulted in desquamation and denudation of the endothelium [73]. In vitro studies showed detachment of cultured venous endothelial cells from their substratum [74]. However, these toxic effects are of little clinical relevance because they occur only at homocysteine concentrations that are much higher than those that are present in hyperhomocysteinemic individuals.

Many subsequent studies have rather focused on more functional aspects of endothelial function, such as endothelium-dependent vasomotor responses. These responses can be assessed non-invasively and they have gained such a wide acceptance and popularity that endothelial dysfunction sometimes is defined by the presence of impaired endothelium-dependent vasodilation. Several methods in and ex vivo have been used to assess arterial endothelium-dependent vasodilation. As NO is a major mediator of endothelium-dependent vasodilation in large arteries and resistance vessels, these methods involve the activation of endothelial NO synthase by stimuli such as acetylcholine, thrombin, bradykinin and shear stress in order to increase the bioavailability of NO. Vessel wall responses to these stimuli are usually compared with the response to an endothelium-independent vasodilator such as nitroprusside or glyceryl trinitrate.

Disturbed endothelium-dependent relaxation of arteries can be demonstrated in patients with atherosclerotic disease and in individuals with cardiovascular risk factors, such as hypertension, smoking, diabetes and hypercholesterolemia. Impaired endothelium-dependent vasodilation of coronary or brachial arteries has also been associated with a higher risk of subsequent vascular events [75–80].

In animal models, it has been demonstrated that monkeys with diet-induced hyperhomocysteinemia (10.6 ± 2.6 vs. 4.0 ± 0.2 μmol/l in controls) exhibited a decreased endothelium-dependent vasodilator response to acetylcholine in the leg [81]. Endothelium-dependent vasodilation of cerebral arterioles was shown to be impaired in hyperhomocysteinemic CBS-, MTHFR- or MS-deficient mice [82].

Most human studies have used the brachial reactive hyperemia model to examine the influence of hyperhomocysteinemia on endothelium-dependent vasodilation. Children with classic homocystinuria who are on vitamin treatment are still hyperhomocysteinemic and show a reduction of flow-mediated vasodilatation by about 70% compared with control subjects, whereas nitroglycerin-mediated vasodilatation is not significantly different [83, 84]. Patients with chronic kidney disease, who have elevated plasma homocysteine levels, exhibit an impaired flow-mediated brachial artery vasodilation independent of traditional risk factors [85–87]. The response to reactive hyperemia in both CBS-deficient and renal failure patients, however, does not correlate with the plasma homocysteine levels.

The results of studies on endothelium-dependent vasodilation and mild hyperhomocysteinemia are conflicting. Two small studies found an impaired endothelium-dependent vasodilation in hyperhomocysteinemic subjects [88, 89], whereas other larger studies did not find a significant relationship between plasma homocysteine level and endothelial function [90–92]. The negative effects of homocysteine on endothelial function have been ascribed to reduced bioavailability of NO due to auto-oxidation of homocysteine in plasma, which leads to oxidative inactivation of NO [93]. Alternatively, by inhibiting dimethylarginine dimethylaminohydrolase, an enzyme which catabolizes asymmetric dimethylarginine, homocysteine may lead to accumulation of this endogenous inhibitor of NO synthase. The effect of homocysteine-lowering treatment with folic acid on brachial endothelium-dependent vasodilation has been examined in different populations [for review, see 94]. In renal failure patients, folic acid treatment was not associated with an improved arterial endothelial response [95, 96]. In asymptomatic hyperhomocysteinemic individuals, some studies found a beneficial effect of folic acid treatment [97, 98] whereas others did not [92]. Most studies in patients with coronary artery disease have shown an improvement of endothelial dysfunction after folate therapy [94]. It is debated whether any beneficial effect of folates on endothelium-dependent vasodilation is the result of the lowering of homocysteine [99] or is to be ascribed to intrinsic effects of folate itself [100].

The relationship between homocysteine and endothelial function markers in plasma is poor [101, 102], and several studies have shown that homocysteine-lowering treatment is not associated with lowering of these markers [58, 63, 95, 103].

Other Mechanisms

Several other biochemical mechanisms than (the induction of endothelial dysfunction by) increased oxidative stress or elevation of asymmetrical dimethylarginine have been proposed to explain the association between homocysteine and atherosclerotic vascular disease.

Hypomethylation. High homocysteine levels may slow down the transmethylation pathway and lead to an impaired methylation and function of important genes and proteins [104].

Protein Homocysteinylation/Acylation. In acylation, homocysteine-thiolactone, a highly reactive compound formed by methionyl-tRNA synthetase, leads to post-translational modification of proteins and protein damage [105].

Endoplasmic Reticulum Stress. The thiol group of homocysteine can undergo disulfide exchange reactions leading to disruption of the folding and the processing of newly synthesized proteins in the endoplasmic reticulum. Consequences of this so-called endoplasmic reticulum stress include an altered lipid metabolism, activation of inflammation and programmed cell death [106].

Is Hyperhomocysteinemia Associated with Increased Arterial Stiffness?

Can Homocysteine Alter Arterial Stiffness?

Arterial stiffness is not only determined by age and blood pressure, but also by other cardiovascular risk factors, notably diabetes mellitus. In this paragraph, the role of hyperhomocysteinemia as a possible determinant of arterial stiffness is discussed.

Epidemiological data have shown that plasma homocysteine is more strongly associated with systolic than with diastolic blood pressure [107, 108]. It can, therefore, be hypothesized that hyperhomocysteinemia increases arterial stiffness. Arterial stiffness is determined by the number and function of smooth muscle cells, by extracellular matrix properties, such as quantity and collagen-to-elastin ratio, and, possibly, by endothelial function. Theoretically, homocysteine might increase arterial stiffness by destroying elastin fibers, increasing collagen production and/or stimulating smooth muscle cell activity.

In vitro and animal studies have demonstrated that moderate to high homocysteine concentrations may lead to smooth muscle cell proliferation, increased collagen production and disruption of elastic fiber formation [reviewed in 109]. An ex vivo study showed that carotid arteries of folate-depleted, hyperhomocysteinemic rats were less elastic than those of control animals [110]. However, homocysteine might also *decrease* arterial stiffness by impairing collagen cross-linking. In a minipig model, diet-induced hyperhomocysteinemia resulted in a 'mega-artery syndrome' with hyperpulsatile arteries, characterized by hypertension, extended reactive hyperemia of conduit arteries and dilatation of the aorta [111]. In these animals, a decreased aortic stiffness was observed in the presence of an increased smooth muscle tension and fragmentation of the arterial wall elastic lamina.

Post-mortem studies of homocystinuric individuals have reported lesions in large, medium-sized, and smaller arteries [2, 112]. There was intimal and medial fibrosis and thickening with fraying and disruption of the internal elastic membranes. Furthermore, focal proliferation of connective tissue of small arteries was found with an increase of fibroblasts, collagen, and elastic fibers. Notably, little or no lipid accumulation was reported.

Biopsies of occluded superficial femoral arteries in patients with peripheral vascular disease showed morphologically similar atherosclerotic lesions in hyper- and normohomocysteinemic individuals, but the smooth muscle cell/extracellular matrix ratio of the medial layer was significantly decreased in those with hyperhomocysteinemia [113]. It remains speculative whether and to which extent a decreased smooth muscle cell/extracellular matrix ratio is involved in altered elastic properties of arteries.

Relationship between Homocysteine and Arterial Stiffness in Humans

In vivo data of the effects of homocysteine on elastic properties of vessel walls in humans have yielded conflicting results (table 3).

In healthy individuals and in high-risk subjects, plasma homocysteine levels were shown to be not or only marginally associated with carotid and femoral artery stiffness [90, 114]. In men without cardiovascular disease, aortic pulse wave velocity was related to homocysteine level univariately, but the association was no longer significant after correction for blood pressure, while systolic blood pressure remained significantly associated with plasma homocysteine [115]. Two studies in patients with end-stage renal disease, who usually are hyperhomocysteinemic, did not find a significant relationship between arterial stiffness and homocysteine [85, 116], whereas another study reported that homocysteine was related to lower-limb, but not upper-limb pulse wave velocity in chronic hemodialysis patients [117]. A significant relationship between homocysteine and aortic stiffness has been described in patients with

Table 3. Studies on the relationship between arterial stiffness and homocysteine in humans

Study	Subjects	Study nature	Stiffness parameter	Outcome
Wilkinson et al. [120]	n = 8, healthy	Methionine loading	Augmentation index timing of reflected pressure wave	No change in aortic and systemic arterial stiffness
Nestel et al. [121]	n = 18, healthy	Methionine loading	Systemic arterial compliance	Increase in central arterial stiffness
Arcaro et al. [122]	n = 12, healthy	Methionine loading	Brachial and femoral DC + CC	Increase in brachial and femoral stiffness
Malinow et al. [115]	n = 174, men without evidence of vascular disease	Cross-sectional	PWV car-fem	Aortic stiffness not associated with Hcy
Van Guldener et al. [85]	n = 28, ESRD n = 28, controls	Cross-sectional	Carotid DC + CC	No significant relationship between carotid stiffness and Hcy
Blacher et al. [117]	n = 74, ESRD n = 57, controls	Cross-sectional	PWV car-fem PWV car-rad PWV fem-tib	Lower-limb stiffness independently associated with Hcy in ESRD patients
Smilde et al. [114]	n = 132, HH, HZ, V, FH, H, S, or C	Cross-sectional	Carotid and femoral DC + CC	Hcy marginally related to carotid and femoral stiffness
Lambert et al. [90]	n = 123, healthy siblings of vascular patients	Cross-sectional	Carotid DC + CC	No significant relationship between carotid stiffness and Hcy
Bortolotto et al. [118]	n = 236, hyper-tension	Cross-sectional	PWV car-fem	Aortic stiffness independently associated with Hcy
Pannier et al. [116]	n = 60, ESRD n = 34, controls	Cross-sectional	Carotid DC	No significant relationship between carotid stiffness and Hcy
Yasmin et al. [119]	n = 115, offspring of hypertensives n = 203, healthy	Cross-sectional	Augmentation index Brachial PWV	Hcy related to aortic and brachial stiffness
Van Guldener et al. [123]	n = 41, ESRD	Randomization to 1 or 5 mg folic acid for 1 year	Carotid DC + CC	No change in carotid stiffness Decrease in systolic and diastolic blood pressure
Van Dijk et al. [124]	n = 124, healthy siblings of vascular patients	Randomization to 5 mg folic acid + 250 mg pyridoxine or placebo for 2 years	Carotid DC + CC	No change in carotid stiffness Decrease in systolic and diastolic blood pressure
Mangoni et al. [125]	n = 24, healthy smokers	Randomization to 5 mg folic acid or placebo for 4 weeks	PWV car-fem	No change in aortic stiffness Decrease in systolic and diastolic blood pressure

Table 3. (continued)

Study	Subjects	Study nature	Stiffness parameter	Outcome
Mangoni et al. [126]	n = 26, DM-2	Randomization to 5 mg folic acid or placebo for 4 weeks	PWV car-fem PWV car-rad	No change in stiffness
Williams et al. [127]	n = 41, normo- or hypertensive men	Randomization to 5 mg folic acid or placebo for 3 weeks	Systemic arterial compliance PWV car-fem PWV fem-ped	Reduction of central arterial stiffness and pulse pressure No change in aortic and lower limb stiffness

ESRD = End-stage renal disease; HH = homozygous cystathionine β-synthase deficiency; HZ = heterozygous cystathionine β-synthase deficiency; V = vascular disease and mild hyperhomocysteinemia; FH = familial hypercholesterolemia; H = hypertension; S = smokers; C = healthy controls; DM-2 = type 2 diabetes mellitus; PWV = pulse wave velocity; DC = distensibility coefficient; CC = compliance coefficient; Hcy = plasma homocysteine concentration.

hypertension [118] and in a combined group of healthy individuals and offspring of hypertensive patients [119].

Conflicting results have also been reported in individuals in whom acute hyperhomocysteinemia was induced by methionine loading (table 3). No significant change in aortic and systemic arterial stiffness was found in healthy individuals in one study [120], whereas others have reported an acute reduction in arterial compliance [121, 122].

The results of homocysteine-lowering interventions on arterial stiffness are rather disappointing (table 3). Homocysteine-lowering therapy had no beneficial effect on carotid distensibility in patients with end-stage renal disease [123], nor in healthy siblings of patients with premature atherosclerosis [124]. Treatment with folic acid was also not associated with an improvement of carotid-femoral pulse wave velocity in smokers [125], patients with type 2 diabetes [126], and a group of normo- and hypertensive men [127]. In the latter study, however, 3 weeks of folic acid therapy led to an increase in systemic compliance as assessed by simultaneous measurements of the ascending aortic blood flow and driving pressure in the ascending aorta [127]. Interestingly, in some studies, a significant lower blood pressure was found after folic acid therapy [123–125].

Conclusion

It can be concluded that the relationship between hyperhomocysteinemia and altered elastic properties of the arterial wall is not clear. One possibility is that the effect of homocysteine on arterial stiffness is relatively small and thus is not picked up by underpowered studies. In this regard, the largest study with

236 hypertensive patients did show a significant relationship between plasma homocysteine and aortic stiffness which was independent of mean arterial pressure [118]. Alternatively, the influence of hyperhomocysteinemia on arterial stiffness may vary in different parts of the vascular tree, being stronger in muscular than in elastic arteries [117], probably depending on the net effect of homocysteine on smooth muscle cell function, endothelial function, and matrix composition. It should be noted that, in humans, the precise sequence and localization of the vascular wall events remain to be established and that the role of homocysteine in these processes is likely to be influenced by other atherogenic factors.

References

1   Mudd SH, Skovby F, Levy HL, Pettigrew KD, Wilcken B, Pyeritz RE, et al: The natural history of homocystinuria due to cystathionine β-synthase deficiency. Am J Hum Genet 1985;37:1–31.
2   McCully KS: Vascular pathology of homocysteinemia: implications for the pathogenesis of arteriosclerosis. Am J Pathol 1969;56:111–128.
3   Wilcken DE, Wilcken B: The pathogenesis of coronary artery disease: a possible role for methionine metabolism. J Clin Invest 1976;57:1079–1082.
4   Stampfer MJ, Malinow R, Willett WC, Newcomer LM, Upson B, Ullmann D, et al: A prospective study of plasma homocysteine and risk of myocardial infarction in US physicians. JAMA 1992; 268:877–881.
5   Verhoef P, Hennekens CH, Malinow R, Kok FJ, Willett WC, Stampfer MJ: A prospective study of plasma homocyst(e)ine and risk of ischemic stroke. Stroke 1994;25:1924–1930.
6   Alfthan G, Pekkanen J, Jauhiainen M, Pitkaniemi J, Karvonen M, Tuomilehto J, et al: Relations of serum homocysteine and lipoprotein concentrations to atherosclerotic disease in a prospective Finnish population-based study. Atherosclerosis 1994;106:9–19.
7   Arnesen E, Refsum H, Bonaa KJ, Ueland PM, Forde OH, Nordrehaug JE: Serum total homocysteine and coronary heart disease. Int J Epidemiol 1995;24:704–709.
8   Perry IJ, Refsum H, Morris RW, Ebrahim SB, Ueland PM, Shaper AG: Prospective study of serum total homocysteine concentration and risk of stroke in middle-aged British men. Lancet 1995: 346:1395–1398.
9   Evans RW, Shaten BJ, Hempel JD, Cutler JA, Kuller LH: Homocysteine and risk of cardiovascular disease in the multiple risk factor intervention trial. Arterioscler Thromb Vasc Biol 1997;17: 1947–1953.
10 Stehouwer CD, Weijenberg MP, van den Berg M, Jakobs C, Feskens EJ, Kromhout D: Serum homocysteine and risk of coronary heart disease and cerebrovascular disease in elderly men: a 10-year follow-up. Arterioscler Thromb Vasc Biol 1998;18:1895–1901.
11 Folsom AR, Nieto J, McGovern PG, Tsai MY, Mallinow MR, Eckfeldt JH, et al: Prospective study of coronary heart disease incidence in relation to fasting total homocysteine, related genetic polymorphisms, and B vitamins: the Atherosclerosis Risk In Communities (ARIC) study. Circulation 1998;98:204–210.
12 Wald NJ, Watt HC, Law MR, Weir DG, McPartlin J, Scott JM: Homocysteine and ischaemic heart disease: results of a prospective study with implications regarding prevention. Arch Intern Med 1998;158:862–867.
13 Bots ML, Launer LJ, Lindemans J, Hoes AW, Hofman A, Witteman JC, et al: Homocysteine and short-term risk of myocardial infarction and stroke in the elderly: the Rotterdam study. Arch Intern Med 1999;159:38–44.

14 Whincup PH, Refsum H, Perry IJ, Morris R, Walker M, Lennon L, et al: Serum total homocysteine and coronary heart disease: prospective study in middle aged men. Heart 1999;82:448–454.

15 Knekt P, Alfthan G, Aromaa A, Heliovaara M, Marniemi J, Rissanen H, et al: Homocysteine and major coronary events: a prospective population study amongst women. J Intern Med 2001;249:461–465.

16 Knekt P, Reunanen A, Alfthan G, Heliovaara M, Rissanen H, Marniemi J, et al: Hyperhomocysteinaemia: a risk factor or a consequence of coronary heart disease? Arch Intern Med 2001;161:1589–1594.

17 Ubbink JB, Fehily AM, Pickering J, Elwood PC, Vermaak WJ: Homocysteine and ischaemic heart disease in the Caerphilly cohort. Atherosclerosis 1998;140:349–356.

18 Ridker PM, Manson JE, Buring JE, Shih J, Matias M, Hennekens CH: Homocysteine and risk of cardiovascular disease among postmenopausal women. JAMA 1999;281:1817–1821.

19 Kark JD, Selhub J, Adler B, Gofin J, Abramson JH, Friedman G, et al: Nonfasting plasma total homocysteine level and mortality in middle-aged and elderly men and women in Jerusalem. Ann Intern Med. 1999;131:321–330.

20 Vollset SE, Refsum H, Tverdal A, Nygard O, Nordrehaug JE, Tell GS, et al: Plasma homocysteine and cardiovascular and noncardiovascular mortality: the Hordaland homocysteine study. Am J Clin Nutr 2001;74:130–136.

21 Bostom AG, Silbershatz W, Rosenberg IH, Selhub J, D'Agostino RB, Wolf PA, et al: Nonfasting plasma total homocysteine levels and all-cause and cardiovascular disease mortality in elderly Framingham men and women. Arch Intern Med 1999;159:1077–1080.

22 Fallon UB, Elwood P, Ben-Shlomo Y, Ubbink JB, Greenwood R, Smith GD: Homocysteine and ischaemic stroke in men: the Caerphilly study. J Epidemiol Community Health 2001;55:91–96.

23 Bostom AG, Rosenberg IH, Silbershatz H, Jacques PF, Selhub J, D'Agostino RB, et al: Nonfasting plasma total homocysteine levels and stroke incidence in elderly persons: the Framingham study. Ann Intern Med 1999;131:352–355.

24 Blacher J, Benetos A, Kirzin JM, Malmejac A, Guize L, Safar ME: Relation of plasma total homocysteine to cardiovascular mortality in a French population. Am J Cardiol 2002;90:591–595.

25 Lind P, Hedblad B, Hultberg B, Stavenow L, Janzon L, Lindgarde F: Risk of myocardial infarction in relation to plasma levels of homocysteine and inflammation-sensitive proteins: a long-term nested case-control study. Angiology 2003;54:401–410.

26 Voutilainen S, Virtanen JK, Rissanen TH, Althan G, Laukkanen J, Nyyssonen K, Mursu J, Valkonen VP, Tuomainen TP, Kaplan GA, Salonen JT: Serum folate and homocysteine and the incidence of acute coronary events: the Kuopio ischaemic heart disease risk factor study. Am J Clin Nutr 2004;80:317–323.

27 Sacco RL, Anand K, Lee HS, Boden-Albala B, Stabler S, Allen R, Paik MC: Homocysteine and the risk of ischemic stroke in a triethnic cohort: the Northern Manhattan Study. Stroke 2004;35:2263–2269.

28 Zylberstein DE, Bengtsson C, Bjorkelund C, Landaas S, Sundh V, Thelle D, Lissner L: Serum homocysteine in relation to mortality and morbidity from coronary heart disease: a 24-year follow-up of the population study of women in Gothenburg. Circulation 2004;109:601–606.

29 Iso H, Moriyama Y, Sato S, Kitamura A, Tanigawa T, Yamagishi K, Imano H, Ohira T, Okamura T, Naito Y, Shimamoto T: Serum total homocysteine concentrations and risk of stroke and its subtypes in Japanese. Circulation 2004;109:2766–2772.

30 Nygard O, Nordrehaug JE, Refsum H, Ueland PM, Farstad M, Vollset SE: Plasma homocysteine levels and mortality in patients with coronary artery disease. N Engl J Med 1997;337:230–236.

31 Anderson JL, Muhlestein JB, Horne BD, Carlquist JF, Bair TL, Madsen TE, Pearson RR: Plasma homocysteine predicts mortality independently of traditional risk factors and C-reactive protein in patients with angiographically defined coronary artery disease. Circulation 2000;102:1227–1232.

32 Omland T, Samuelsson A, Hartford M, Herlitz J, Karlsson T, Christensen B, Caidahl K: Serum homocysteine concentration as an indicator of survival in patients with acute coronary syndromes. Arch Intern Med 2000;160:1834–1840.

33   Stubbs PJ, Al-Obaidi MK, Conroy RM, Collinson PO, Graham IM, Noble MI: Effect of plasma homocysteine concentration on early and late events in patients with acute coronary syndromes. Circulation 2000;102:605–610.

34   Tanne D, Haim M, Goldbourt U, Boyko V, Doolman R, Adler Y, Brunner D, Behar S, Sela BA: Prospective study of serum homocysteine and risk of ischemic stroke among patients with pre-existing coronary heart disease. Stroke 2003;34:632–636.

35   Boysen G, Brander T, Christensen H, Gideon R, Truelsen T: Homocysteine and risk of recurrent stroke. Stroke 2003;34:1258–1261.

36   Stehouwer CDA, Gall MA, Hougaard P, Jakobs C, Parving HH: Plasma homocysteine concentration predicts mortality in non-insulin-dependent diabetic patients with and without albuminuria. Kidney Int 1999;55:308–314.

37   Kark JD, Selhub J, Bostom A, Adler B, Rosenberg IH: Plasma homocysteine and all-cause mortality in diabetes. Lancet 1999;353:1936–1937.

38   Hoogeveen EK, Kostense PJ, Jakobs C, Dekker JM, Nijpels G, Heine RJ, Bouter LM, Stehouwer CD: Hyperhomocysteinemia increases risk of death, especially in type 2 diabetes: 5-year follow-up of the Hoorn Study. Circulation 2000;101:1506–1511.

39   Soinio M, Marniemi J, Laakso M, Lehto S, Ronnemaa T: Elevated plasma homocysteine level is an independent predictor of coronary heart disease events in patients with type 2 diabetes mellitus. Ann Intern Med 2004;140:94–100.

40   Bostom AG, Shemin D, Verhoef P, et al: Elevated fasting total plasma homocysteine levels and cardiovascular disease outcomes in maintenance dialysis patients. Arterioscler Thromb Vasc Biol 1997;17:2554–2558.

41   Moustapha A, Naso A, Nahlawi M, et al: Prospective study of hyperhomocysteinemia as an adverse cardiovascular risk factor in end-stage renal disease. Circulation 1998;97:138–141. Erratum in: Circulation 1998;97:711.

42   Ducloux D, Motte G, Challier B, Gibey R, Chalopin JM: Serum total homocysteine and cardiovascular disease occurrence in chronic, stable renal transplant recipients: a prospective study. J Am Soc Nephrol 2000;11:134–137.

43   Mallamaci F, Zoccali C, Tripepi G, et al: Hyperhomocysteinemia predicts cardiovascular outcomes in hemodialysis patients. Kidney Int 2002;61:609–614.

44   Suliman ME, Qureshi R, Barany P, et al: Hyperhomocysteinemia, nutritional status, and cardiovascular disease in hemodialysis patients. Kidney Int 2000;57:1727–1735.

45   Kalantar-Zadeh K, Block G, Humphreys MH, McAllister CJ, Kopple JD: A low, rather than a high, total plasma homocysteine is an indicator of poor outcome in hemodialysis patients. J Am Soc Nephrol 2004;15:442–453.

46   Suliman ME, Stenvinkel P, Qureshi R, et al: Hyperhomocysteinemia in relation to plasma free amino acids, biomarkers of inflammation and mortality in patients with chronic kidney disease starting dialysis therapy. Am J Kidney Dis 2004;44:455–465.

47   Petri M, Roubenoff R, Dallal GE, Nadeau MR, Selhub J, Rosenberg IH: Plasma homocysteine as a risk factor for atherothrombotic events in systemic lupus erythematosus. Lancet 1996;348:1120–1124.

48   Boushey CJ, Beresford SA, Omenn GS, Motulsky AG: A quantitative assessment of plasma homocysteine as a risk factor for vascular disease. Probable benefits of increasing folic acid intakes. JAMA 1995;274:1049–1057.

49   Wald DS, Law M, Morris JK: Homocysteine and cardiovascular disease: evidence on causality from a meta-analysis. BMJ 2002;325:1202–1206.

50   Yap S, Boers GH, Wilcken B, Wilcken DE, Brenton DP, Lee PJ, et al: Vascular outcome in patients with homocystinuria due to cystathionine β-synthase deficiency treated chronically: a multi-center observational study. Arterioscler Thromb Vasc Biol 2001;21:2080–2085.

51   Homocysteine Studies Collaboration: Homocysteine and risk of ischemic heart disease and stroke: a meta-analysis. JAMA 2002;288:2015–2022.

52   Verhoef P, Kok FJ, Kruyssen DA, Schouten EG, Witteman JC, Grobbee DE, Ueland PM, Refsum H: Plasma total homocysteine, B vitamins, and risk of coronary atherosclerosis. Arterioscler Thromb Vasc Biol 1997;17:989–995.

Homocysteine and Large Arteries

53   Jacques PF, Bostom AG, Williams RR, Ellison RC, Eckfeldt JH, Rosenberg IH, et al: Relation between folate status, a common mutation in methylenetetrahydrofolate reductase, and plasma homocysteine concentrations. Circulation 1996;93:7–9.

54   Casas JP, Bautista LE, Smeeth L, Sharma P, Hingorani AD: Homocysteine and stroke: evidence on a causal link from mendelian randomisation. Lancet 2005;365:224–232.

55   Van Guldener C, Stehouwer CDA: Homocysteine-lowering treatment: an overview. Expert Opin Pharmacother 2001;2:1449–1460.

56   Homocysteine Lowering Trialists' Collaboration: Lowering blood homocysteine with folic acid based supplements: meta-analysis of randomised trials. BMJ 1998;316:894–898.

57   Vermeulen EG, Stehouwer CD, Twisk JW, van den Berg M, de Jong SC, Mackaay AJ, et al: Effect of homocysteine-lowering treatment with folic acid plus vitamin B_6 on progression of subclinical atherosclerosis: a randomised, placebo-controlled trial. Lancet 2000;355:517–522.

58   Vermeulen EG, Rauwerda JA, van den Berg M, de Jong SC, Schalkwijk C, Twisk JW, et al: Homocysteine-lowering treatment with folic acid plus vitamin B_6 lowers urinary albumin excretion but not plasma markers of endothelial function or C-reactive protein: further analysis of secondary end-points of a randomized clinical trial. Eur J Clin Invest 2003;33:209–215.

59   Vermeulen EG, Stehouwer CD, Valk J, van der Knaap M, van den Berg M, Twisk JW, et al: Effect of homocysteine-lowering treatment with folic acid plus vitamin B_6 on cerebrovascular atherosclerosis and white matter abnormalities as determined by MRA and MRI: a placebo-controlled, randomized trial. Eur J Clin Invest 2004;34:256–261.

60   Schnyder G, Roffi M, Pin R, Flammer Y, Lange H, Eberli FR, et al: Decreased rate of coronary restenosis after lowering of plasma homocysteine levels. N Engl J Med 2001;345:1593–1600.

61   Schnyder G, Roffi M, Flammer Y, Pin R, Hess OM: Effect of homocysteine-lowering therapy with folic acid, vitamin B_{12}, and vitamin B_6 on clinical outcome after percutaneous coronary intervention. JAMA 2002;288:973–979.

62   Lange H, Suryapranata H, De Luca G, Borner C, Dille J, Kallmayer K, et al: Folate therapy and in-stent restenosis after coronary stenting. N Engl J Med 2004;350:2673 2681.

63   Dusitanond P, Eikelboom JW, Hankey GJ, Thom J, Gilmore G, Loh K, et al: Homocysteine-lowering treatment with folic acid, cobalamin, and pyridoxine does not reduce blood markers of inflammation, endothelial dysfunction, or hypercoagulability in patients with previous transient ischemic attack or stroke: a randomized substudy of the VITATOPS trial. Stroke 2005;36:144–146.

64   Durga J, van Tits LJ, Schouten EG, Kok FJ, Verhoef P: Effect of lowering of homocysteine levels on inflammatory markers: a randomized controlled trial. Arch Intern Med 2005;165:1388–1394.

65   Liem A, Reynierse-Buitenwerf GH, Zwinderman AH, Jukema JW, van Veldhuisen DJ: Secondary prevention with folic acid: effects on clinical outcomes. J Am Coll Cardiol 2003;41:2105–2113.

66   Toole JF, Malinow MR, Chambless LE, Spence JD, Pettigrew LC, Howard VJ, et al: Lowering homocysteine in patients with ischemic stroke to prevent recurrent stroke, myocardial infarction, and death: the Vitamin Intervention for Stroke Prevention (VISP) randomized controlled trial. JAMA 2004;291:565–575.

67   Wrone EM, Hornberger JM, Zehnder JL, McCann LM, Coplon NS, Fortmann SP: Randomized trial of folic acid for prevention of cardiovascular events in end-stage renal disease. J Am Soc Nephrol 2004;15:420–426.

68   Watanabe M, Osada J, Aratani Y, Kluckman K, Reddick R, Malinow MR, et al: Mice deficient in cystathionine β-synthase: animal models for mild and severe homocyst(e)inemia. Proc Natl Acad Sci USA 1995;92:1585–1589.

69   Chen Z, Karaplis AC, Ackerman SL, Pogribny IP, Melnyk S, Lussier-Cacan S, et al: Mice deficient in methylenetetrahydrofolate reductase exhibit hyperhomocysteinemia and decreased methylation capacity, with neuropathology and aortic lipid deposition. Hum Mol Genet 2001;10:433–443.

70   Hofmann MA, Lalla E, Lu Y, Ryu Gleason M, Wolf BM, Tanji N, et al: Hyperhomocysteinemia enhances vascular inflammation and accelerates atherosclerosis in a murine model. J Clin Invest 2001;107:675–683.

71   Troen AM, Lutgens E, Smithe DE, Rosenberg IH, Selhub J: The atherogenic effect of excess methionine intake. Proc Natl Acad Sci USA 2003;100:15089–15094.

72   Wang H, Jiang X, Yang F, Gaubatz JW, Ma L, Magera MJ, et al: Hyperhomocysteinemia accelerates atherosclerosis in cystathionine β-synthase and apolipoprotein E double knock-out mice with and without dietary perturbation. Blood 2003;101:3901–3907.

73   Harker LA, Ross R, Slichter SJ, Scott CR: Homocystine-induced arteriosclerosis: the role of endothelial cell injury and platelet response in its genesis. J Clin Invest 1976;58:731–741.

74   Wall RT, Harlan JM, Harker LA, Striker GE: Homocysteine-induced endothelial cell injury in vitro: a model for the study of vascular injury. Thromb Res 1980;18:113–121.

75   Al Suwaidi J, Hamasaki S, Higano ST, Nishimura RA, Holmes DR, Lerman A: Long-term follow-up of patients with mild coronary artery disease and endothelial dysfunction. Circulation 2000; 101:948–954.

76   Schachinger V, Britten MB, Zeiher AM: Prognostic impact of coronary vasodilator dysfunction on adverse long-term outcome of coronary heart disease. Circulation 2000;101:1899–1906.

77   Halcox JP, Schenke WH, Zalos G, Mincemoyer R, Prasad A, Waclawiw MA, et al: Prognostic value of coronary vascular endothelial dysfunction. Circulation 2002;106:653–658.

78   Perticone F, Ceravolo R, Pujia A, Ventura G, Iacopino S, Scozzafava A, et al: Prognostic significance of endothelial dysfunction in hypertensive patients. Circulation 2001;104:191–196.

79   Heitzer T, Schlinzig T, Krohn K, Meinertz T, Munzel T: Endothelial dysfunction, oxidative stress, and risk of cardiovascular events in patients with coronary artery disease. Circulation 2001;104: 2673–2678. Erratum in: Circulation 2003;108:500.

80   Neunteufl T, Heher S, Katzenschlager R, Wolfl G, Kostner K, Maurer G, et al: Late prognostic value of flow-mediated dilation in the brachial artery of patients with chest pain. Am J Cardiol 2000;86:207–210.

81   Lentz SR, Sobey CG, Piegors DJ, Bhopatkar MY, Faraci FM, Malinow MR, et al: Vascular dysfunction in monkeys with diet-induced hyperhomocyst(e)inemia. J Clin Invest 1996;98:24–29.

82   Dayal S, Devlin AM, McCaw RB, Liu ML, Arning E, Bottiglieri T, et al: Cerebral vascular dysfunction in methionine synthase-deficient mice. Circulation 2005;112:737–744.

83   Celermayer DS, Sorensen K, Ryalls M, Robinson J, Thomas O, Leonard JV, et al: Impaired endothelial function occurs in the systemic arteries of children with homozygous homocystinuria but not in their heterozygous parents. J Am Coll Cardiol 1993;22:854–858.

84   Pullin CH, Bonham JR, McDowell IF, Lee PJ, Powers HJ, Wilson JF, et al: Vitamin C therapy ameliorates vascular endothelial dysfunction in treated patients with homocystinuria. J Inherit Metab Dis 2002;25:107–118.

85   Van Guldener C, Lambert J, Janssen MJ, Donker AJ, Stehouwer CD: Endothelium-dependent vasodilatation and distensibility of large arteries in chronic haemodialysis patients. Nephrol Dial Transplant 1997;12(suppl 2):14–18.

86   Van Guldener C, Janssen MJ, Lambert J, Steyn M, Donker AJ, Stehouwer CD: Endothelium-dependent vasodilatation is impaired in peritoneal dialysis patients. Nephrol Dial Transplant 1998; 13:1782–1786.

87   Thambyrajah J, Landray MJ, McGlynn FJ, Jones HJ, Wheeler DC, Townend JN: Abnormalities of endothelial function in patients with predialysis renal failure. Heart 2000;83:205–209.

88   Tawakol A, Omland T, Gerhard M, Wu JT, Creager MA: Hyperhomocyst(e)inemia is associated with impaired endothelium-dependent vasodilation in humans. Circulation 1997;95:1119–1121.

89   Woo KS, Chook P, Lolin YI, Cheung AS, Chan LT, Sun YY, et al: Hyperhomocyst(e)inemia is a risk factor for arterial endothelial function in humans. Circulation 1997;96:2542–2544.

90   Lambert J, van den Berg M, Steyn M, Rauwerda JA, Donker AJ, Stehouwer CD: Familial hyperhomocysteinaemia and endothelium-dependent vasodilatation and arterial distensibility of large arteries. Cardiovasc Res 1999;42:743–751.

91   De Valk-de Roo GW, Stehouwer CD, Lambert J, Schalkwijk CG, van der Mooren MJ, Kluft C, et al: Plasma homocysteine is weakly correlated with plasma endothelin and von Willebrand factor but not with endothelium-dependent vasodilatation in healthy postmenopausal women. Clin Chem 1999;45:1200–1205.

92   Woodman RJ, Celermajer DE, Thompson PL, Hung J: Folic acid does not improve endothelial function in healthy hyperhomocysteinaemic subjects. Clin Sci 2004;106:353–358.

93 Welch GN, Loscalzo J: Homocysteine and atherothrombosis. N Eng J Med 1998;338:1042–1050.

94 Moat SJ, Lang D, McDowell IF, Clarke ZL, Madhavan AK, Lewis MJ, Goodfellow J: Folate, homocysteine, endothelial function and cardiovascular disease. J Nutr Biochem 2004;15:64–79.

95 Van Guldener C, Janssen MJ, Lambert J, ter Wee PM, Jakobs C, Donker AJ, et al: No change in impaired endothelial function after long-term folic acid therapy of hyperhomocysteinaemia in haemodialysis patients. Nephrol Dial Transplant 1998;13:106–112.

96 Thambyrajah J, Landray MJ, McGlynn FJ, Jones HJ, Wheeler DC, Townend JN: Does folic acid decrease plasma homocysteine and improve endothelial function in patients with predialysis renal failure? Circulation 2000;102:871–875.

97 Bellamy MF, McDowell IF, Ramsey MW, Brownlee M, Newcombe RG, Lewis MJ: Oral folate enhances endothelial function in hyperhomocysteinaemic subjects. Eur J Clin Invest 1999;29:659–662.

98 Woo KS, Chook P, Cheung AS, Fung WH, Qiao M, Lolin YI, et al: Long-term improvement in homocysteine levels and arterial endothelial function after 1-year folic acid supplementation. Am J Med 2002;112:535–539.

99 Chambers JC, Ueland PM, Obeid OA, Wrigley J. Refsum H, Kooner JS: Improved vascular endothelial function after oral B-vitamins: an effect mediated through reduced concentrations of free plasma homocysteine. Circulation 2000;102:2479–2483.

100 Verhaar MC, Wever RM, Kastelijn JJ, van Dam T, Koomans HA, Rabelink TJ: 5-Methyltetrahydrofolate, the active form of folic acid restores endothelial dysfunction in familial hypercholesterolemia. Circulation 1998;97:237–241.

101 De Jong SC, Stehouwer CD, van den Berg M, Vischer UM, Rauwerda JA, Emeis JJ: Endothelial markers proteins in hyperhomocysteinemia. Thromb Haemost 1997;78:1332–1337.

102 Becker A, van Hinsbergh VW, Kostense PJ, Jager A, Dekker JM, Nijpels G, Heine RJ, Bouter LM, Stehouwer CD: Serum homocysteine is weakly associated with von Willebrand factor and soluble vascular cell adhesion molecule 1, but not with C-reactive protein in type 2 diabetic and non-diabetic subjects – the Hoorn Study. Eur J Clin Invest 2000;30:763–770.

103 Peeters AC, van der Molen EF, Blom HJ, den Heijer M: The effect of homocysteine reduction by B-vitamin supplementation on markers of endothelial dysfunction. Thromb Haemost 2004;92:1086–1091.

104 Van Guldener C, Stehouwer CD: Hyperhomocysteinemia and vascular disease – a role for DNA hypomethylation? Lancet 2003;361:1668–1669.

105 Jakubowski H: Homocysteine-thiolactone and S-nitroso-homocysteine mediate incorporation of homocysteine into protein in humans. Clin Chem Lab Med 2003;41:1462–1466.

106 Hossain GS, van Thienen JV, Werstuck GH, Zhou J, Sood SK, Dickhout JG, et al: TDAG51 is induced by homocysteine, promotes detachment-mediated programmed cell death, and contributes to the development of atherosclerosis in hyperhomocysteinemia. J Biol Chem 2003;278:30317–30327.

107 Lim U, Cassano PA: Homocysteine and blood pressure in the Third National Health and Nutrition Examination Survey, 1988–1994. Am J Epidemiol 2002;156:1105–1113.

108 Van Guldener C, Nanayakkara PW, Stehouwer CD: Homocysteine and blood pressure. Curr Hypertens Rep 2003;5:26–31.

109 Van Guldener C, Stehouwer CD: Hyperhomocysteinemia, vascular pathology, and endothelial dysfunction. Semin Thromb Hemost 2000;26:281–289.

110 Symons JD, Mullick AE, Ensunsa JL, Ma AA, Rutledge JC: Hyperhomocysteinemia evoked by folate depletion: effects on coronary and carotid arterial function. Arterioscler Thromb Vasc Biol 2002;22:772–780.

111 Rolland PH, Friggi A, Barlatier A, Piquet P, Latrille V, Faye MM, et al: Hyperhomocysteinemia-induced vascular damage in the minipig. Captopril-hydrochlorothiazide combination prevents elastic alterations. Circulation 1995;91:1161–1174.

112 Gibson JB, Carson NA, Neill DW. Pathological findings in homocystinuria. J Clin Pathol 1964;17:427–437.

113 Vermeulen EG, Niessen HW, Bogels M, Stehouwer CD, Rauwerda JA, van Hinsbergh VW: Decreased smooth muscle cell/extracellular matrix ratio of media of femoral artery in patients with atherosclerosis and hyperhomocysteinemia. Arterioscler Thromb Vasc Biol 2001;21:573–577.

114 Smilde TJ, van den Berkmortel FW, Boers GH, Wollersheim H, de Boo T, van Langen H, et al: Carotid and femoral artery wall thickness and stiffness in patients at risk for cardiovascular disease, with special emphasis on hyperhomocysteinemia. Arterioscler Thromb Vasc Biol 1998;18: 1958–1963.

115 Malinow MR, Levenson J, Giral P, Nieto FJ, Razavian M, Segond P, et al: Role of blood pressure, uric acid, and hemorheological parameters on plasma homocyst(e)ine concentration. Atherosclerosis 1995;114:175–183.

116 Pannier B, Guerin AP, Marchais SJ, Metivier F, Safar ME, London GM: Postischemic vasodilation, endothelial activation, and cardiovascular remodeling in end-stage renal disease. Kidney Int 2000;57:1091–1099.

117 Blacher J, Demuth K, Guerin AP, Safar ME, Moatti N, London GM: Influence of biochemical alterations on arterial stiffness in patients with end-stage renal disease. Arterioscler Thromb Vasc Biol 1998;18:535–541.

118 Bortolotto LA, Safar ME, Billaud E, Lacroix C, Asmar R, London GM, et al: Plasma homocysteine, aortic stiffness, and renal function in hypertensive patients. Hypertension 1999;34:837–842.

119 Yasmin, Falzone R, Brown MJ: Determinants of arterial stiffness in offspring of families with essential hypertension. Am J Hypertens 2004;17:292–298.

120 Wilkinson IB, Megson IL, MacCallum T, Rooijmans DF, Johnson SM, Boyd JL, et al: Acute methionine loading does not alter arterial stiffness in humans. J Cardiovasc Pharmacol 2001;37: 1–5.

121 Nestel PJ, Chronopoulos A, Cehun M: Arterial stiffness is rapidly induced by raising the plasma homocysteine concentration with methionine. Atherosclerosis 2003;171:83–86.

122 Arcaro G, Fava C, Dagradi R, Faccini G, Gaino S, Degan M, et al: Acute hyperhomocysteinemia induces a reduction in arterial distensibility and compliance. J Hypertens 2004;22:775–781.

123 Van Guldener C, Lambert J, ter Wee PM, Donker AJ, Stehouwer CD: Carotid artery stiffness in patients with end-stage renal disease: no effect of long-term homocysteine-lowering therapy. Clin Nephrol 2000;53:33–41.

124 Van Dijk RA, Rauwerda JA, Steyn M, Twisk JW, Stehouwer CD: Long-term homocysteine-lowering treatment with folic acid plus pyridoxine is associated with decreased blood pressure but not with improved brachial artery endothelium-dependent vasodilation or carotid artery stiffness: a 2-year, randomized, placebo-controlled trial. Arterioscler Thromb Vasc Biol 2001;21:2072–2079.

125 Mangoni AA, Sherwood RA, Swift CG, Jackson SH: Folic acid enhances endothelial function and reduces blood pressure in smokers: a randomized controlled trial. J Intern Med 2002;252:497–503.

126 Mangoni AA, Sherwood RA, Asonganyi B, Swift CG, Thomas S, Jackson SH: Short-term oral folic acid supplementation enhances endothelial function in patients with type 2 diabetes. Am J Hypertens 2005;18:220–226.

127 Williams C, Kingwell BA, Burke K, McPherson J, Dart AM: Folic acid supplementation for 3 weeks reduces pulse pressure and large artery stiffness independent of MTHFR genotype. Am J Clin Nutr 2005;82:26–31.

Dr. Coen D.A. Stehouwer
Department of Internal Medicine, University Hospital Maastricht
PO Box 5800, NL–6202 AZ Maastricht (The Netherlands)
Tel. +31 43 387 7006, Fax +31 43 387 5006
E-Mail Csthe@sint.azm.nl

Safar ME, Frohlich ED (eds): Atherosclerosis, Large Arteries and Cardiovascular Risk.
Adv Cardiol. Basel, Karger, 2007, vol 44, pp 302–314

························

Nitrates, Arterial Function, Wave Reflections and Coronary Heart Disease

Harold Smulyan

Department of Medicine, Upstate Medical University, Syracuse, N.Y., USA

Abstract

This chapter traces the history of nitroglycerin from the initial nitration of glycerol
to its widespread clinical use. The pharmacologic differences between nitroglycerin and
nitric oxide are described, as well as their similar mechanisms of action. The vasoactivity
of nitroglycerin requires a biochemical transformation, the nature of which remains incompletely understood. This poorly defined mechanism probably also relates to the phenomenon of nitroglycerin tolerance. By increasing the distensibility of muscular arteries,
nitroglycerin slows pulse wave velocity, reduces wave reflections and alters the shape of
the aortic pulse. This alteration reduces the systolic blood pressure and left ventricular
after load and helps to explain the usefulness of nitroglycerin in angina pectoris, congestive heart failure and isolated systolic hypertension.

History

An Italian chemist, Ascanio Sobrero, working in Paris under the tutelage
of a French chemist, Theophile-Jules Pelouse, accomplished the nitration of
glycerol in 1847. They found that, unless cooled, the compound would deto-
nate. Sobrero also reported that a minute quantity placed on the tongue would
produce a violent headache for several hours. Four years later, Alfred Nobel
visited Pelouse's laboratory and took the compound back to Stockholm, where
he and his father, Immanuel, invented a method to control its detonation. As

is now well known, this invention became a huge commercial success and some of the proceeds were used to found the prize bearing his name. It is ironic that in 1890, Alfred Nobel developed angina pectoris, but refused to take nitroglycerin (NTG) as advised by his physician [1].

After some animal experimentation, the clinical use of nitrates began in 1867, when a Scotsman, Thomas Lauder Brunton, tried it on himself. Experience in the use of NTG in patients grew slowly and was then described for the treatment of angina pectoris by a number of physicians, among them a Londoner, William Murrell [2]. Within a few years, NTG had become accepted as an effective form of therapy. Brunton's seminal work in this field was reviewed in his *Textbook of Pharmacology and Therapeutics* in 1885. The history of NTG and nitric oxide (NO) was well described in greater detail by Marsh and Marsh [1] in 2000.

Mechanism of Action

Although used for more than a century as a treatment for angina pectoris, the mechanism of action of NTG went undiscovered. A near-chance observation, and one that at the time appeared to have little relevance to NTG, was published by Furchgott and Zawadski [3] in 1980. They observed that acetylcholine-induced relaxation of rabbit aortic strips only occurred if the endothelium of these strips was intact. If the endothelium was removed (rubbed off), acetylcholine induced contraction (rather than relaxation) mediated by muscarinic receptors. The requirement for an intact endothelium for acetylcholine to induce smooth muscle relaxation led to the belief that the endothelium had been stimulated to release a relaxing substance. Since the nature of this substance was unknown, it was called endothelium-derived relaxing factor or EDRF. Near-simultaneous investigations by Ignarro et al. [4] and by Palmer et al. [5] later identified EDRF as NO. These fundamental observations had subsequent far-reaching consequences in physiology and medicine that led to the awarding of the Nobel Prize. This award closed a historical/scientific loop that began with the invention of dynamite.

The discovery of the endothelium as an organ with a paracrine function that influenced vascular control led to an explosion of investigations of other physiological functions and pathological disturbances of the endothelium. As far as NO was concerned, it was found that NO was generated by the action of NO synthase, an endothelial enzyme (eNOS) on L-arginine, converting it to L-citrulline. The identification of both the substrate for NO production and a competitive inhibitor of eNOS, N^G-monomethyl-L-arginine, permitted many studies that either stimulated or inhibited the formation of NO in a variety of

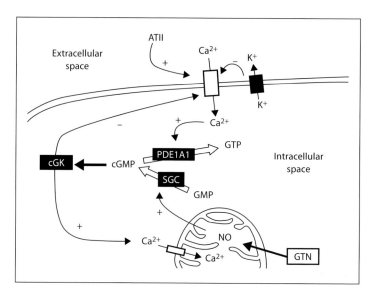

Fig. 1. Mechanisms of action of GTN. GTN is metabolized to NO which stimulates the synthesis of cGMP. In turn, cGMP reduces cytoplasmic Ca2+ by inhibiting inflow and stimulating mitochondrial uptake, causing relaxation of smooth muscle cells. PDE1A1 = Phosphodiesterase 1A1; GTP = guanosine triphosphate; cGMP = cyclic guanosine monophosphate; ATII = angiotensin II; K^+ = potassium currents [7].

vascular beds [6]. Subsequent work also showed that NO produced in the endothelium could diffuse into nearby smooth muscle, where the NO stimulated the synthesis of soluble guanylate cyclase that, in turn, increased the synthesis of cyclic guanosine monophosphate from guanosine triphosphate. It is the guanosine monophosphate that finally leads to smooth muscle relaxation by reducing cytoplasmic calcium. This is accomplished by inhibiting inflow of calcium into the cell and stimulating the uptake of calcium by the mitochondria (fig. 1) [7].

Although the mechanism of action of endogenous NO is now well understood and accepted, the same cannot be said for the biotransformation of NTG and other similar therapeutic drugs into pharmacologically active agents. Since both NTG and nitroprusside (NTP) have vasodilator activity similar to that of NO, it is reasonable to believe that in some way, each contributes NO, or an NO intermediary, to the vasodilation process, but the mechanism(s) by which this takes place is not clear. Initially it was believed that these nitrate donors reacted with cysteine to form unstable intermediate S-nitrosothiols that in turn activated guanylate cyclase [8]. This has not been completely ac-

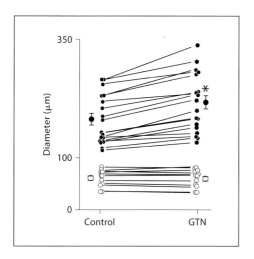

Fig. 2. Coronary arteriolar responses to 10 μM nitroglycerin (GTN). Large symbols represent means for groups with control diameters <100 μm (open circles) and >100 μm (filled circles) ± SEM. GTN dilated large vessels from 183 ± 12 to 218 ± 15 μm but had no effect on small vessels (58.5 ± 5 to 58.9 ± 5 μm). * Different from control value, $p <$ 0.05 [13].

cepted [9] and alternative possibilities have been proposed [10]. The release of NO from the non-organic NTP appears to be less complex and related only to a single electron transfer [9]. These differences in the biotransformation of NTG and NTP help explain some of the other differences in the behavior of these two drugs and from endogenous NO.

Endothelial function may be disturbed either locally or systemically by a variety of clinical conditions such as hypertension, diabetes mellitus or coronary atherosclerosis. This dysfunction of the endothelium reduces the amount and the influence of endogenous NO on vascular tone. But the therapeutically administered nitrate donors bypass endothelium and stimulate smooth muscle relaxation more directly. Although the vasorelaxation induced by both endogenous NO and the nitrate donors are similar, the mechanisms for the release of the active principle from the donor molecules induce some differences in behavior. For example, NO is a potent vasodilator of resistance microvessels of all sizes. But NTG, while successfully dilating microvessels >100 μm in diameter, does not dilate vessels <100 μm (fig. 2). This has been attributed to a suspected relative deficiency of available sulfhydryl groups in the small vessels and their resulting inability to process NTG to an active form – possibly that of nitrosothiols [11–13]. In contrast to NTG, the release of an active principle from NTP is simpler, permitting it to be active in the small microvessels.

Another difference between endothelium-derived NO and therapeutically administered NTG is the development of NTG tolerance. There is no tolerance to NO alone. Initially, tolerance to NTG was attributed to reduced availability of local thiols for the biotransformation of NTG. Since then, many other explanations have been proposed [7, 14]. Of these, two seem more promising than the others. NTG tolerance is associated with increased levels of angiotensin II and some investigators have described the relief of tolerance with both angiotensin-converting enzyme inhibitors and angiotensin receptor blockers. The other plausible explanation for NTG tolerance involves the link with oxidative stress [15]. NO as well as NTG react readily with superoxide radicals to form peroxynitrite – a mystery molecule with both beneficial and harmful effects [15–17]. This binding of therapeutically useful nitrates may explain the reduced endothelial function induced by oxidative stress and the reduced vasodilator effects of continued NTG use. Whether or not antioxidants are useful in the relief of NTG tolerance remains controversial.

Clinical Use

Nitrate donors in frequent clinical use are displayed in figure 3. From a clinical perspective, the circulatory effects of NTG can be viewed in two ways – venous and arterial. As a venodilator, NTG induces venous pooling and reduces venous return. The resulting reduction in ventricular preload has found an important place in the treatment of heart failure [18] – in acute heart failure with intravenous NTG and in chronic heart failure with oral preparations. The venodilatory effect of NTG also plays a role in the relief of angina pectoris by reducing left ventricular end-diastolic pressure, ventricular wall tension and improving subendocardial blood flow. Long-term use of organic nitrates for heart failure has been limited because of nitrate tolerance.

The use of NTG for more than a century in the treatment of angina pectoris has long been attributed to its effects on the arterial side of the circulation. NTG has a powerful dilating effect on muscular arteries. Coronary arteriographic studies have shown increased diameter of normal coronary segments and reduction in the narrowing of coronary stenoses, with a resultant decrease in the resistance to blood flow across these stenoses (fig. 4) [19, 20]. NTG also improves the function of collateral vessels distal to proximal stenoses (fig. 5) [21]. In contrast to inorganic nitrates, as described earlier, NTG must undergo biotransformation before it becomes active. Resistance vessels <100 μm in diameter in the coronary circulation lack the biochemical machinery to activate NTG and are therefore not dilated by the drug. Larger microvessels (>200 μm) are able to biotransform NTG and these vessels are therefore responsive to the

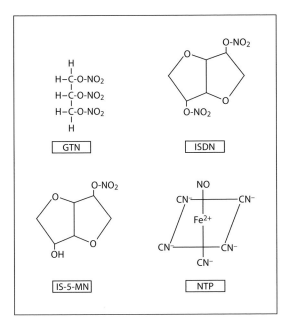

Fig. 3. Chemical structure of selected nitrovasodilators. GTN = Glyceryl trinitrate; ISDN = isosorbide dinitrate; IS-5-MN = isosorbide 5-mononitrate; NTP = nitroprusside [9].

action of NTG. By contrast, NO can dilate all arteriolar sizes [11]. This differential effect of NTG on arterioles of different sizes may play an important role in how NTG relieves angina pectoris. Because the small resistance vessels are not responsive to NTG, the resistance to flow in unobstructed coronary arteries is little changed. But the effect of NTG on flow in stenosed vessels is enhanced by its effect on the larger arterioles and on the epicardial stenoses themselves. This combination acts to reduce or eliminate any 'coronary steal' from affected to unaffected arteries. Such an advantage is not available from the non-organic nitrates.

Effects on Large Arteries

NTG also has differential effects on other parts of the arterial tree. Because the central aortic walls have little in the way of smooth muscle, the effect of NTG in this part of the arterial tree is small [22, 23]. In the walls of the large peripheral arteries however, smooth muscle is abundant and NTG is not only

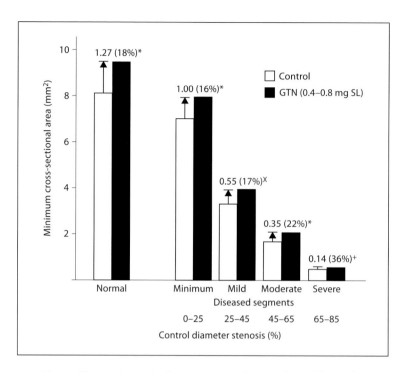

Fig. 4. Change in luminal cross-sectional area after sublingual GTN. The normal lumens are the relatively smooth segments proximal and distal to the stenosis. Narrowed segments are characterized as having minimum, mild, moderate or severe disease, depending on their percent diameter reduction (% stenosis). Each bar represents the average value of all luminal areas in each of the five groups, either before or after GTN. The percent changes reflect the average increase in area for all luminal areas in each of the five groups. [X] $p < 0.05$; * $p < 0.01$; [+] $p < 0.005$ [20].

effective in increasing their diameter but increases their compliance as well (fig. 6) [23, 24]. Therefore, in the central aorta there is little change in pulse wave velocity or stiffness, while in the periphery, pulse wave velocity is reduced and distensibility increased.

These changes in the behavior of the peripheral arterial walls alter the way in which the arterial pulse is transmitted and reflected. Studies in the frequency domain have shown no change in the impedance modulus of the aorta at zero frequency (systemic vascular resistance) from administered NTG, probably due to its lack of effect in the smallest resistance vessels. There was also no change in the characteristic impedance, as indicated above, but there were consistent decreases in the lowest frequency components of the impedance

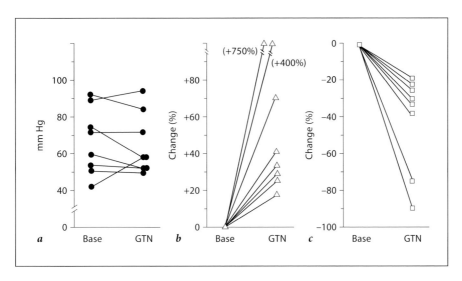

Fig. 5. Aortic pressure (*a*), retrograde flow (*b*) and calculated coronary collateral resistance (*c*) before (Base) and after GTN when aortic pressure decrease is mechanically prevented. In the absence of significant associated aortic pressure drop, GTN induced a uniform and a dramatic rise in retrograde flow and fall in collateral resistance (geometric mean decrease: 50%). Thus a decrease in aortic pressure was not requisite to demonstrate GTN-induced salutary effect on collateral function [21].

modulus, indicating a reduction in the amplitude and delay in the timing of the reflected waves [25, 26]. The results of these changes can be easily seen on the aortic pulse wave itself (fig. 7) [25] where the reflected wave after NTG is of lower amplitude and peaks later in systole. This salutary effect of NTG on the aortic pulse may not be readily observed in the brachial artery pulse. Here, closer to the periphery, the reflected wave more markedly augments the primary systolic wave than it does in the aorta. The result is a higher brachial systolic blood pressure (SBP) than in the aorta (pulse amplification) and indicates to the clinician a smaller reduction in the SBP than that which has occurred centrally [23]. The functional effect of these changes in aortic pulse shape is to lower the SBP with little change in the mean blood pressure. Of the three major determinants of left ventricular afterload, systemic vascular resistance, aortic distensibility and reflected waves, NTG is able to lighten the load on the left ventricle by reducing the effect of reflected waves with little alteration in the other two. The explanation for the reduction in the reflected waves is speculative since the wave reflection sites are multiple and not well defined. If the primary waves are reflected from physiologically abrupt changes in small

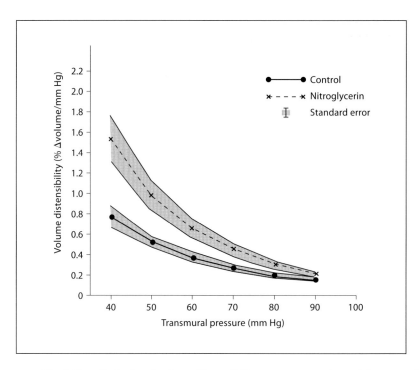

Fig. 6. Plot of calculated volume distensibility vs. transmural arterial pressure before and during nitroglycerin infusion [24].

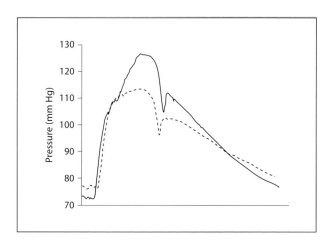

Fig. 7. Effect of sublingual GTN (0.3 mg) on ascending aortic pressure. There is a 15 mm Hg reduction of peak systolic pressure due to a diminution of the late systolic pressure peak. Continuous line denotes control, broken line values after GTN [25].

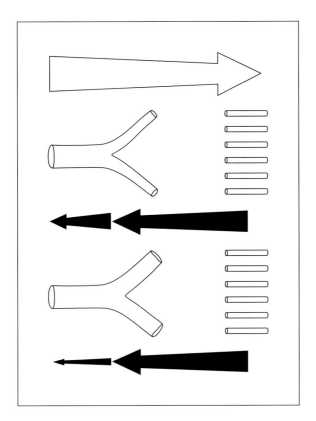

Fig. 8. The proposed mechanism for reduction in peripheral reflection coefficient with GTN. The forward traveling wave is shown above, reflected at the peripheral arterioles indicated at right. The backward traveling reflected wave (dark arrow) is shown in the top panel under control conditions, and in the bottom panel after GTN. Wave reflection at peripheral arterioles is quite unchanged, but amplitude of the backward traveling reflected wave as observed centrally is decreased by negative ('open-ended') reflection at the junctions of parent artery with disproportionately dilated daughter branches [27].

arterial caliber, NTG-induced vasodilation could move those sites distally and help explain the time delay for the reflected wave to return to the central aorta (fig. 8) [27]. Reduced pulse wave velocity in the muscular arteries could also play a role. Relaxation of the larger arterioles (>200 μm) could also reduce the reflection coefficient and thus the magnitude of the reflected wave. Whatever the explanation, NTG effectively reduces left ventricular afterload with little change in mean blood pressure.

Effects in Hypertension

Isolated systolic hypertension in the elderly has been related to the age-induced increase in aortic stiffness. Although the benefits of calcium channel blockers and diuretics have been demonstrated in this disease [28, 29], clinical experience has shown that it is often difficult to lower the brachial artery SBP to the therapeutic target without using uncomfortably large doses. These doses may also induce excessive reductions in diastolic pressures that relate to total and cardiovascular mortality [30]. Greater decreases in diastolic blood pressure than in SBP stress the importance of pulse pressure during therapy as a risk factor. Although organic nitrates may not be able to combat the aortic stiffness of aging, they have a vasorelaxing effect on the peripheral arteries and ameliorate the deleterious effects of strong reflected waves into the aorta. Several small observational studies support this possibility as clinically useful [31–33]. Although the use of nitrates in patients with isolated systolic hypertension whose SBPs are difficult to control seems reasonable, there are no large randomized, controlled trials to support it. Nitrate tolerance could be a problem, but oral administration, once or twice daily, or even 12-hourly nitrate patches might ameliorate this problem. At present, isosorbide might be added with benefit to a conventional regimen in those patients with isolated systolic hypertension who are difficult to treat.

Conclusions

Although organic nitrates have been in clinical use for many years, it is only more recently that their mechanisms of action have been clarified. The complexity of these mechanisms account, in part, for the multiplicity of its clinical activity and the variety of clinical situations in which they find use. These vary from heart failure to angina pectoris, to isolated systolic hypertension. Rather than being supplanted by newer, safer and more effective medications, the nitrates appear firmly established and widely used in their present roles.

References

1   Marsh N, Marsh A: A short history of nitroglycerin and nitric oxide in pharmacology and physiology. Clin Exp Pharmacol Physiol 2000;27:313–319.
2   Murrell W: Nitroglycerin as a remedy for angina pectoris. Lancet 1879;1:80–81.
3   Furchgott RF, Zawadski JV: The obligatory role of endothelial cells in the relaxation of arterial smooth muscle by acetylcholine. Nature 1980;288:373–376.

4   Ignarro LJ, Byrns RE, Buga GM, Wood KS: Endothelium-derived relaxing factor from pulmonary artery and vein possesses pharmacologic and chemical properties identical to those of nitric oxide. Circ Res 1987;61:866–879.

5   Palmer RMJ, Ferrige AG, Moncada S: Nitric oxide release accounts for the biological activity of endothelium-derived relaxing factor. Nature 1987;327:524–526.

6   Moncada S, Higgs A: The L-arginine-nitric oxide pathway. N Engl J Med 1993;329:2002–2012.

7   Gori T, Parker JD: Nitrate tolerance. A unifying hypothesis. Circulation 2002;106:2510–2513.

8   Ignarro LJ: Biological actions and properties of endothelium-derived nitric oxide formed and released from artery and vein. Circ Res 1989;65:1–21.

9   Anderson TJ, Meredith IT, Ganz P, Selwyn AP, Yeung AC: Nitric oxide and nitrovasodilators: similarities, differences and potential interactions. J Am Coll Cardiol 1994;24:555–566.

10 Chen Z, Zhang J, Stamler JS: Identification of the enzymatic mechanism of nitroglycerin bioactivation. Proc Natl Acad Sci USA 2002;99:8306–8311.

11 Sellke FW, Myers PR, Bates JN, Harrison DG: Influence of vessel size on the sensitivity of porcine coronary microvessels to nitroglycerin. Am J Physiol 1990;258:H515–H520.

12 Wheatley RM, Dockery SP, Kurz MA, Sayegh HS, Harrison DG: Interactions of nitroglycerin and sulfhydryl-donating compounds in coronary microvessels. Am J Physiol 1994;266:H291–H297.

13 Kurz MA, Lamping KG, Bates JN, Eastham CL, Marcus ML, Harrison DG: Mechanisms responsible for the heterogeneous coronary microvascular response to nitroglycerin. Circ Res 1991;68:847–855.

14 Gori T, Parker JD: The puzzle of nitrate tolerance: pieces smaller than we thought? Circulation 2002;106:2404–2408.

15 Fayers KE, Cummings MH, Shaw KM, Laight DW: Nitrate tolerance and the links with endothelial dysfunction and oxidative stress. Br J Clin Pharmacol 2003;56:620–628.

16 Liaudet L, Soriano FG, Szabo C: Biology of nitric oxide signaling. Crit Care Med 2000;28:N37–N52.

17 Ronson RS, Nakamura M, Vinten-Johansen J: The cardiovascular effects and implications of peroxynitrite. Cardiovasc Res 1999;44:47–59.

18 Natarajan D, Khurana TR, Karhade V, Nigam PD: Sustained hemodynamic effects with therapeutic doses of intravenous nitroglycerin in congestive heart failure. Am J Cardiol 1988;62:319–321.

19 Feldman RL, Pepine CJ, Conti CR: Magnitude of dilation of large and small coronary arteries by nitroglycerin. Circulation 1981;64:324–333.

20 Brown BG, Bolson E, Petersen RB, Pierce CD, Dodge HT: The mechanisms of nitroglycerin action: stenosis vasodilation as a major component of the drug response. Circulation 1981;64:1089–1097.

21 Goldstein RF, Stinson EB, Scherer JL, Seningen RP, Grehl TM, Epstein SE: Intraoperative coronary collateral function in patients with coronary occlusive disease. Circulation 1974;49:298–308.

22 Latson TW, Hunter WC, Katoh N, Sagawa K: Effect of nitroglycerin on aortic impedance, diameter, and pulse-wave velocity. Circ Res 1988;62:884–890.

23 Nichols WW, O'Rourke MF: Therapeutic strategies; in McDonald's Blood Flow in Arteries, ed 5. London, Hodder Arnold, 2005, chapt 24, pp 435–450.

24 Smulyan H, Mookherjee S, Warner RA: The effect of nitroglycerin on forearm arterial distensibility. Circulation 1986;73:1264–1269.

25 Fitchett DH, Simkus GJ, Beaudry JP, Marpole DG: Reflected pressure waves in the ascending aorta: effect of glyceryl trinitrate. Cardiovasc Res 1988;22:494–500.

26 Soma J, Angelsen BA, Aakhus S, Skjaerpe T: Sublingual nitroglycerin delays arterial wave reflections despite increased aortic 'stiffness' in patients with hypertension: a Doppler echocardiography study. J Am Soc Echocardiogr 2000;13:1100–1108.

27 Yaginuma T, Avolio A, O'Rourke M, Nichols W, Morgan JJ, Roy P, Baron D, Branson J, Feneley M: Effect of glyceryl trinitrate on peripheral arteries alters left ventricular hydraulic load in man. Cardiovasc Res 1986;20:153–160.

28   SHEP Cooperative Research Group: Prevention of stroke by antihypertensive drug treatment in older persons with isolated systolic hypertension. Final results of the Systolic Hypertension in the Elderly Program (SHEP). JAMA 1991;265:3255–3264.

29   Staessen JA, Fagard R, Thijs L, Celis H, Arabidze GG, Birkenhager WH, Bulpitt CJ, de Leeuw PW, Dollery CT, Fletcher AE, Forette F, Leonetti G, Nachev C, O'Brien ET, Rosefeld J, Rodicio JL, Tuomilehto J, Zanchetti A, for the Systolic Hypertension in Europe (SYST-EUR) Trial Investigators. Lancet 1997;350:757–764.

30   Staessen JA, Gasowski J, Wang JG, Thijs L, Den Hond E, Biossel JP, Coope J, Ekbom T, Gueyffier F, Liu L, Kerlikowske K, Pocock S, Fagard RH: Risks of untreated and treated isolated systolic hypertension in the elderly: meta-analysis of outcome trials. Lancet 2000;355:865–872.

31   Duchier J, Iannascoli F, Safar M: Antihypertensive effect of sustained-release isosorbide dinitrate for isolated systolic hypertension in the elderly. Am J Cardiol 1987;60:99–102.

32   Stokes GS, Ryan M, Brnabic A, Nyberg G: A controlled study of the effects of isosorbide mononitrate on arterial blood pressure and pulse wave form in systolic hypertension. J Hypertens 1999;17:1767–1773.

33   Stokes GS, Barin ES, Gilfillan KL: Effects of isosorbide mononitrate and AII inhibition on pulse wave reflection in hypertension. Hypertension 2003;41:297–301.

Harold Smulyan
Department of Medicine, Upstate Medical University, Health Science Center
Syracuse, NY 13210 (USA)
Tel. +1 315 464 56 63, Fax +1 315 464 5797
E-Mail smulyanh@upstate.edu

Safar ME, Frohlich ED (eds): Atherosclerosis, Large Arteries and Cardiovascular Risk.
Adv Cardiol. Basel, Karger, 2007, vol 44, pp 315–330

······················

Modulation of Atherosclerosis, Blood Pressure and Arterial Elasticity by Statins

Anjan K. Sinha   *Jawahar L. Mehta*

Division of Cardiovascular Medicine, University of Arkansas for Medical Sciences
and Central Arkansas Veterans Healthcare Center, Little Rock, Ark., USA

Abstract

It is well known that dyslipidemia and hypertension frequently coexist. There is increasing recognition of a mutually facilitative interaction between dyslipidemia and renin-angiotensin system (RAS) activation in the development of atherosclerosis. Both of
these systems share many of the same properties in terms of activation of pro-inflammatory, pro-oxidant and pro-atherosclerosis pathways. Statins in particular have been shown
to influence the biology of endothelial cells, vascular smooth muscle cells and constituents
of the interstitial matrix, particularly fibroblasts. It is no wonder that concurrent therapy
of dyslipidemia with statins enhances the effects of RAS inhibitors. Although the effects
of statins on the regulation of determinants of vascular stiffness are not well defined, it is
quite likely that these regulatory pathways will be influenced by dyslipidemia therapy,
especially statins.

Introduction

Cardiovascular disease is the most common cause of morbidity and mortality in developed countries. This is related mainly to atherosclerotic disease
in the arterial system. Anatomically speaking, the arterial wall becomes thick-
ened with an inward narrowing, while physiologically speaking, the arterial
wall loses its elasticity.

Atherosclerosis is an ongoing process that continues to develop and re-
model over time, ranging from macroscopically intact arteries in the early
stages to ruptured atherosclerotic plaque resulting in an acute event. The
pathogenesis of atherosclerosis comprises various steps, including endothelial

activation or dysfunction, expression of adhesion molecules, monocyte adhesion and migration, foam cell formation, development of fatty streak, smooth muscle cell (SMC) migration and plaque formation, and, finally, plaque rupture or intraplaque hemorrhage. The rupture occurs in part because of the break in the fibrous plaque covering the lipid-filled plaque. Since thrombus formation is the most important event in the evolution of an acute vascular event, the process has become known as atherothrombosis.

In recent years, atherosclerosis has been recognized as a chronic inflammatory process. The atherosclerotic vessel expresses a variety of pro-inflammatory genes, proteins, and growth factors as seen in chronic inflammation. Inflammatory cells, such as monocytes, are found in early atherosclerotic lesions, while the more advanced lesions contain a large number of T and B lymphocytes reminiscent of an immune response [1]. There is convincing clinical and experimental evidence that there is a state of oxidative stress during the entire process of atherogenesis due to an imbalance between synthesis of oxidants and availability of neutralizing anti-oxidants [2]. Both inflammatory and oxidative processes are intimately involved in determining the elasticity of the vessel as well as formation of the fibrous cap over the atherosclerotic plaque.

HMG-CoA reductase inhibitors (commonly known as statins) have evolved to be viewed as potent antiatherosclerotic agents, and their use is now the cornerstone of therapy for patients with atherosclerotic disease. The aim of this review is to discuss the role of statins as it relates to atherosclerosis, blood pressure and arterial elasticity.

Pleiotropic Effects of Statins

The word 'pleiotropic' usually is applied to genetics, referring to the multiple actions of a single gene. With regard to statin therapy for dyslipidemia, the term has become synonymous with clinical benefits of statins beyond the effects on lipoproteins.

Hypercholesterolemia is strongly associated with coronary and vascular atherosclerotic disease. Atherosclerosis is mediated, in part, by the uptake of modified low-density lipoprotein (LDL) into the vessel wall. The predominant mechanism underlying the beneficial effects of statins is the inhibition of the enzyme HMG-CoA, thus blocking the early rate-limiting step in cholesterol biosynthesis. Therapeutic doses of statins reduce serum total and LDL cholesterol levels markedly in humans.

Several large primary and secondary prevention trials have demonstrated that these agents decrease the incidence of cardiovascular events in hypercholesterolemic individuals [3]. However, this benefit is also evident in individuals without a significantly high cholesterol level. This has led to the hypothesis that statins may exert protective effects beyond cholesterol reduction. This was first noted in the subgroup analyses of the West of Scotland Coronary Prevention Study (WOSCOPS) [4], which suggested that statin-treated subjects had a significantly lower risk of coronary heart disease events than seen in the age-matched, placebo-treated individuals, despite comparable serum cholesterol levels. Further, meta-analyses of past clinical trials have revealed that the risk of cardiovascular events in individuals treated with statins is significantly less than in individuals treated with other cholesterol-lowering agents or modalities, despite similar reduction in serum cholesterol levels in both groups.

Mechanistic Basis of the Efficacy of Statins in Atherothrombosis

In addition to their well-documented effects on serum lipid levels, there are several other postulated mechanisms by which statins exert a variety of beneficial effects on the determinants of atherothrombosis. These effects are summarized in table 1. Most of these effects have been attributed to the modification of the altered biology of endothelial cells and vascular SMCs as well as coagulation and platelet activation pathways. In particular, statins enhance the activity of endothelial nitric oxide synthase (eNOS) and thereby the biosynthesis of the potent vasodilator and platelet inhibitor NO in vascular endothelial cells [5]. Statins also prevent degradation of NO by inhibiting the generation of oxidant species. Statins inhibit pre-proET-1 mRNA expression and reduce ET-1 release in bovine endothelial cells [6]. Recent studies show that statins decrease angiotensin II type 1 receptor expression in SMCs which is another potent vasoconstrictor and pro-fibrotic stimulus [7]. In addition, statins promote vasculogenesis and bone formation [8] and inhibit SMC proliferation and migration. Many of these effects are unrelated to the lowering of LDL cholesterol and may involve reduction in the prenylation of proteins.

It is well known that the enzyme HMG-CoA reductase catalyzes the conversion of HMG-CoA into mevalonate, the rate-limiting step in cholesterol synthesis. Mevalonate is not only the precursor of cholesterol, but also of the isoprenoids farnesyl-pyrophosphate and geranylgeranyl-pyrophosphates. Isoprenoids play an important role in the post-translational lipid modification of regulatory proteins such as G proteins, Ras, Rho, and Rab [9]. Covalently linked to these proteins, isoprenoids allow their membrane localization and function. Thus, besides inhibiting the synthesis of cholesterol, statins may also reduce the prenylation of proteins involved in cell signaling, cell proliferation and intracellular trafficking. Recently, a new immunomodulatory effect of statins was described which, in contrast to previously described effects, is not

Table 1. Non-lipid-lowering effects of statins

Anti-thrombotic effects	Reduction in PAI-1 Increase in t-PA Increase in NOS expression and activity Reduction in tissue factor expression Reduction in fibrinogen Decreased platelet aggregation Increase in thrombomodulin
Effects on endothelial cell biology	Enhanced eNOS expression and activity Reduction in genes for leukocyte adhesion and inflammatory signals Reduction in endothelial permeability Increased endothelial growth Increase in endothelial progenitor cells/angiogenesis Reduction in pre-pro-ET-1 expression
Effects on vascular smooth muscle cells	Reduction in VSMC growth and migration Decrease in expression of AT1 receptor in response to injurious stimuli
Miscellaneous effects	Reduction in generation of oxidant species Increase in gene expression of antioxidants Decrease in fibroblast growth and collagen formation Inhibition of LDL oxidation and ox-LDL uptake Inhibition of mitogen-stimulated T- and B-lymphocyte proliferation Inhibition of expression of class II MHC Blockade of the effects of angiotensin II Inhibitor of natural killer cell cytotoxicity Stimulation of bone formation

mediated by the blockade of HMG-CoA reductase [10]. This statin effect involves the inhibition of the integrin lymphocyte function-associated antigen-1 (LFA-1, αLβ2, CD11a/CD18).

Studies from our and other laboratories indicate that the expression of a lectin-like receptor for ox-LDL (LOX-1) is upregulated in atherosclerotic lesions [11, 12], and the increased expression of LOX-1 promotes the pathobiological effects of ox-LDL and lysophosphatidylcholine [12, 13]. Li et al. [14] showed that statins inhibit the uptake of ox-LDL in human coronary artery endothelial cells and thereby the expression of LOX-1. Enhanced activity of protein kinase B (PKB/Akt), a cell survival kinase, appears to be relevant in the effect of statins in the expression of LOX-1 in HCAECs [14]. Inhibition of LOX-1 may also be the mechanism by which statins upregulate eNOS expression [15]. Other studies from our laboratory [15] show that LOX-1 expression and activation result in the release of metalloproteinases (MMPs) and the expression of pro-inflammatory signals such as CD40 and CD40L. Cola et al. [16], from our laboratory, showed that endothelium, when exposed to atherogenic stimuli, ox-LDL in particular, regulates the process of calcification by enhancing the expression of the bone inhibitory matrix gla-protein (MGP), a potent inhibitor of calcification, while the expression of core binding factor-α_1 (Cbfa1/Runx2), a pivotal transcriptional regulator of osteogenesis, remains unchanged. The effect of pro-atherogenic stimuli appears to be mediated by LOX-1 activation. It is likely that the modification of bone-forming proteins is an important activity of the statin group of drugs.

Plasminogen activator inhibitor type-1 (PAI-1) is an endogenous inhibitor of tissue plasminogen activator (t-PA) which is crucial in the regulation of fibrinolysis, atherosclerosis, and tissue remodeling. PAI-1 expression has been shown to be enhanced in human atherosclerotic lesions, and PAI-1 knockout mice have diminished formation of atherosclerotic lesions [17]. These data suggest a powerful role of PAI-1 in the pro-atherogenic and pro-thrombotic processes. A decrease in PAI-1 and an increase in t-PA have been observed after treatment of endothelial cells with statins. These agents have also been shown to reduce tissue factor and fibrinogen availability, and enhance thrombomodulin secretion [18]. Platelets are also key elements in the pathophysiology of acute coronary syndrome. Platelet aggregation is reduced by administration of statins. All these effects may participate in inhibiting the thrombosis part of atherothrombosis.

SMC proliferation is seen in several vascular processes, such as post-angioplasty restenosis, transplant arteriosclerosis and saphenous vein graft occlusion. Statins appear to attenuate vascular proliferative disease in post-transplant settings. Coupled with the effects described above, inhibition of SMC proliferation and inhibition of the coagulation cascade is a major component of the benefits of statins.

Reactive oxygen species (ROS) affect vascular function. Statins attenuate the Ang II-induced ROS production in vascular smooth cells [19]. Statins decrease the number of inflammatory cells in atherosclerotic plaques and thereby exert anti-inflammatory effects on the vascular wall.

Relevant Vascular Effects of Statins

Endothelial Function

Endothelium is a key element in the pathophysiology of coronary and vascular atherosclerotic disease processes. Endothelial function is altered early during the atherosclerotic process into an activated state. Endothelial activation involves a pro-inflammatory, pro-proliferative, and pro-coagulant state which promotes inflammation and thrombosis.

High cholesterol levels initiate endothelial activation followed by its dysfunction, which is observed even before plaque formation. Endothelial activation and dysfunction may relate to the decreased bioavailability of vasodilators such as NO, and/or excess of vasoconstrictors such as endothelin. High cholesterol concentrations are responsible for endothelial activation, since endothelial function promptly improves after plasma LDL aphaeresis. This may explain the beneficial effects of statins which have a potent LDL-lowering property.

However, in some studies restoration of endothelial function occurred even before a significant reduction in serum cholesterol levels was evident, suggesting that there are also cholesterol-independent effects of statins by which endothelial function improves [20].

Improvement in NO release with statins is associated with upregulation of eNOS mRNA and improvement of endothelial function. Since statins also increase NO production in humans at clinically relevant doses, this effect of statins on endothelial function has been studied in hyper- and normocholesterolemic individuals. In randomized, placebo-controlled, double-blind studies, statins alone or with anti-oxidant therapy significantly increased the bioavailability of NO in hypercholesterolemic patients [21, 22]. The improvement in endothelial function occurred as early as within 1 month of treatment.

Inflammation

A wide array of inflammatory cells such as monocytes, macrophages, and T lymphocytes are observed in atheroma, which suggests complex inflammatory process in atherosclerosis. These inflammatory cells secrete cytokines, thereby modifying endothelial function, SMC proliferation, collagen degradation, and thrombosis. Statins possess anti-inflammatory properties because of their ability to reduce the number of inflammatory cells in atherosclerotic plaques. Inhibition of adhesion molecules, such as intercellular adhesion molecule-1 (ICAM-1), by statins is one mechanism which leads to a reduced recruitment of inflammatory cells under statin treatment. Expression of LOX-1, which is observed to be upregulated early during atherogenesis, is also a potent pro-inflammatory signal, since it is associated with the upregulation of a variety of other pro-inflammatory signals. LOX-1 expression and its activation are both suppressed by statins [23]. High levels of C-reactive protein (CRP), released from the liver in response to the inflammatory cytokine IL-6, are often observed in the setting of coronary and vascular atherosclerotic disease. In hypercholesterolemic patients, statin therapy lowers CRP levels. In cultured endothelial cells, all statins reduce the mRNA and protein for CRP, showing an independent effect of statins on CRP release [24]. In clinical studies involving thousands of patients (CARE and AFCAPS/TexCAP) [25, 26], statins were shown to be effective in reducing clinical events in patients with previous events as well as in those at risk of developing events. Importantly, statins were particularly effective in those who had elevated cholesterol as well as CRP levels, suggesting that part of the benefit of statins may be derived from their anti-inflammatory effect.

Role of Fibroblasts

There is renewed interest in the biology of fibroblasts in atherogenesis. Since fibroblasts generate collagen and the matrix-degrading MMPs, these cells play a powerful role in the regulation of the structural integrity of the vessel wall. There is only scant data on the effects of statins on fibroblast biology. Recent data from our laboratory suggest that statins can reduce the expression of pro-collagen without a significant effect on the release of MMPs in cultured mice fibroblasts exposed to Ang II [Chen et al., unpubl. data]. Fukumoto et al. [27] showed that statins can reduce MMP expression in atheroma and that cell-permeant statins can decrease SMC number and collagen gene expression in the rabbit atheroma. These observations support the contention of Bauersachs et al. [28] that statin use improves left ventricular function and collagen I synthesis in rats with experimental myocardial infarction and subsequent cardiac remodeling. On the other hand, Maeda et al. [29] observed that simvastatin slightly increased the type I collagen mRNA abundance throughout the osteoblast cell line, and markedly inhibited the gene expression of collagenase-1 between days 14 and 22 of culture. The latter effect may be salutary in bone formation.

Statins and Blood Pressure

Interaction of Dyslipidemia and Renin-Angiotensin System (RAS)

Interactions between dyslipidemia and activation of neurohumoral systems, such as RAS, may not only explain the frequent coexistence of hypertension and dyslipidemia, but also play an important role in the pathogenesis of atherosclerosis. Experimental data suggest that the effects of Ang II and lipoproteins on atherogenic risk are not independent and that the pathways by which Ang II and dyslipidemia lead to vascular disease may frequently overlap. There is a suggestion that the combined use of cholesterol-lowering drugs along with agents that modulate RAS may have additive benefits in the prevention and treatment of coronary artery disease, hypertension, and heart failure.

Keidar et al. [30] harvested macrophages from the peritoneum after injection of Ang II in the rat, and observed that Ang II dramatically increased macrophage cellular cholesterol biosynthesis with no significant effect on blood pressure or on plasma cholesterol levels. Fosinopril and the AT1 receptor blocker (losartan) decreased cholesterol biosynthesis in response to Ang II. Further, in cells that lack the AT1 receptor (RAW macrophages), Ang II did not increase cellular cholesterol synthesis, thereby confirming the role of AT1 receptor in Ang II-mediated cholesterol synthesis by macrophages.

Increased oxidative stress is regarded an important feature of hypercholesterolemic atherosclerosis. LDL enhances Ang II AT1 receptor expression in cultured SMCs, and atherosclerotic lesions are associated with increased angiotensin-converting enzyme (ACE) expression, which may serve as a source of local production of Ang II and ultimately increased stimulation of superoxide anion production. Experimental studies have shown that dyslipidemia activates RAS. All components of increased RAS activation have been identified in hyperlipidemic atherosclerotic lesions. These include, in particular, increased expression of ACE and AT1 receptor [31]. A number of recent studies in human atherosclerotic tissues have confirmed the upregulation of ACE and AT1 receptors, particularly in the regions that are prone to plaque rupture. Importantly, these same areas show extensive inflammatory cell deposits, macrophage accumulation, and apoptosis.

In vitro studies have shown that incubation of vascular SMCs with LDL increases expression of the AT1 receptors. Li et al. [32] in our laboratory examined the expression of Ang II receptors in human coronary artery endothelial cells and observed that ox-LDL increases the mRNA and protein for AT1, but not AT2, receptors, implying that ox-LDL increases AT1 expression at the transcriptional level. In this process, activation of the redox-sensitive transcription factor NF-κB plays a critical role. In recent studies, we showed that ox-LDL also enhances ACE expression in human coronary artery endothelial cells.

The association of hypertension with hyperlipidemia has been noted in population studies as well. The prevalence of hypertension is greater in populations with high cholesterol. Sung et al. [33] examined the blood pressure response to a standard mental arithmetic test in 37 healthy normotensive subjects with hypercholesterolemia and 33 normotensive subjects with normal cholesterol levels. The blood pressure response during the arithmetic test was significantly higher in the hypercholesterolemic group compared to the normocholesterolemic group. In a double-blind, crossover design, treatment with statins was associated with lower mean systolic blood pressure prior to and during the arithmetic test. These observations suggest that individuals with hypercholesterolemia have exaggerated systolic blood pressure responses to mental stress, and the lipid lowering improves systolic blood pressure response to stress. Nazzaro et al. [34] made an interesting observation of combined and distinct effects of ACE inhibitors and statins on blood pressure. They examined the effects of lipid lowering on blood pressure in a study of 30 subjects with coexisting hypertension and hypercholesterolemia. The combination of statins and ACE inhibitor achieved greater blood pressure reduction than either alone.

To define the relationship of RAS and lipids in humans, Nickenig et al. [35] administered Ang II in normocholesterolemic and hypercholesterolemic men and found that blood pressure was exaggerated in the hypercholesterolemic group and this response could be blunted by LDL cholesterol-lowering agents. Further, these investigators found that there was a linear relationship between AT1 receptor density on platelets and LDL cholesterol concentration in plasma. Further, treatment with statins decreased AT1 receptor density. Statin-mediated downregulation of AT1 receptor expression has also been shown in vascular SMCs. A recent study has indeed shown that statins directly decrease AT1 receptor expression in endothelial cells.

Atherosclerosis is inhibited by fosinopril and losartan in animal studies, suggesting that the antiatherosclerotic effects of RAS inhibitors may be due, at least in part, to direct inhibition of LDL oxidation and other actions of Ang II in the vessel wall. In order to examine the direct contribution of RAS in dyslipidemic atherosclerosis, we recently conducted a study in apoE knockout mice fed a high cholesterol diet. Treatment of these animals with candesartan, an AT1 receptor blocker, decreased the extent of atherosclerosis as did the treatment with the potent HMG-CoA reductase inhibitor rosuvastatin. More importantly, we observed that concurrent therapy with candesartan and rosuvastatin almost completely abolished atherogenesis. In concert with prevention of atherogenesis, the animals treated with the combination of anti-hypertensive and anti-dyslipidemic therapy had ablation of inflammatory signals – ICAM-1, VCAM-1, MCP-1, CD40/CD40L and expression of LOX-1.

These findings unarguably suggest a mutually facilitative interaction between dyslipidemia and RAS in relation to atherogenesis and development of hypertension. These observations also suggest that inflammatory signals are also related to dyslipidemia and RAS activation. Notably, a similar interaction between altered biosynthesis of NO as well as vasoconstrictor autacoids, such as endothelin-1 and leukotrienes, has also been implicated in this vascular dysfunction [36, 37].

Clinical Evidence of Cross-Talk between Dyslipidemia and RAS Activation

O'Callaghan et al. [38] examined the effects of pravastatin in the setting of background antihypertensive therapy with ACE inhibitors and calcium antagonists. They treated 25 hypertensive hypercholesterolemic patients with 12 weeks of either pravastatin or placebo in this double-blind, placebo-controlled parallel group study. Placebo treatment did not alter plasma lipids, whereas 12 weeks of treatment with pravastatin reduced total cholesterol by 27% and LDL cholesterol by 35%. There was no change in systolic or diastolic blood pressure following 12 weeks of treatment or 3 weeks of withdrawal of pravastatin. Sposito et al. [39] demonstrated an additional effect of statins on blood pressure reduction by comparing patients receiving ACE inhibitors alone with those receiving these medications plus statins after 3 months of dietary intervention. Although blood pressure was similarly reduced at week 4, the statin-treated group had a greater reduction in blood pressure and total cholesterol levels at week 16, suggesting a synergistic effect between cholesterol-lowering with statins and ACE inhibitor treatment for hypertensive patients. Borghi et al. [40] compared the extent of blood pressure changes in 41 patients with hypertension and hypercholesterolemia taking antihypertensive drugs and treated for 3 months with statins (pravastatin or simvastatin) with matched controls with high or normal serum cholesterol undergoing antihypertensive treatment combined with dietary treatment alone. After 3 months of follow-up, a greater reduction of systolic and diastolic blood pressure values was observed in the statin recipients. In the statin-treated patients, a slight linear relation was found between changes in diastolic blood pressure and those in plasma total cholesterol. This study demonstrated that the use of statins in combination with antihypertensive drugs can improve blood pressure control in patients with uncontrolled hypertension and high serum cholesterol levels. The additional blood pressure reduction observed in patients treated with statins is clinically relevant and only partially related to the lipid-lowering effect [40]. Several other small studies have also shown that lipid-lowering treatment with statins may have a blood pressure-lowering effect. Some of the important studies are summarized in table 2.

Effects of Statins on Vascular Elasticity

Determinant of Vascular Elasticity and Compliance
Vascular elasticity or compliance or stiffness is a major determinant of vascular resistance. The elasticity is determined by all components of the vessel wall, including the endothelium, SMCs, and the interstitium composed primarily of fibroblasts.

Table 2. Evidence for blood pressure-lowering effect of statins

Author	Study outline	Statin used	Outcome
Abetel et al. [49]	23 patients with hypertension and hyperlipidemia	Fluvastatin 40 mg for 3 months	Fluvastatin lowered blood pressure by 8–16 mm Hg
Borghi et al. [40]	Patients with hypertension and hyperlipidemia	Statins (pravastatin or simvastatin) in addition to antihypertensive treatment	Additive benefit of statins in lowering blood pressure
Glorioso et al. [50]	25 patients with hypertension and hyperlipidemia	Pravastatin 20–40 mg vs. placebo for 32 weeks	Pravastatin decreased systolic blood pressure by 8 mm Hg
O'Callaghan et al. [38]	25 patients with hypertension and hyperlipidemia	Pravastatin vs. placebo for 12 weeks	Pravastatin did not lower blood pressure
Sposito et al. [39]	Patients with hypertension and hyperlipidemia	ACE inhibitor (enalapril or lisinopril) alone or with statin (lovastatin or pravastatin)	Additive blood pressure-lowering effect of the combination compared to ACE inhibitor alone
Tonolo et al. [51]	26 microalbuminuric hypertensive type 2 diabetic patients	Simvastatin in addition to antihypertensive treatment	Simvastatin exerted additional blood pressure-lowering effect and also reduced 24-hour urinary albumin excretion
Ferrier et al. [53]	22 normolipidemic patients with stage I isolated systolic hypertension	Atorvastatin therapy (80 mg/day) and placebo for 3 months in cross-over design	Intensive cholesterol reduction with atorvastatin reduced large artery stiffness and blood pressure in normo-cholesterolemic patients with stage I isolated systolic hypertension

The effects of statins on endothelium have been amply described, and include an increase in eNOS expression (and activity). Statins also reduce the generation of oxidant species in endothelial cells. These effects appear to be dose-dependent and are shared by all statins with minor inter-statin variability. Schmalfuss et al. [41], in our laboratory, examined the effects of different statins on vascular endothelial cell growth. Whereas atorvastatin and simvastatin reduced endothelial cell growth in culture, pravastatin did not affect it.

Increase in endothelial progenitor cells or neovascularization has been described with all statins with increasing regularity. How this phenomenon correlates with alteration in elasticity is not clear. Cooke [42] suggested that lower dosages of statins may be pro-angiogenic whereas the higher doses may be anti-angiogenic. The precise mechanism of increase in vascularity with statins is not known, but activation of protein kinase B/Akt, the cell survival signal related to generation of NO, has been thought to be responsible for this phenomenon.

Increased formation and activity of NO may influence arterial SMC contractile activity and proliferation. The reduction in vascular SMC proliferation and disarrayed growth may also be involved in salutary effects of statins on vascular compliance. In this regard, decrease in AT1R expression may also contribute to the improvement of the contractile response of vascular SMCs.

The interstitium, consisting primarily of fibroblasts, affects vascular compliance by generation of collagen and collagen-degrading enzymes. Reduced vascular elasticity (and loss of compliance) is often observed in hypertension, diabetes mellitus and aging. Dechend et al. [43] showed that cerivastatin reduced pro-fibrotic response in the hearts of rats made transgenic for human renin and angiotensinogen. Patel et al. [44] also showed reduced fibrosis in response to simvastatin in β-myocyte heavy-chain transgenic mice. The studies on improvement in cardiac diastolic as well as systolic function, a reflection of cardiovascular system compliance with statins, were reviewed recently by Reddy et al. [45].

Although there are very few studies relating to arterial compliance and elasticity with statins, one study is particularly noteworthy. Dougherty et al. [46] examined the effect of Ang II infusion on aortic anatomical changes in the aorta and noted formation of microaneurysms. Interesting, the formation of microaneurysms was greater in hypercholesterolemic mice, showing the importance of cross-talk between dyslipidemia and RAS.

The effects of statins on elasticity are not as well studied, and there is paucity of literature in this area. Ichihara et al. [47] recently reported the differential effect of statins on aortic stiffness. In this single-blind, randomized prospective study, 85 hyperlipidemic, hypertensive patients were followed for 12 months. Aortic stiffness was assessed by measuring pulse wave velocity every 3 months. Patients were randomly allocated to groups treated with pravastatin, simvastatin, fluvastatin, or a non-statin antihyperlipidemic drug. During the 12-month treatment period, pulse wave velocity did not change in the pravastatin group or the non-statin group, but it was transiently reduced in the simvastatin group and significantly decreased in the fluvastatin group. Notably, the doses of the statins used in this study were lower than the usually prescribed dose. All four antihyperlipidemic drugs significantly decreased serum cholesterol levels without affecting blood pressure, ankle brachial index, or serum triglyceride levels. These results suggest that long-term use of statins in hyperlipidemic, hypertensive patients is associated with a significant reduction in aortic stiffness without any effect on blood pressure.

Raison et al. [48] assessed arterial stiffness in 23 patients, aged 32–70 years, who had hypertension and hypercholesterolemia. Subjects received either atorvastatin or a placebo. Aortic stiffness was measured from aortic pulse wave velocity after a 12-week treatment. The results revealed that atorvastatin did not change blood pressure; however, it significantly lowered plasma total and LDL cholesterol and increased aortic pulse wave velocity by +8 vs. 2% under placebo. The percentage changes in plasma total and LDL cholesterol and in pulse wave velocity were significantly and negatively correlated, independent of blood pressure level. These results support the possibility that statins might contribute to a change in arterial stiffness independent of blood pressure level.

Kontopoulos et al. [52] assessed the effect of atorvastatin on aortic stiffness in hypercholesterolemic patients free of arterial hypertension and diabetes mellitus. Thirty-six patients (18 with coronary artery disease and 18 without coronary artery disease) received atorvastatin for a 2-year period. As expected, total cholesterol, LDL cholesterol, triglycerides and high-density lipoprotein cholesterol levels changed favorably. Aortic stiffness was assessed by transthoracic echocardiography at baseline and 2 years later. After 2-years' treatment with atorvastatin, aortic stiffness was significantly reduced by 14% (p = 0.019) which was similar in patients with or without coronary artery disease. Ferrier et al. [53] investigated the effect of high-dose atorvastatin on large artery stiffness and blood pressure in normolipidemic patients with isolated systolic hypertension. Atorvastatin 80 mg/day and placebo were used for 3 months in a randomized, double-blind, cross-over study design. Systemic arterial compliance was measured non-invasively using carotid applanation tonometry and Doppler velocimetry of the ascending aorta. Systemic arterial compliance was higher after treatment (placebo vs. atorvastatin: 0.36 ± 0.03 vs. 0.43 ± 0.05 ml/mm Hg, p = 0.03) whereas brachial systolic, mean and diastolic blood pressures were lower after treatment.

Conclusion

It is quite evident that dyslipidemia and hypertension frequently coexist. There is increasing recognition of a mutually facilitative interaction between dyslipidemia and RAS activation in the development of atherosclerosis. Both share many of the same properties in terms of activation of pro-inflammatory, pro-oxidant, and pro-atherosclerosis pathways. It is no wonder that the concurrent therapy of dyslipidemia with statins enhances the effects of RAS inhibitors. Although the effects of statins on regulation of determinants of vascular stiffness are not well defined, it is quite likely that these regulatory pathways will be influenced by dyslipidemia therapy, especially statins.

References

1 Frostegard J, Ulfgren AK, Nyberg P, Hedin U, Swedenborg J, Andersson U, Hansson GK: Cytokine expression in advanced human atherosclerotic plaques: Dominance of pro-inflammatory (Th1) and macrophage-stimulating cytokines. Atherosclerosis 1999;145:33–43.

2 McEwen JE, Zimniak P, Mehta JL, Reis RJ: Molecular pathology of aging and its implications for senescent coronary atherosclerosis. Curr Opin Cardiol 2005;20:399–406.

3 Scandinavian Simvastatin Survival Study (4S): Randomised trial of cholesterol lowering in 4,444 patients with coronary heart disease. Lancet 1994;344:1383–1389.

4 West of Scotland Coronary Prevention Study (WOSCOPS): Influence of pravastatin and plasma lipids on clinical events in the WOSCOPS. Circulation 1998;97:1440–1445.

5 Mehta JL, Li DY, Chen HJ, Joseph J, Romeo F: Inhibition of LOX-1 by statins may relate to up-regulation of eNOS. Biochem Biophys Res Commun 2001;289:857–861.

6 Hernandez-Perera O, Perez-Sala D, Navarro-Antolin J, Sanchez-Pascuala R, Hernandez G, Lamas S: Effects of the 3-hydroxy-3-methylglutaryl-CoA reductase inhibitors, atorvastatin and simvastatin, on the expression of endothelin-1 and endothelial nitric oxide synthase in vascular endothelial cells. J Clin Invest 1998;101:2711–2719.

7 Nickenig G, Baumer AT, Temur Y, Kebben D, Jockenhovel F, Bohm M: Statin-sensitive dysregulated AT1 receptor function and density in hypercholesterolemic men. Circulation 1999;100:2131–2134.

8 Mundy G, Garrett R, Harris S, Chan J, Chen D, Rossini G, Boyce B, Zhao M, Guttierrez G: Stimulation of bone formation in vitro and in rodents by statins. Science 1999;286:1946–1949.

9 Holstein SA, Wohlford-Lenane CL, Hohl RJ: Consequences of mevalonate depletion. Differential transcriptional, translational, and post-translational up-regulation of Ras, Rap1a, RhoA, and RhoB. J Biol Chem 2002;277:10678–10682.

10 Weitz-Schmidt G, Welzenbach K, Brinkmann V, Kamata T, Kallen J, Bruns C, Cotten S, Takada Y, Hommel U: Statins selectively inhibit leukocyte function antigen-1 by binding to a novel regulatory integrin site. Nat Med 2001;7:687–692.

11 Kume N, Murase T, Moriwaki H, Aoyama T, Sawamura T, Masaki T, Kita T: Inducible expression of lectin-like oxidized LDL receptor-1 in vascular endothelial cells. Circ Res 1998;83:322–327.

12 Mehta JL, Li DY: Identification, regulation and function of LOX-1, a novel receptor for ox-LDL. J Am Coll Cardiol 2002;39:1429–1435.

13 Aoyama T, Chen M, Fujiwara H, Masaki T, Sawamura T: LOX-1 mediates lysophosphatidylcholine-induced oxidized LDL uptake in smooth muscle cells. FEBS Lett 2000;467:217–220.

14 Li DY, Chen HJ, Mehta JL: Statins inhibit oxidized-LDL-mediated LOX-1 expression, uptake of oxidized-LDL and reduction in PKB phosphorylation. Cardiovasc Res 2001;52:130–135.

15 Li D, Liu L, Chen H, Sawamura T, Ranganathan S, Mehta JL: LOX-1 mediates oxidized low-density lipoprotein-induced expression of matrix metalloproteinases in human coronary artery endothelial cells. Circulation 2003;107:612–617.

16 Cola C, Almeida M, Li D, Romeo F, Mehta JL: Regulatory role of endothelium in the expression of genes affecting arterial calcification. Biochem Biophys Res Commun 2004;320:424–427.

17 Eitzman DT, Westrick RJ, Xu Z, Tyson J, Ginsburg D: Plasminogen activator inhibitor-1 deficiency protects against atherosclerosis progression in the mouse carotid artery. Blood 2000;96:4212–4215.

18 Shi J, Wang J, Zheng H, Ling W, Joseph J, Li D, Mehta JL, Ponnappan U: Statins increase thrombomodulin expression and function in human endothelial cells by a nitric oxide-dependent mechanism and counteract tumor necrosis factor-α-induced thrombomodulin downregulation. Blood Coagul Fibrinolysis 2003;14:575–585.

19 Delbosc S, Cristol JP, Descomps B, Mimran A, Jover B: Simvastatin prevents angiotensin II-induced cardiac alteration and oxidative stress. Hypertension 2002;40:142–147.

20 Wolfrum S, Jensen KS, Liao JK: Endothelium-dependent effects of statins. Arterioscler Thromb Vasc Biol 2003;23:729–736.

21 Treasure CB, Klein JL, Weintraub WS, Talley JD, Stillabower ME, Kosinski AS, Zhang J, Boccuzzi SJ, Cedarholm JC, Alexander RW: Beneficial effects of cholesterol-lowering therapy on the coronary endothelium in patients with coronary artery disease. N Engl J Med 1995;332:481–487.

22 Anderson TJ, Meredith IT, Yeung AC, Frei B, Selwyn AP, Ganz P: The effect of cholesterol-lowering and antioxidant therapy on endothelium-dependent coronary vasomotion. N Engl J Med 1995;332:488–493.

23 Li DY, Chen HJ, Romeo F, Sawamura T, Saldeen T, Mehta JL: Statins modulate ox-LDL-mediated adhesion molecule expression in human coronary artery endothelial cells: role of LOX-1. J Cardiovasc Pharmacol Ther 2002;302:601–605.

24 Jialal I, Stein D, Balis D, Grundy SM, Adams-Huet B, Devaraj S: Effect of hydroxymethyl glutaryl coenzyme A reductase inhibitor therapy on high sensitive C-reactive protein levels. Circulation 2001;103:1933–1935.

25 Sacks FM, Pfeffer MA, Moyé LA, Rouleau JL, Rutherford JD, Cole TG, Brown L, Warnica JW, Arnold JMO, Wun C, Davis BR, Braunwald E: The effect of pravastatin on coronary events after myocardial infarction in patients with average cholesterol levels: Cholesterol and Recurrent Events Trial Investigators. N Engl J Med 1996;335:1001–1009.

26 Gotto AM Jr, Whitney E, Stein EA, Shapiro DR, Clearfield M, Weis S, Jou JY, Langendorfer A, Beere PA, Watson DJ, Downs JR, de Cani JS: Relation between baseline and on-treatment lipid parameters and first acute major coronary events in the Air Force/Texas Coronary Atherosclerosis Prevention Study (AFCAPS/TexCAPS). Circulation 2000;101:477–484.

27 Fukumoto Y, Libby P, Rabkin E, Hill CC, Enomoto M, Hirouchi Y, Shiomi M, Aikawa M: Statins alter smooth muscle cell accumulation and collagen content in established atheroma of Watanabe heritable hyperlipidemic rabbits. Circulation 2001;103:993–999.

28 Bauersachs J, Galuppo P, Fraccarollo D, Christ M, Ertl G: Improvement of left ventricular remodeling and function by hydroxymethylglutaryl coenzyme A reductase inhibition with cerivastatin in rats with heart failure after myocardial infarction. Circulation 2001;104:982–985.

29 Maeda T, Matsunuma A, Kawane T, Horiuchi N: Simvastatin promotes osteoblast differentiation and mineralization in MC3T3-E1 cells. Biochem Biophys Res Commun 2001;280:874–877.

30 Keidar S, Heinrich R, Kaplan M, Aviram M: Oxidative stress increases the expression of the angiotensin-II receptor type 1 in mouse peritoneal macrophages. J Renin Angiotensin Aldosterone Syst 2002;3:24–30.

31 Singh BK, Sinha AK, Mehta JL: Statins in the primary prevention of atherosclerosis-related events; in Mehta JL (ed): Statins: Understanding Clinical Use. Philadelphia, Saunders 2004.

32 Li DY, Zhang YC, Philips MI, Sawamura T, Mehta JL: Upregulation of endothelial receptor for oxidized low-density lipoprotein (LOX-1) in cultured human coronary artery endothelial cells by angiotensin II type 1 receptor activation. Circ Res 1999;84:1043–1049.

33 Sung BH, Izzo JL Jr, Wilson MF: Effects of cholesterol reduction on BP response to mental stress in patients with high cholesterol. Am J Hypertens 1997;10:592–599.

34 Nazzaro P, Manzari M, Merlo M, Triggiani R, Scarano A, Ciancio L, Pirrelli A: Distinct and combined vascular effects of ACE blockade and HMG-CoA reductase inhibition in hypertensive subjects. Hypertension 1999;33:719–725.

35 Nickenig G, Baumer AT, Temur Y, Kebben D, Jockenhovel F, Bohm M: Statin-sensitive dysregulated AT1 receptor function and density in hypercholesterolemic men. Circulation 1999;100: 2131–2134.

36 Vidal F, Colome C, Martinez-Gonzalez J, Badimon L: Atherogenic concentrations of native low-density lipoproteins down-regulate nitric oxide synthase mRNA and protein levels in endothelial cells. Eur J Biochem 1998;252:378–384.

37 Kotchen TA, Talwalkar RT: Increased enzymatic activity of renin and hyperlipidemia. Am J Physiol 1981;240:E60–E64.

38 O'Callaghan CJ, Krum H, Conway EL, Lam W, Skiba MA, Howes LG, Louis WJ: Short-term effects of pravastatin on blood pressure in hypercholesterolaemic hypertensive patients. Blood Press 1994;3:404–406.

39 Sposito AC, Mansur AP, Coelho OR, Nicolau JC, Ramires JA: Additional reduction in blood pressure after cholesterol-lowering treatment by statins (lovastatin or pravastatin) in hypercholesterolemic patients using angiotensin-converting enzyme inhibitors (enalapril or lisinopril). Am J Cardiol 1999;83:1497–1499.

40 Borghi C, Prandin MG, Costa FV, Bacchelli S, Degli Esposti D, Ambrosioni E: Use of statins and blood pressure control in treated hypertensive patients with hypercholesterolemia. J Cardiovasc Pharmacol 2000;35:549–555.

41   Schmalfuss CM, Chen LY, Bott JN, Staples ED, Mehta JL: Superoxide anion generation, superoxide dismutase activity, and nitric oxide release in human internal mammary artery and saphenous vein segments. J Cardiovasc Pharmacol Ther 1999;4:249–257.
42   Cooke JP: NO and angiogenesis. Atheroscler Suppl 2003;4:53–60.
43   Dechend R, Fiebeler A, Park JK, Muller DN, Theuer J, Mervaala E, Bieringer M, Gulba D, Dietz R, Luft FC, Haller H: Amelioration of angiotensin II-induced cardiac injury by a 3-hydroxy-3-methylglutaryl coenzyme A reductase inhibitor. Circulation 2001;104:576–581.
44   Patel R, Nagueh SF, Tsybouleva N, et al: Simvastatin induces regression of cardiac hypertrophy and fibrosis and improves cardiac function in a transgenic rabbit model of human hypertrophic cardiomyopathy. Circulation 2001;104:317–324.
45   Reddy R, Chahoud G, Mehta JL: Modulation of cardiovascular remodeling with statins: fact or fiction? Curr Vasc Pharmacol 2005;3:69–79.
46   Daugherty A, Cassis L: Chronic angiotensin II infusion promotes atherogenesis in low density lipoprotein receptor –/– mice. Ann NY Acad Sci 1999;892:108–118.
47   Ichihara A, Hayashi M, Koura Y, Tada Y, Kaneshiro Y, Saruta T: Long-term effects of statins on arterial pressure and stiffness of hypertensives. J Hum Hypertens 2005;19:103–109.
48   Raison J, Rudnichi A, Safar ME: Effects of atorvastatin on aortic pulse wave velocity in patients with hypertension and hypercholesterolaemia: a preliminary study. J Hum Hypertens 2002;16:705–710.
49   Abetel G, Poget PN, Bonnabry JP: Hypotensive effect of an inhibitor of cholesterol synthesis (fluvastatin). A pilot study. Schweiz Med Wochenschr 1998;128:272–277.
50   Glorioso N, Troffa C, Filigheddu F, Dettori F, Soro A, Parpaglia PP, Collatina S, Pahor M: Effect of the HMG-CoA reductase inhibitors on blood pressure in patients with essential hypertension and primary hypercholesterolemia. Hypertension 1999;34:1281–1286.
51   Tonolo G, Ciccarese M, Brizzi P, Puddu L, Secchi G, Calvia P, Atzeni MM, Melis MG, Maioli M: Reduction of albumin excretion rate in normotensive microalbuminuric type 2 diabetic patients during long-term simvastatin treatment. Diabetes Care 1997;20:1891–1895.
52   Kontopoulos AG, Athyros VG, Pehlivanidis AN, Demitriadis DS, Papageorgiou AA, Boudoulas H: Long-term treatment effect of atorvastatin on aortic stiffness in hypercholesterolaemic patients. Curr Med Res Opin 2003;19:22–27.
53   Ferrier KE, Muhlmann MH, Baguet JP, Cameron JD, Jennings GL, Dart AM, Kingwell BA: Intensive cholesterol reduction lowers blood pressure and large artery stiffness in isolated systolic hypertension. J Am Coll Cardiol 2002;39:1020–1025.

J.L. Mehta, MD, PhD
Division of Cardiovascular Medicine, University of Arkansas for Medical Sciences
4301 W. Markham St., Slot 532
Little Rock, AR 72205 (USA)
Tel. +1 501 296 1401, Fax +1 501 686 6180, E-Mail mehtajl@uams.edu

Safar ME, Frohlich ED (eds): Atherosclerosis, Large Arteries and Cardiovascular Risk.
Adv Cardiol. Basel, Karger, 2007, vol 44, pp 331–351

······················

Atherosclerosis, Arterial Stiffness and Antihypertensive Drug Therapy

Michel E. Safar[a]   *Harold Smulyan*[b]

[a]The Diagnosis Center, Hôtel-Dieu Hospital, Paris, France, and
[b]Department of Medicine, Upstate Medical University, Syracuse, N.Y., USA

Abstract

Increased aortic stiffness is a consequence of cardiovascular (CV) aging and may be observed in the elderly with or without hypertension. Hypertension and arterial stiffness are independent risk factors for CV events, but such events may also be complicated by atherosclerosis, especially in the older population. The purpose of this chapter is to determine whether, in the presence of atherosclerosis, systolic hypertension in the elderly requires specific drug therapy. It will be shown that, in addition to the targeted drug treatment of associated hypercholesterolemia and/or hyperglycemia, the major problem nowadays is to find specific antihypertensive drugs causing a selective reduction of systolic blood pressure (SBP).

Before presenting antihypertensive agents acting selectively on systolic blood pressure (SBP), a brief overview of past therapeutic trials and meta-analyses is needed.

Antihypertensive Drug Therapy: A Simplified Overview of Past Therapeutic Trials and Their Meta-Analyses

In recent years, therapeutic trials and meta-analyses have become the major guidelines for the management of patients with hypertension. Before analyzing their results, it is important to briefly review their historical background.

A Brief Historic Overview

From 1950 to 1980, the effectiveness of antihypertensive drug therapy was demonstrated for the first time in men in the Veterans Administration trials [1, 2]. Later, both men and women were studied [1, 2]. The effect of drug therapy on CV risk was easy to demonstrate in relatively small populations with severe or malignant hypertension, but much larger populations and longer follow-up times were needed for subjects with mild to moderate hypertension. The defined goal of these early studies was to reduce CV risk exclusively through reduction of diastolic blood pressure (DBP). DBP was the single entry criterion for the hypertensive population and the only criterion used to determine drug effectiveness [1, 2]. Changes in SBP were frequently not published. During this period, therapeutic trials never included old subjects with isolated systolic hypertension, defined as DBP ≤90 mm Hg but SBP >160 mm Hg.

Circa 1990, it was shown that antihypertensive drugs reduced CV risk in subjects with isolated systolic hypertension or with systolic-diastolic hypertension and a disproportionate increase of SBP over DBP [3, 4]. These trials included much older patients (>65 years) of both sexes and emphasized the importance of including women in study cohorts. As a consequence, results were frequently focused on SBP but the effects of drug treatment were also related to DBP, although in many trials, baseline DBP values were already normal or even low.

More recently, comparisons of the effectiveness of various antihypertensive agents have been performed [5, 6]. In most studies, it was not possible to clearly identify any difference between the effects of various antihypertensive agents at similar levels of BP reduction. In these trials, the target of antihypertensive drug therapy had become both SBP and DBP reduction. However, there was no consistent improvement in the reduction of CV events, when compared to the earlier primary trials. To test such conclusions, Staessen et al. [6] compared new and old antihypertensive drugs and computed pooled odds ratios from stratified tables. Compared with early drugs (diuretics and β-blockers), calcium-channel blockers, angiotensin-converting enzyme inhibitors and angiotensin II antagonists provided similar overall CV protection. However, some published results suggested that dihydropyridine calcium-channel blockers might offer a selective benefit in the prevention of stroke and inhibitors of the renin-angiotensin system in the prevention of heart failure [5, 6]. For prevention of myocardial infarction, the results were more equivocal. However, the prevention of myocardial infarction by antihypertensive therapy had been constantly the object of debate since the early phases of antihypertensive therapy. Finally, taken together, these results suggested that all antihypertensive drugs provided similar overall CV protection.

Effects of Antihypertensive Drug Treatment on CV Risk

During the 30-year evolution of therapeutic trials and meta-analyses, it is evident that (1) the clinical face of hypertension has considerably changed, from severe and malignant to milder forms of hypertension, including systolic hypertension in the aged; (2) the number of classes of antihypertensive agents has also increased, as a function of the discovery and commercialization of new antihypertensive agents; (3) the concomitant use of non-antihypertensive agents, such as statins, has also markedly increased, and (4) no consistent differences have been sought in the strategy of drug treatment between men and women despite the well-established lower CV risk in women [7].

During all these remarkable changes over time, the effects of drug treatment on CV risk remained quite stable [1, 2] (fig. 1). The major results over the years were the reduction of stroke and congestive heart failure, both clearly demonstrated from the initial studies. Another salutary result was the stabilization or even the improvement of renal function, although relatively few large therapeutic trials were performed on this subject. Finally, the beneficial effects of drug treatment on the prevention of myocardial infarction continued to be more difficult to demonstrate than that of stroke and undoubtedly remained lower than expected from the initial epidemiological predictions.

Effect of Drug Treatment on Brachial BP

An important aspect of all these therapeutic trials was the effect of antihypertensive agents on brachial BP determinations. Despite the heterogeneity of the different classes of antihypertensive agents, the resulting changes in BP were quite homogeneous for all trials. DBP was lowered to ≤ 90 mm Hg in approximately 80% of treated patients but SBP remained ≥ 140 mm Hg in approximately 60% [8–10] (fig. 2). These findings in many patients resulted in an increase in pulse pressure (PP), above that which rises normally and substantially with aging. This increased PP became a possible index of residual CV risk during therapy and therefore represented an important factor in the total evaluation of antihypertensive drug therapy (see chapter by Verdecchia and Angeli, pp 150–159). Finally, for most authors, the consistent reduction of CV risk and the homogeneity of the changes in BP under various treatments contrasted with the heterogeneity of the classes of antihypertensive agents. This disparity suggested a substantial cause-effect relationship between the reduction of BP (mainly SBP) and CV events [11–13].

To test whether such conclusions were valid, Staessen et al. [6] considered new outcome trials published in recent years (2005). For these trials, Staessen et al. [13] predicted outcome from achieved SBP using their previously published meta-regression models. The main finding of the overview was that re-

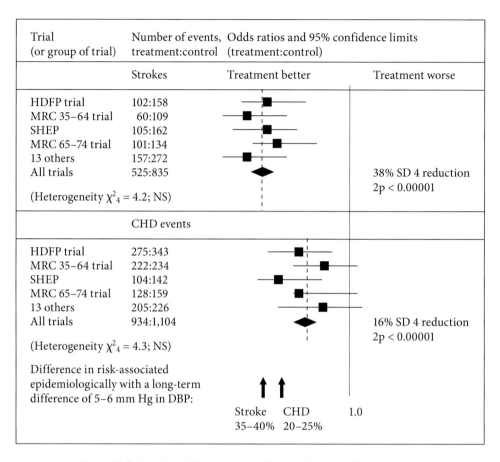

Trial (or group of trial)	Number of events, treatment:control	Odds ratios and 95% confidence limits (treatment:control)		
		Strokes	Treatment better	Treatment worse
HDFP trial	102:158			
MRC 35–64 trial	60:109			
SHEP	105:162			
MRC 65–74 trial	101:134			
13 others	157:272			
All trials	525:835			38% SD 4 reduction 2p < 0.00001
(Heterogeneity $\chi^2_4 = 4.2$; NS)				
		CHD events		
HDFP trial	275:343			
MRC 35–64 trial	222:234			
SHEP	104:142			
MRC 65–74 trial	128:159			
13 others	205:226			
All trials	934:1,104			16% SD 4 reduction 2p < 0.00001
(Heterogeneity $\chi^2_4 = 4.3$; NS)				
Difference in risk-associated epidemiologically with a long-term difference of 5–6 mm Hg in DBP:		Stroke CHD 1.0 35–40% 20–25%		

Fig. 1. Global results of therapeutic trials according to references 1 and 2. Note that the effectiveness is much more pronounced for stroke than for coronary heart disease (CHD). SD = Standard deviation. Acronyms of trials are explained in references 1 and 2.

duction in brachial SBP largely explained CV outcomes in the recently published actively controlled trials in hypertensive patients and in placebo-controlled secondary prevention trials (fig. 3). The hypothesis that new antihypertensive drugs might influence CV prognosis over and beyond their antihypertensive effect was considered to be unproven and a need for a better BP control seemed evident.

Using a different epidemiological approach, Benetos et al. [14] published similar conclusions. These authors observed that treated but persistently hypertensive subjects not only had higher SBPs and DBPs, but also had a higher prevalence of associated CV risk factors when compared to untreated subjects,

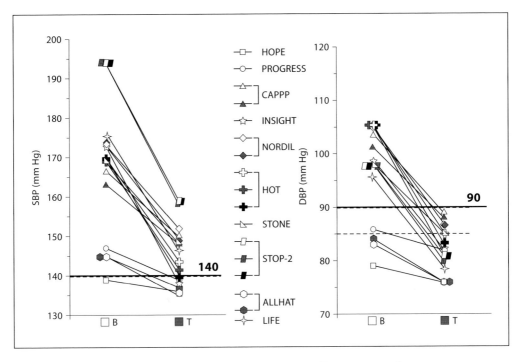

Fig. 2. Results of therapeutic trials [as described in 10] of hypertension: drug treatment tends to normalize DBP but not SBP. B = Before treatmen; T = under treatment. Acronyms of trials are indicated in reference 10.

some of whom were normotensive. Treated hypertensives compared to these controls presented a twofold increase in the risk ratio (RR) for CV mortality (RR 1.96; 95% confidence interval (CI) 1.74–2.22) and coronary mortality (RR 1.99; 95% CI 1.63–2.44). Adjustment for unmodifiable risk factors (height etc.) decreased the excess CV risk observed in treated subjects only slightly: RR 1.77; 95% CI 1.56–2.00 for CV mortality, and RR 1.76; 95% CI 1.44–2.16 for coronary mortality. After additional adjustment for modifiable associated CV risk factors (plasma glucose, cholesterol etc.), the increased mortality in treated subjects persisted: RR 1.52; 95% CI 1.33–1.74 for CV mortality, and RR 1.49; 95% CI 1.19–1.86 for coronary mortality. Only after additional adjustment for SBP were CV mortality and coronary mortality similar in the two groups of subjects: RR 1.06; 95% CI 0.92–1.23, and RR 1.06; 95% CI 0.85–1.35, respectively. Finally, such results indicated again that there is a need for a tight SBP control in treated hypertensive subjects.

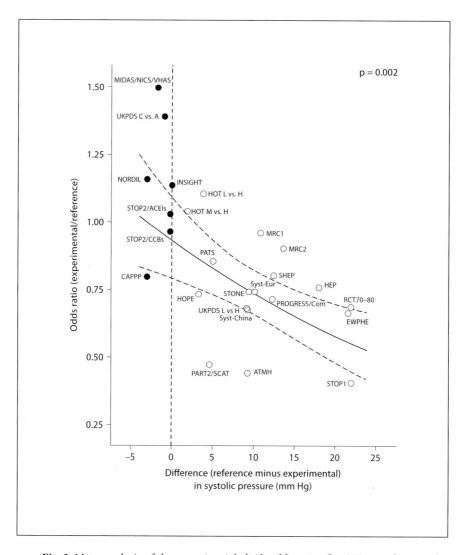

Fig. 3. Meta-analysis of therapeutic trials [13]: odds ratios for CV mortality in relation to corresponding differences in SBP. Odds ratios were calculated for experimental versus reference treatment. BP differences were obtained by subtracting achieved levels in experimental groups from those in reference groups. Negative values indicate tighter BP on control than on reference treatment. The regression lines were plotted with 95% CI and were weighted for the inverse of the variance of the individual odds ratios. Open symbols denote placebo-controlled studies or trials with an untreated control group. Closed symbols indicate actively controlled trials. Acronyms of trials are explained in reference 13.

Atherosclerosis, Arterial Stiffness and Antihypertensive Therapy

As shown earlier in this book, the links between atherosclerosis, arterial stiffness, age and high BP are often difficult to establish, particularly according to age. Many atherosclerotic alterations (AA) are subclinical and difficult to define in routine clinical investigations. On the other hand, many markers have been proposed, such as defects in vascular relaxation, alterations in endothelium-dependent flow dilatation and/or presence of atherosclerotic plaques (see chapter by Baldewsing et al., pp 35–61, and chapter by Hayoz and Mazzolai, pp 62–75). Within the framework of antihypertensive drug therapy, it seems likely that the links between atherosclerosis and arterial stiffness should primarily be explored through a simple clinical description of CV events clearly related to AA. The principal AA are those responsible for peripheral arterial disease (see chapter by Safar, pp 199–211), coronary ischemic disease (see chapter by Kingwell and Ahimastos, pp 125–138) and carotid atherosclerotic disease (mainly stenosis of the carotid artery) (see chapter by Agabiti-Rosei and Muiesan, pp 173–186). The relation of such CV events to arterial stiffness, and potentially age and high BP, are evaluated in the following paragraphs.

In clinical medicine, the best examples associating hypertension and AA are represented by subjects with atherosclerosis of the lower limbs [15, 16]. Increased SBP and PP are commonly observed in these patients, whereas mean arterial pressure, systemic vascular resistance and ventricular ejection remain usually within the normal range. Arterial stiffness is significantly increased (see chapter by Safar, pp 199–211). This increase is exaggerated in the presence of high sodium intake and acute non-selective β-blockade. The increased PP is significantly and independently associated with the limitation of the vasodilating arteriolar properties of the diseased limbs [17]. This suggests that atherosclerosis, through increased arterial stiffness and wave reflections, might contribute to the elevated SBP and PP even when vascular resistance and DBP are normal. In vessels of the lower limbs, non-fibrous and non-calcified plaques contribute little to increase arterial stiffness. By contrast, in more advanced disease, atherosclerosis may contribute greatly to increased collagen content and calcifications of the arterial wall and accentuate arterial rigidity, especially in the presence of advanced age and/or hypertension.

Coronary ischemic disease has been found to be almost constantly associated with increased aortic stiffness [18] (see chapter by Kingwell and Ahimastos, pp 125–138). Although an increased incidence of elevated SBP has not been widely reported in populations of subjects with ischemic heart diseases, these subjects often display an increased PP and a decreased diastolic pressure-time index, probably due to aortic stiffening. Experimentally, increased aortic stiffness, which reduces DBP, participates in and aggravates the myocardial ischemia observed in the presence of stenosis of coronary arteries [19]. Finally, even in the absence of systolic hypertension, increased stiffness is a major contributor to the evolution of coronary heart disease and predicts myocardial ischemia (see chapter by Danchin and Mourad, pp 139–149, chapter by Verdecchia and Angeli, pp 150–159, and chapter by McEniery and Cockcroft, pp 160–172).

In contrast, with narrowed coronary arteries, stenosis of the internal carotid artery is frequently associated with systolic hypertension [20]. In subjects with carotid endarterectomy, a significant increase of SBP variability is also observed, particularly during the night [21]. Atherosclerotic plaques of the common carotid artery and of the carotid bifurcation are classical features of hypertensive subjects, particularly over 50 years of age [22]. Decreased carotid distensibility, increased arterial wall thickness and calcifications are observed in uncomplicated hypertensive subjects for the same age and gender as normotensive controls [22]. Such populations have been also the object of specific therapeutic trials (see chapter by Mackey et al., pp 234–244) [22, 23].

Finally, whatever the clinical aspects of AA may be, the links of atherosclerosis with age, increased arterial stiffness and hypertension are similar in the different vascular territories and are all related by the presence of increased SBP. There is only one exception to this description, coronary ischemic disease, where the increased arterial stiffness and SBP are frequently masked by an associated reduction of ventricular ejection. Thus, the therapeutic links between AA and increased arterial stiffness are now easy to understand. The more difficult issue is how to treat systolic hypertension in the elderly. It is increased SBP. This problem must be approached cautiously. First, the principal goal of drug treatment, SBP reduction, involves a common denominator that combines several associated parameters: arterial stiffness, atherosclerosis, age and high BP. Second, to be valid in terms of AA, the reduction of SBP by drug treatment should be accompanied by the reduction of biomarkers of atherosclerosis, such as modifications in atherosclerotic plaques.

Target Trials Showing Selective SBP Reduction

Any antihypertensive drug reducing arteriolar tone, and therefore mean arterial pressure, may decrease SBP through a passive reduction of arterial stiffness and change in the timing of wave reflections (see chapter by Safar, pp 1–18) [24, 25]. However, in the case of subjects with a disproportionate increase of SBP over DBP, the target mechanisms are rather a decrease of ventricular ejection, an active decrease of arterial stiffness or a change in wave reflections. Regarding ventricular ejection, the decrease in stroke volume, observed with ventricular pacing and treatment of atrioventricular block [24], will not be detailed in this book. The change in wave reflection is the main objective of this chapter. We have shown that some drugs, such as nitrates, may act predominantly on large artery structure and function independent of mean blood pressure (MBP) changes [26–28], particularly in the elderly [29–31] (chapter by Smulyan, pp 302–314). Here it will be also shown that prolongation of survival in hypertensive subjects requires reduction not only of BP but also of arterial stiffness and/or wave reflections.

The main therapeutic trial demonstrating the role of arterial stiffness and wave reflections in the control of SBP and PP was performed in hypertensive patients with end-stage renal disease (ESRD) undergoing hemodialysis [32]. Many studies have shown that the clinical and hemodynamic profile of these patients is very similar to those described in systolic hypertension in the elderly [30, 33]. The primary objective of the trial in ESRD patients was to reduce CV morbidity and mortality through a therapeutic regimen involving first salt and water depletion by hemodialysis, then, after randomization, angiotensin-converting enzyme inhibition or calcium-entry blockade, and finally the combination of the two agents and their association with a β-blocker. Using this design, it was possible to evaluate over a long-term follow-up (51 months) whether the drug-induced MBP reduction was or was not associated with a parallel decrease of arterial stiffness and the resulting consequences on CV risk [32]. During the follow-up, it was clear that MBP, PP and aortic pulse wave velocity (PWV) were reduced in parallel in the surviving population. In contrast, in subjects who died from CV events, MBP was lowered to the same extent as in survivors, but neither PP nor PWV were significantly modified by drug treatment (fig. 4). From the results of this trial, it seemed likely that a failure of the aortic PWV to fall, despite a significant drug-induced MBP reduction, was a significant predictor of CV death in subjects with ESRD.

In elderly subjects with systolic hypertension the Syst-Eur trial provided similar results to those observed in ESRD subjects. The predictive value of conventional and ambulatory PP for CV morbidity and mortality was studied during follow-up of the Syst-Eur after adjustment for all significant confounding covariables [34]. In the placebo group, conventional and mostly ambulatory PP – but not MBP – predicted total and CV mortality, all CV events, stroke and cardiac events. In the group treated with calcium channel antagonists compared with those who received placebo, the relation between clinical outcomes and ambulatory (and conventional) PP was significantly attenuated and even reached non-significant levels. Furthermore, at any given level of 24-hour SBP, a lower 24-hour DBP was shown to be significantly associated with a worsening of CV risk. Finally, the results of the Syst-Eur trial clearly confirmed that PP in

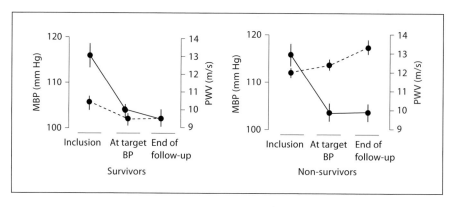

Fig. 4. Therapeutic trial in subjects with chronic renal failure undergoing hemodialysis [32]: BP reduction is observed both in survivors and non-survivors (—●—). The main difference is that non-survivors have no reduction of PWV (−−●−−).

the elderly is a significant CV risk factor and that its lowering is a necessary goal in elderly hypertensive subjects to improve CV morbidity and mortality.

Taken together, all these studies have shown the need in hypertensive subjects, particularly in the elderly, to develop drugs acting specifically on the large artery wall, i.e. either on arterial stiffness or on wave reflections or on a combination of both, to produce improvements of AA and CV risk [35]. The recent finding of aortic PWV as an independent predictor of CV risk has confirmed this conceptual approach.

Pharmacological Basis of Selective SBP Reduction

Many antihypertensive agents, such as dihydralazine, propanolol and diuretics in middle age [24, 33], have been shown to have no effect on arterial stiffness or wave reflections and cannot target the above-mentioned mechanisms. What follows is focused on antihypertensive drugs that have a potential direct effect on large artery structure and function.

Changes in Stiffness and Wave Reflections Induced by Nitrates
Two double-blind randomized placebo-controlled studies [31, 36] have investigated the effect of chronic isosorbide dinitrate (ISDN) in elderly subjects with isolated systolic hypertension. In one study, ISDN caused a significant decrease of SBP, from the 8th to the 12th week of treatment: −27 mm Hg with ISDN and −13 mm Hg with placebo. DBP and heart rate did not differ from

placebo. The other study confirmed the reduction in office PP with ISDN after 8 weeks of treatment (ISDN: –18%; placebo: –5%) without a reduction in DBP (ISDN: 0%; placebo: –6%). In addition, ambulatory PP was also reduced with ISDN, while it did not change during placebo [36]. During this study, no nitrate tolerance was observed. Similar findings have been reported in hypertensive subjects of middle age using transdermal nitroglycerin or the long-acting agent molsidomine [37, 38]. The fact that nitrates decrease PP without decreasing DBP suggests that these compounds act mainly on muscular conduit arteries without a substantial effect on small resistance vessels.

Investigations with the NO donor sinitrodil in young healthy volunteers [39] showed a dose-dependent increase in brachial artery compliance after a single oral dose. With sinitrodil 40 mg, brachial artery compliance increased by 27% while compliance was only increased 8% after ISDN 20 mg. In contrast, total peripheral resistance decreased by 11% after ISDN and only 7% after sinitrodil. It therefore appears possible to develop drugs that act even more selectively on large arteries than nitrates. Drugs like the NO donor sinitrodil are presumed to be suitable candidates to decrease PP, thereby decreasing SBP without decreasing, or even increasing, DBP.

Apart from NO donors, enhancers of NO production/release might be of interest in the treatment of systolic hypertension in the elderly. Recent studies suggest that some compounds like the diuretic agent cicletanine [40, 41], the selective β_1-blocker nebivolol [42] and even the selective atrial natriuretic peptides [43] act as enhancers of NO production and/or release with a resulting decrease of arterial stiffness. These examples offer some prospective views on the development of drugs acting specifically on systolic hypertension in the elderly. Recent studies in old hypertensive rats support the concept that NO dysfunction and/or related endothelial alterations involving oxidative stress may be important target mechanisms in the development of the age-related increase of PP and arterial stiffness [44]. In addition, clinical interference with gene polymorphisms related to NO synthase has been reported in humans to modulate the age-PP relationship [45].

Stiffness and Wave Reflection Changes Associated with Sodium and the Renin-Angiotensin System

Since angiotensin II stimulates the production of various types of collagen fibers [46] together with a number of growth factors [47], converting enzyme inhibition and angiotensin II type I AT_1 receptor blockade have been used as pharmacological tools to show that in vivo, the chronic inhibition of the effects of angiotensin II prevents the aortic accumulation of collagen in spontaneously hypertensive rats (SHRs) [48]. Antihypertensive doses of converting-enzyme inhibitor were shown to prevent the chronic accumulation of aortic collagen, whereas this result was not observed with the non-specific vasodilator hydralazine for the same BP reduction. The collagen reduction was noted even with non-antihypertensive doses of converting enzyme inhibitor and paralleled the decrease of angiotensin-converting enzyme measured in the aortic tissue, but not in the plasma [48]. Further experiments clearly indicated that the collagen effects were not due to bradykinin but involved specifically the blockade of AT_1 receptors of angiotensin II [49]. Finally, such findings were observed exclusively on a normal, but not a high sodium diet [50], a situation in which the production of transforming growth factor-β_1 is increased [51]. Furthermore, when a diuretic and a converting enzyme inhibitor were studied in SHRs, the combination of the two agents was able to consistently prevent carotid collagen accumulation and, at the same time, decrease isobaric carotid stiffness [52]. Thus, it is important now to re-evaluate the possible links between sodium, diuretics, blockers of the renin-angiotensin system, and changes of extracellular matrix of arterial vessels in humans and rat models of hypertension.

Experimental data on sodium-induced changes of arterial structure and function have been mostly obtained in genetic strains of hypertensive rats, such as stroke-sensitive and -resistant SHRs and Dahl salt-sensitive rats [50, 53, 54]. In these models, increased sodium intake does not significantly modify intra-arterial BP (with the exception of Dahl salt-sensitive rats), but is associated with reduced isobaric carotid stiffness, increased aortic wall thickness and collagen accumulation. Such alterations are prevented by reduced sodium diet or administration of diuretics, without concomitant change of the intra-arterial BP level. Numerous findings in molecular biology have demonstrated the pressure-independent effect of sodium and/or diuretic compounds on the aortic and carotid vessel wall, leading to a loss or a reduction in the contractile properties of vascular smooth muscle cells and to an increase in their secretory properties [55].

In the clinical investigation of hypertensive humans, substantial links between arterial stiffness, sodium and blockade of the renin-angiotensin system have been reported. As in hypertensive rats, converting enzyme inhibitors are able to produce a pressure-independent increase of diameter, compliance and distensibility of peripheral muscular arteries [56]. Such changes are observed even in the presence of diuretic compounds. By contrast, diuretics alone, given to middle-aged hypertensive patients, cause little changes in arterial diameter and stiffness [57, 58]. The REASON study in hypertensive patients [59] has shown that the combination of perindopril (Per) and indapamide (Ind) decreases brachial SBP and PP more than the β-blocking agent atenolol for the same reduction of DBP (fig. 5). This result is even more obvious when BP is measured centrally, in the carotid artery and the thoracic aorta, and not in the

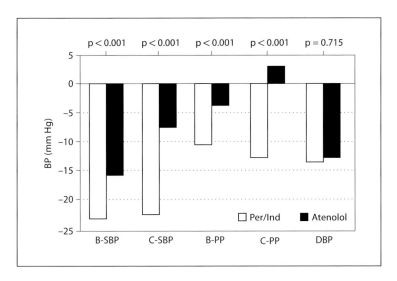

Fig. 5. REASON study [64]: in middle-aged hypertensive subjects, the indapamide/perindopril combination reduces more SBP than the β-blocking agent atenolol for the same DBP reduction. Subsequently, PP is more reduced with the combined drug treatment, particularly at the site of central (carotid) arteries. B = Brachial; C = carotid; BP = blood pressure.

brachial artery. After 6 months of therapy, the hemodynamic pattern showed a change in central wave reflections, and at 1 year, a pressure-independent reduction of aortic stiffness. These findings, observed with Per/Ind, but not atenolol, strongly suggest that structural changes of the vessels occur after 1 year of drug treatment, because, in the long term, drug treatment has limited effect on the thickness of elastic arteries [60], but does better on the structure of muscular arteries and arterioles [61, 62]. Therefore, the weight of evidence suggests a parallelism between the reduction of SBP and PP under Per/Ind and the regression of arteriolar structural changes, commonly observed under blockade of the renin-angiotensin system, but not with atenolol. The validity of this observation is strengthened by two modifications previously noted under drug treatment by converting enzyme inhibition (but not with β-blocking agents): a reduction in arteriolar peripheral reflection coefficients [63] and in the timing and/or amplitude of backward pressure wave [64, 65], responsible for the observed selective decrease in central SBP and PP (fig. 5). This interpretation is compatible with the finding by Rizzoni et al. [66] that, in hypertensive subjects, structural alterations of small resistance arteries predict CV risk, as well as increased PP level. Finally, taken together, these results suggest that drug treatment of hypertension to selectively reduce SBP and PP requires complex interactions between structure and function of small and large arteries.

Stiffness Changes Induced by Aldosterone Antagonists

In recent years, experimental studies in rats have shown that chronic aldosterone administration might act on the mechanical properties of large vessels as well as on myocardial stiffness [67]. Immunohistochemical methods have shown that the intensity of staining of mineralocorticoid receptors within the vascular wall predominates in the aorta and decreases with the size of the arteries [68]. Endogenous vascular synthesis of aldosterone occurs in the rat mesenteric artery, even after adrenalectomy, and requires the presence of an intact endothelium [69, 70]. In this line of evidence, Benetos et al. [71, 72] have observed that, both in younger and older hypertensive rats, spironolactone prevents in vivo both myocardial and aortic collagen accumulation with minimal changes of intra-arterial BP. Conversely, long-term aldosterone infusion in the presence of high sodium intake increases the intrinsic rigidity of the aortic wall in rats [67]. This increased aortic rigidity is reversed in the presence of the selective aldosterone antagonist eplerenone [67]. In contrast, in hypertensive patients, studies of spironolactone administration for 2 weeks never produced a change in brachial artery stiffness [33], suggesting that long-term treatments may be needed to limit aortic stiffness.

Interestingly, in untreated hypertensive subjects, increased aortic stiffness and increased plasma aldosterone have been shown to be statistically associated [73]. In addition, in hypertensive subjects, a polymorphism of the aldosynthase gene has been found to be associated with a pressure-independent increase of aortic stiffness with age [74]. Long-term studies are needed in subjects with hypertension, particularly in the elderly, to demonstrate a reduction of arterial stiffness and SBP following aldosterone antagonism, since recently it is commonly used in subjects with congestive heart failure.

Stiffness Changes and Mechanotransduction Mechanisms

Mechanical properties of the large arteries may be modified independently of mean arterial pressure not only through structural modifications of elastin and collagen, but also through the specific effects of interstitial molecules of the extracellular matrix, which are implicated in the cell-cell and cell-matrix attachments and thus in mechanotransduction [75]. In rats and in man, aminoguanidine and collagen breakers such as ALT711 decrease isobaric carotid stiffness without changing mean arterial pressure or the elastin and collagen contents of the arterial wall [76–78]. The stiffness improvement seems to be the consequence of blockade of collagen glycation with resulting changes in collagen cross-linking. On the other hand, diuretic compounds, such as inda-

pamide, have been shown to reduce aortic stiffness and to modify wave reflections in SHRs and in man, in association with changes in the proteoglycan-
labeling patterns of the arterial wall [79, 80]. Finally, other antihypertensive
compounds, as calcium-entry blockers (see p. 146) or mostly converting enzyme inhibitors, whether or not associated with atrial peptides, act mostly on
fibronectin [81], a major component with integrins of mechanotransduction
mechanisms within the arterial wall.

Finally, numerous substances, such as estrogens, have been proposed in
the future to improve the mechanical properties of hypertensive large arteries
independently of MBP changes.

Prospective Views for the Drug Treatment of Hypertension in Old Subjects with Atherosclerosis

Nowadays, the standard treatment of hypertension in middle age aims to
decrease SBP, DBP and MBP and therefore to shift the age-BP curve towards
lower values of SBP, DBP and MBP. The findings discussed in this chapter
clearly indicate that, over 60 years of age, a novel objective of treatment should
be not only a shift of the BP curve but also a reduction of the normal increase
of SBP and decrease of DBP with aging, thereby reducing the slope of the age-
PP curve (fig. 6) [82]. This goal may be achieved only through a specific action
on large (and not small) arteries, thus modifying arterial stiffness and wave
reflections and normalizing not only SBP and DBP, but also PP.

A first approach consists of the use of standard antihypertensive drugs,
since some of them have noticeable effects on the mechanical properties of
large arteries. For example, from experimental studies, it appears that aortic
collagen accumulation may be prevented independent of mean arterial pressure by converting enzyme inhibition and/or aldosterone antagonism [54].
However, for this purpose, there is no evidence in hypertensive humans that
the doses of these drugs may be the same as those required for conventional
antihypertensive drug therapy. Studies in clinical pharmacology, particularly
those done with the calcium-entry blocker mibefradil [35], have shown that
the most effective dosages commonly used for the lowering of SBP and DBP
may be inadequate for reducing the PP. Moreover, the level of brachial PP reduction may differ from that of aortic PP reduction (see chapter by Safar,
pp 1–18) [22]. Further investigations are needed to resolve these new aspects
of clinical CV pharmacology.

The second approach is to develop antihypertensive agents that influence
vasomotor tone and the structural composition of the vessel wall of both small
and large arteries. The goal is to identify agents that act on the secretory prop-

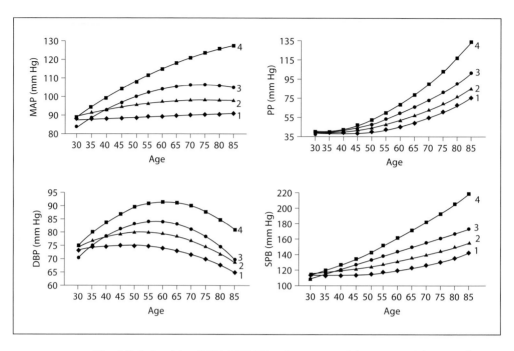

Fig. 6. Relationship of SBP, DBP, PP and mean arterial pressure with age in the untreated subjects of the Framingham population [35]: because the relationship of SBP and DBP with age is non-linear, it is not sufficient to simply shift the age-BP curves toward lower values. It is necessary to reduce the slope of the age-BP relationship, particularly for SBP. Groups examined at index examination: (1) SBP <120; (2) SBP 120–139; (3) SBP 140–159, and (4) SBP 160+.

erties rather than on the contractile properties of vascular smooth muscle cells. These agents might particularly operate via mechanotransduction mechanisms acting on cell-cell and cell-matrix attachments of the vessel wall [75–77]. From these new approaches for the drug treatment of hypertension, therapeutic trials should to be developed to detect a reduction in CV morbidity and mortality through specific changes of arterial stiffness and wave reflections, as begun in the REASON study [83] and continued by the CAFE study [84] (see p. 146).

A third approach should be considered. In hypertensive populations, there is extreme interindividual variability for the increase of SBP and PP and the decrease of DBP with age. Thus, selection of hypertensive subjects at risk, based on screening of the associated environmental and/or genetic factors responsible for this variability, should be taken into account for the choice of drug treatment.

Finally, in clinical practice, an important approach should be to modify extensively the guidelines of hypertension that currently ignore the importance of the interactions between small and large arteries as well as the concepts of pulsatility, SBP and PP amplification within the CV system.

References

1   MacMahon S, Peto R, Cutler J, Collins R, Sorlie P, Neaton J, Abbott R, Godwin J, Dyer A, Stamler J: Blood pressure, stroke, and coronary heart disease. 1. Prolonged differences in blood pressure: prospective observational studies corrected for the regression dilution bias. Lancet 1990; 335:765–774.
2   Collins R, Peto R, MacMahon S, Hebert P, Fiebach NH, Everley KA, Godwin J, Quizilbash N, O'Taylor J: Blood pressure, stroke, and coronary heart disease. 2. Short-term reductions in blood pressure: overview of randomized drug trials in their epidemiological context. Lancet 1990;335: 827–838.
3   SHEP Cooperative Research Group: Prevention of stroke by antihypertensive drug treatment in older persons with isolated systolic hypertension: final results of the Systolic Hypertension in the Elderly Program (SHEP). JAMA 1991;265:3255–3264.
4   Staessen JA, Fagard R, Thijs L Celis H, Arabidze GG, Birkenhager WH, Bulpitt CJ, de Leeuw PW, Dollery CT, Fletcher AE, Foette F, Leonetti G, Nacheve C, O'Brien ET, Rosenfeld J, Rodicio JL, Tuomilehto J, Zanchetti A, and for the Systolic Hypertension in Europe (Syst-Eur) Trial Investigators: Randomized double-blind comparison of placebo and active treatment for older patients with isolated systolic hypertension. Lancet 1997;350:757–764.
5   Blood Pressure Lowering Treatment Trialists' Collaboration: Effects of different blood-pressure-lowering regimens on major cardiovascular events: results of prospectively-designed overviews of randomized trials. Lancet 2003;362:1527–1535.
6   Staessen JA, Wang JG, Thijs L: Cardiovascular protection and blood pressure reduction: a meta-analysis. Lancet 2001;358:1305–1315.
7   Hansson L: Are these benefits from any antihypertensive agent additional to blood pressure lowering per se? In Birkenhäger H, Robertson JL, Zanchetti A (eds): Handbook of Hypertension. Amsterdam, Elsevier, 2004, pp 526–540.
8   Kannel WB: Hypertension as a risk factor: the Framingham contribution; in Birkenhäger H, Robertson JL, Zanchetti A (eds): Handbook of Hypertension. Amsterdam, Elsevier, 2004, pp 129–142.
9   Black HR, Yi JY: A new classification scheme for hypertension based on relative and absolute risk with implications for treatment and reimbursement. Hypertension 1996;28:719–724.
10   Mancia G, Seravalle G, Grassi G: Systolic blood pressure: an underestimated cardiovascular risk factor. J Hypertens 2002;20:S21–S27.
11   Guidelines Committee: 2003 European Society of Hypertension-European Society of Cardiology guidelines for the management of arterial hypertension. J Hypertens 2003;21:1011–1053.
12   Zanchetti A: Blood pressure: from systolic to diastolic and back to systolic values as guides to prognosis and treatment; in Birkenhäger H, Robertson JL, Zanchetti A (eds): Handbook of Hypertension. Amsterdam, Elsevier, 2004, pp 143–150.
13   Staessen JA, Li Y, Thijs L, Wang JG: Changing concepts on the role of blood pressure reduction in cardiovascular prevention; in O'Rourke MF, Safar ME (eds): Handbook of Hypertension. Amsterdam, Elsevier, 2006, pp 485–502.
14   Benetos A, Thomas F, Bean KE, Guize L: Why cardiovascular mortality is higher in treated hypertensive versus subjects of the same age, in the general population. J Hypertens 2003;21:1635–1640.
15   Levenson JA, Simon AC, Fiessinger JN, Safar ME, London GM, Housset EM: Systemic arterial compliance in patients with arteriosclerosis obliterans of the lower limbs: observations on the effect of intravenous propanolol. Arteriosclerosis 1982;2:266–271.

16   Farrar DI, Malindzak GS, Johnson G: Large vessel impedance in peripheral atherosclerosis. Cardiovscular Surg 1977;II-56:170–178.

17   Safar ME, Toto Moukouo JJ, Asmar RA, Laurent S: Increase pulse pressure in patients with atherosclerosis obliterans of the lower limbs. Arteriosclerosis 1987;7:232–237.

18   Stefanidis C, Wooley CF, Bush CA, Kolibash AJ, Boudoulas J: Aortic distensibility abnormalities in coronary artery disease. Am J Cardiol 1987;59:1300–1304.

19   Cruickshank JM: Coronary flow reserve and the J curve relation between diastolic blood pressure and myocardial infarction. Br Med 1988;297:1227–1230.

20   Kelly R, Tunin R, Kass D: Effect of reduced aortic compliance on left ventricular contractile function and energetics in vivo. Circ Res 1992;71:490–502.

21   Asmar RG, Julia PL, Mascarel VL, Fabiani JN, Benetos A, Safar ME: Ambulatory blood pressure profile after carotid endarterectomy in patients with ischemic arterial disease. J Hypertens 1994; 12:697–702.

22   Zanchetti A, Bond MG, Hennig M, Neiss A, Mancia G, Dal Palu C, Hansson L, Magnani B, Rahn KH, Reid JL, Rodicio J, Safar M, Eckes L, Ravinetto R on behalf of the ELSA Investigators: Risk factors associated with alterations in carotid intima-media thickness in hypertension. Baseline data from the European Lacidipine Study on Atherosclerosis. J Hypertens 1998;16:949–961.

23   Zanchetti A, Bond MG, Hennig M, Neiss A, Mancia G, Dal Palu C, Hansson L, Magnani B, Rahn KH, Reid JL, Rodicio J, Safar M, Eckes L, Rizzini P, European Lacidipine Study on Atherosclerosis Investigators: Calcium antagonist lacidipine slows down progression of asymptomatic carotid atherosclerosis: principal results of the European Lacidipine Study on Atherosclerosis (ELSA), a randomized double-blind, long-term trial. Circulation 2002;106:2422–2427.

24   Nichols WW, O'Rourke M: McDonald's Blood Flow in Arteries. Theoretical, Experimental and Clinical Principles, ed 4. London, Arnold, 1998, pp 54–113, 201–222, 284–292, 347–401.

25   Milnor WR: Hemodynamics, ed 2. Baltimore, Wilkins, 1989, pp 211–241.

26   Safar ME: Antihypertensive effects of nitrates in chronic human hypertension. J Appl Cardiol 1990;5:69–81.

27   Simon AC, Safar ME, Levenson JA, Kheder AM, Levy BI: Systolic hypertension: hemodynamic mechanism and choice of antihypertensive treatment. Am J Cardiol 1979;44:505–511.

28   Taylor MG: Wave travel in arteries and the design of the cardiovascular system; in Attinger EO (ed): Pulsatile Blood Flow. New York, McGraw-Hill, 1964, pp 343–347.

29   Stokes GS, Ryan M, Brnabic A, Nyberg G: A controlled study of the effects of isosorbide mononitrate on arterial blood pressure and pulse wave form in systolic hypertension. J Hypertens 1999;17:1767–1773.

30   Safar ME, Blacher J, Mourad JJ, London GM: Stiffness of carotid artery wall material and blood pressure in humans: application to antihypertensive therapy and stroke prevention. Stroke 2000; 31:782–790.

31   Duchier J, Iannascoli F, Safar M: Antihypertensive effect of sustained-release isosorbide dinitrate for isolated systolic hypertension in the elderly. Am J Cardiol 1987;60:99–102.

32   Guerin AP, Blacher J, Pannier B, Marchais SJ, Safar ME, London GM: Impact of aortic stiffness attenuation on survival of patient in end-stage renal failure. Circulation 2001;103:987–992.

33   Safar ME, London GM: The arterial system in human hypertension; in Swales JD (ed): Textbook of Hypertension. London, Blackwell Scientific, 1994, pp 85–102.

34   Staessen JA, Thijs L, O'Brien ET, Bulpitt CJ, de Leeuw PW, Fagard RH, Nachev C, Palatini P, Parati G, Tuomilehto J, Webster J, Safar ME, and for the Syst-Eur Trial Investigators: Ambulatory pulse pressure as predictor of outcome in older patients with systolic hypertension. Am J Hypertens 2002;15:835–843.

35   Safar ME, London GM, for the Clinical Committee of Arterial Structure and Function: Therapeutic studies and arterial stiffness in hypertension: recommendations of the European Society of Hypertension. J Hypertens 2000;18:1527–1535.

36   Starmans-Kool MJF, Kleinjans HAJ, Lustermans FAT, Kragten JA, Breed JS, Van Bortel LMAB: Treatment of elderly patients with isolated systolic hypertension with isosorbide dinitrate in an asymmetric dosing schedule. J Hum Hypertens 1998;12:557–561.

37   Simon G, Wittig VJ, Cohn JN: Transdermal nitroglycerin as a step 3 antihypertensive drug. Clin Pharmacol Ther 1986;40:42–45.

38   Milei J, Vasquez A, Lemus J: Double-blind controlled trial of molsidomine in hypertension. Eur J Clin Pharmacol 1980;18:231–235.

39   Kool MJ, Spek JJ, Struijker Boudier HAJ, Hoeks AP, Reneman RS, Van Herwaarden RH, Van Bortel LMAB: Acute and subacute effects of nicorandil and isosorbide dinitrate on vessel wall properties of large arteries and hemodynamics in healthy volunteers. Cardiovasc Drugs Ther 1995;9:331–337.

40   Chamiot-Clerc P, Choukri N, Legrand M, Droy-Lefay MT, Safar ME, Renaud JF: Relaxation of vascular smooth muscle by cicletanine in aged Wistar aorta under stress conditions. Am J Hypertens 2000;13:208–213.

41   Levy BI, Curmi P, Poitevin P, Safar ME: Modifications of arterial mechanical properties of normotensive and hypertensive rats without arterial pressure changes. J Cardiovasc Pharmacol 1989;14:253–259.

42   Cockcroft JR, Chowienczyk PJ, Brett SE, Chen CP, Dupont AG, Van Nueten L, Wooding SJ, Ritter JM: Nebivolol vasodilates human forearm vasculature: evidence for an L-arginine/NO-dependent mechanism. J Pharmacol Exp Ther 1995;274:1067–1071.

43   Costa M, Gonzalez LV, Majowicz MP, Vidal NA, Balaszczuk AM, Arranz CT: Atrial natriuretic peptide modifies arterial blood pressure through nitric oxide pathway in rats. Hypertension 2000;35:1119–1123.

44   Chamiot-Clerc P, Renaud JF, Safar ME: Pulse pressure, aortic reactivity and endothelium dysfunction in old hypertensive rats. Hypertension 2001;37:313–321.

45   Philip I, Plantfeve G, Vuillaumier-Barrot S, Vicaut E, Le Marie C, Henrion D, Poirier O, Levy BI, Desmonts JM, Durand G, Benessiano J: G894T polymorphism in the endothelial nitric oxide synthase gene is associated with an enhanced vascular responsiveness to phenylephrine. Circulation 1999;22:3096–3098.

46   Kato H, Suzuki H, Tajima S, Ogata Y, Tominaga T, Sato A, Saruta T: Angiotensin II stimulates collagen synthesis in cultured vascular smooth muscle cells. J Hypertens 1991;9:17–22.

47   Gibbons GH, Pratt RE, Dzau VJ: Vascular smooth muscle cell hypertrophy vs. hyperplasia: autocrine transforming growth factor-β_1 expression determines growth response to angiotensin II. J Clin Invest 1992;90:456–461.

48   Albaladejo P, Bouaziz H, Duriez M, Gohlke P, Levy B, Safar M, Benetos A: Angiotensin-converting enzyme inhibition prevents the increase in aortic collagen in rats. Hypertension 1994;23: 74–82.

49   Benetos A, Levy BI, Lacolley P, Taillard F, Duriez M, Safar ME: Role of angiotensin II and bradykinin on aortic collagen following converting enzyme inhibition in spontaneously hypertensive rats. Arterioscler Thromb Vasc Biol 1997;17:3196–3201.

50   Labat C, Lacolley P, Lajemi M, De Gasparo M, Safar ME, Benetos A: Effects of valsartan on mechanical properties of the carotid artery in spontaneously hypertensive rats under high-salt diet. Hypertension 2001;38:439–443.

51   Ying WZ, Sanders PW: Dietary salt increases endothelial nitric oxide synthase and TGF-β_1 in rat aortic endothelium. Am J Physiol 1999;277:H1293–H1298.

52   Richard V, Joannides R, Henry JP, Mulder P, Mace B, Guez D, Schiavi P, Thuillez C: Fixed-dose combination of perindopril with indapamide in spontaneously hypertensive rats: hemodynamic, biological and structural effects. J Hypertens 1996;14:1447–1454.

53   Limas C, Westrum B, Limas CJ, Cohn JN: Effect of salt on the vascular lesions of spontaneously hypertensive rats. Hypertension 1980;2:477–489.

54   Safar ME, Thuillez C, Richard V, Benetos A: Pressure-independent contribution of sodium to large artery and function in hypertension. Cardiovasc Res 2000;46:269–276.

55   Contard F, Glukova M, Marotte F, Narcisse G, Schatz C, Swynghedauw B, Guez D, Samuel JL, Rappaport L: Diuretic effects on cardiac hypertrophy in the stroke-prone spontaneously hypertensive rat. Cardiovasc Res 1993;27:429–434.

56   Safar M, Van Bortel L, Struijker Boudier H: Resistance and conduit arteries following converting enzyme inhibition in hypertension. J Vasc Res 1997;81:34–67.

57   Asmar R, Benetos A, Chaouche-Teyara K, Raveau-Landon C, Safar M: Comparison of effects of felodipine versus hydrochlorothiazide on arterial diameter and pulse-wave velocity in essential hypertension. Am J Cardiol 1993;72:794–798.

58   Benetos A, Lafleche A, Asmar R, Gautier S, Safar A, Safar ME: Arterial stiffness, hydrochloro-thiazide and converting enzyme inhibition in essential hypertension. J Hum Hypertens 1996;10: 77–82.

59   Asmar RG, London GM, O'Rourke MF, Safar ME and for the REASON Project Coordinators and Investigators: Improvement in blood pressure, arterial stiffness and wave reflections with a very-low-dose perindopril/indapamide combination in hypertensive patients: a comparison with atenolol. Hypertension 2001;38:922–926.

60   Safar M, Van Bortel L, Struijker Boudier H: Resistance and conduit arteries following converting enzyme inhibition in hypertension. J Vasc Res 1997;81:34–67.

61   Intengan HD, Thibault G, Li JS, Schiffrin EL: Resistance artery mechanics, structure, and extra-cellular components in spontaneously hypertensive rats: effect of angiotensin receptor antago-nism and converting enzyme inhibition. Circulation 1999;100:2267–2275.

62   Girerd X, Giannattasio C, Moulin C, Safar M, Mancia G, Laurent S: Regression of radial artery wall hypertrophy and improvement of carotid artery compliance after long-term antihyperten-sive treatment in elderly patients. J Am Coll Cardiol 1998;31:1064–1073.

63   Ting CT, Chen CH, Chang MS, Yin FC: Short- and long-term effects of antihypertensive drugs on arterial reflections compliance and impedance. Hypertension 1995;26:524–530.

64   London GM, Asmar RG, O'Rourke MF, Safar ME, on behalf of the REASON Project Investiga-tors: Mechanism(s) of selective systolic blood pressure reduction after a low-dose combination of perindopril/indapamide in hypertensive subjects: comparison with atenolol. J Am Coll Car-diol 2004;43:92–99.

65   Chen CH, Ting CT, Lin SJ, Hsu TL, Yin FC, Siu CO, Chou P, Wang SP, Chang MS: Different ef-fects of fosinopril and atenolol on wave reflections in hypertensive patients. Hypertension 1995; 25:1034–1041.

66   Rizzoni D, Porteri E, Boari GE, De Ciucies C, Sleiman I, Muiesan M, et al: Prognostic signifi-cance of small-artery structure in hypertension. Circulation 2003;108:2230–2235.

67   Lacolley P, Labat C, Pujol A, Delcayre C, Benetos A, Safar M: Increased carotid wall elastic mod-ulus and fibronectin in aldosterone-salt treated rats – effects of eplerenone. Circulation 2002; 106:2848–2853.

68   Lombes M, Oblin ME, Gasc JM, Baulieu EE, Farman N, Bonvallet JP: Immunohistochemical and biochemical evidence of a cardiovascular mineralocorticoid receptor. Circ Res 1992;71:503–510.

69   Lockett MF: Hormonal actions of the heart and the lungs on the isolated kidney. J Physiol 1967; 193:661–669.

70   Kornel L, Kanamariapudi N, Travers T, Taff DJ, CC Patel W, Baum RM, Raynor WJ: Studies on high affinity binding of mineralo- and glucocorticoids in rabbit aorta cytosol. J Steroid Biochem 1983;16:245–264.

71   Benetos A, Lacolley P, Safar ME: Prevention of aortic fibrosis by spironolactone in spontane-ously hypertensive rats. Arterioscler Thromb Vasc Biol 1997;17:1152–1156.

72   Lacolley P, Safar ME, Lucet B, Le Dudal K, Labat C, Benetos A: Prevention of aortic and cardiac fibrosis by spironolactone in old normotensive rats. J Am Coll Cardiol 2001;37:662–667.

73   Blacher J, Amah G, Girerd X, Kheder A, Ben Maiz H, London GM, Safar ME: Association be-tween increased plasma levels of aldosterone and decreased systemic arterial compliance in sub-jects with essential hypertension. Am J Hypertens 1997;10:1326–1334.

74   Pojoga L, Gautier S, Blanc H, Guyene TT, Poirier O, Cambien F, Benetos A: Genetic determina-tion of plasma aldosterone levels in essential hypertension. Am J Hypertens 1998;11:856–860.

75   Davies PF: Flow-mediated endothelial mechanotransduction. Physiol Rev 1995;75:519–560.

76   Corman B, Duriez M, Poitevin P, Heudes D, Bruneval P, Tedgui A, Levy BI: Aminoguanidine prevents age-related arterial stiffening and cardiac hypertrophy. Proc Natl Acad Sci USA 1998; 95:1301–1306.

77   Vaitkevicius PV, Lane M, Spurgeon HA, Ingram DK, Roth GS, Egan JJ, Vasan S, Wagle DR, Ul-rich R, Brines M, Wuerth JP, Cerami A, Lakata EG: A cross-link breaker has sustained effects on arterial and ventricular properties in older rhesus monkeys. Proc Natl Acad Sci USA 2001;98: 1171–1175.

78   Kass DA, Shapiro EP, Kawaguchi M, Capriotti AR, Scuteri A, Degroof RC, Lakatta EG: Improved arterial compliance by a novel advanced glycation end-product crosslink breaker. Circulation 2001;104:1464–1470.

79   Et-Taouil K, Schiavi P, Levy BI, Plante GE: Sodium intake, large artery stiffness and proteoglycans in the SHR. Hypertension 2001;38:1172–1176.

80   Intengan HD, Thibault G, Li JS, Schiffrin EL: Resistance artery mechanics, structure, and extracellular components in spontaneously hypertensive rats: effects of angiotensin receptor antagonism and converting enzyme inhibition. Circulation 1999;100:2267–2275.

81   Koffi I, Lacolley P, Kichengaast M, Pomies JP, Laurent S, Benetos A: Prevention of arterial structural alterations with verapamil and trandolapril and consequences for mechanical properties in spontaneously hypertensive rats. Eur J Pharmacol 1998;361:51–60.

82   Franklin S, Gustin IV W, Wong ND, Larson MG, Weber M, Kannel WB, Levy D: Hemodynamic patterns of age-related changes in blood pressure. The Framingham Heart Study. Circulation 1997;96:308–315.

83   de Luca N, Asmar RG, London GM, O'Rourke MF, Safar ME, REASON Project Investigators: Selective reduction of cardiac mass and central blood pressure on low-dose combination perindopril/indapamide in hypertensive subjects. J Hypertens 2004;22:1623–1630.

84   Williams B, Lacy PS, Thom SM, Cruickshank K, Stanton A, Collier D, Hughes AD, Thurston H, O'Rourke M; CAFE Investigators; Anglo-Scandinavian Cardiac Outcomes Trial Investigators; CAFE Steering Committee and Writing Committee: Differential impact of blood pressure-lowering drugs on central aortic pressure and clinical outcomes: principal results of the Conduit Artery Function Evaluation (CAFE) Study. Circulation 2006;113:1213–1225.

Prof. Michel Safar
Centre de Diagnostic, Hôtel-Dieu Hospital
1, place du Parvis Notre-Dame
FR–75181 Paris Cedex 04 (France)
Tel. +33 1 4234 8025, Fax +33 1 4234 8632, E-Mail michel.safar@htd.ap-hop-paris.fr

Author Index

Subject Index

Laser Doppler iontophoresis, endothelial
function testing 64
LOX-1, statin effects 318, 319

Marfan syndrome, fibrillin defects 110
Matrix metalloproteinases (MMPs)
arterial stiffness studies 87
cholesterol and arterial stiffness 271
cyclic strain response 225
regulation 80, 81
types 80
Mechanical stress, *see* Stress, mechanical
Metabolic syndrome
arterial stiffness 246, 247
cholesterol relationship 267, 268
Microalbuminuria, endothelial function
testing 65

Nicorandil, arterial stiffness effects 132
Nitrates
arterial stiffness effects 131, 182, 183
clinical use 306, 307
historical perspective 302, 303
hypertension response 312
large artery effects 307–309, 311
mechanism of action 303–306
nitroglycerine tolerance 306
peripheral arterial disease response
204, 205
selective systolic blood pressure
reduction 340, 341
Nitric oxide (NO), *see also* Endothelial
function
age-related arterial stiffness role 70–72
endothelial function and
atherosclerosis role 66, 168, 169
function 66
history of study 303
insulin response 254
mechanical stress effects 70
synthesis 303, 304

Omapatrilat, arterial stiffness effects 122
Oxidative stress
chronic kidney disease patients
189–191
end-stage renal disease 189–191
statin effects 319

Peripheral arterial disease (PAD)
ankle-brachial index for screening 200
arterial stiffness
endothelial dysfunction 204
nervous system alterations 206
structural changes 203, 204
blood pressure and systemic
hemodynamic findings 200–202,
206, 207
coronary heart disease risks 207, 208
nitrate response 204, 205
pulse wave velocity findings 202, 203
Pioglitazone, carotid atherosclerosis
effects 179, 180
Plaque
animal models 102
elasticity imaging with intravascular
ultrasound
modulus elastography
implementation 51, 52
material deformation model 54
minimization algorithm 54
motivation 50, 51
parametric finite element model
geometry 53
patient findings 54–56
overview 41, 42
prospects 56, 57
strain elastography/palpography
animal studies 48, 49
correlation-based elastography 44,
46
envelope-based technique 44
patient findings 49, 50
principles 42–44
radiofrequency–based technique
44
validation in humans 46–48
histology 37, 39
pulse pressure relationship 216, 218
vulnerable plaque
identification
calcified nodule 40
erosion–prone plaque 40
rupture–prone plaque 39, 40
terminology 36
Plasminogen activator inhibitor-I
(PAI-I), statin effects 319